MEDICINE ... MENT

THE WELLCOME INSTITUTE SERIES IN THE HISTORY OF MEDICINE

Forthcoming Titles

The History of Medical Education in Britain
Edited by Vivian Nutton and Roy Porter

The Health of Prisoners: Historical Essays
Edited by W. F. Bynum

The Science and Culture of Nutrition 1840–1940
Edited by H. Kamminga and A. Cunningham

Academic inquiries regarding the series should be addressed
to the editors W. F. Bynum and Roy Porter at
the Wellcome Institute for the History of Medicine,
183 Euston Road, London NW1 2BE, UK

MEDICINE IN THE ENLIGHTENMENT

Edited by
Roy Porter

Rodopi

Amsterdam – Atlanta GA 1995

First published in 1995
by Editions Rodopi B. V., Amsterdam – Atlanta, GA 1995.

Design and Typesetting by Christine Lavery, the Wellcome Trust.
Printed and bound in The Netherlands by Editions Rodopi B. V.,
Amsterdam – Atlanta, GA 1995.

British Library Cataloguing in Publication Data
A catalogue record for this book is available from the British Library
ISBN 90-5183-562-0 (Bound)

Medicine
Medicine in the Enlightenment – Amsterdam – Atlanta, GA
Rodopi. – ill.
(Clio Medica 29/The Wellcome Institute Series in the
History of Medicine)

CIP-GEGEVENS KONINKLIJKE BIBLIOTHEEK, DEN HAAG

Front cover: MONR· LE MEDICIN. Pubd. accords. to Act of Parllt,
June 13th: 1771 by MDarly 39 Strand.

Met index lit. opg.
ISBN 90-5183-562-0 (Bound)
Trefw.: geneeskunde; geschiedenis; Verlichting, (Tijdperk).

Printed in The Netherlands

Contents

Preface

This volume takes its inspiration from a lively one-day symposium held in May 1992 at the Wellcome Institute for the History of Medicine, London. Lawrence Brockliss, Isobel Grundy, Johanna Geyer-Kordesch, Andreas-Holger Maehle, Mary Lindemann and Rosalind Rey all gave earlier versions of the papers here published to that meeting. I am delighted additionally to have recruited contributions from Jonathan Andrews, Mark Jackson, Ludmilla Jordanova, Francis McKee, David Shuttleton, Akihito Suzuki and Philip Wilson. Taken together, these papers constitute a broad and rich coverage of Britain and the Continent in the eighteenth century, integrating explorations of medicine, literature, philosophy and politics. After many years during which the Enlightenment was widely viewed as a lost era or as an arid desert in medical history, today's historians are now becoming conscious, almost for the first time, of the multi-faceted role that medical thinking played in the eighteenth-century processes of criticism and modernization. This volume should contribute to the revaluation of Enlightenment medicine.

For helping to make the editing of this book so speedy, trouble-free and pleasurable, my thanks to Frieda Houser, Christine Lavery and Michael Wilcox.

Roy Porter

Notes on Contributors

Jonathan Andrews is a Research Fellow at the Wellcome Unit for the History of Medicine, at the University of Glasgow. He is currently engaged in research on Gartnavel Royal Hospital, Glasgow, and psychiatry in the West of Scotland during the nineteenth and twentieth centuries. His Ph.D thesis was a study of Bethlem Hospital in the seventeenth and eighteenth centuries. He has edited a book on Gartnavel Royal Hospital and published articles on Bethlem and the history of psychiatry.

L. W. B. Brockliss was born in 1950 and educated at the University of Cambridge. For ten years he taught history at the University of Hull, until he moved to Oxford in 1984 and became a Fellow and Tutor in Modern History at Magdalen College. For 20 years he has worked on the history of education, science and medicine in early modern France and has published widely in the field. From 1985 to 1992 he was also editor of the annual publication *History of Universities.* His most important work to date is *French Higher Education in the Seventeenth and Eighteenth Centuries: A cultural history* (Oxford, 1987). At present he is completing a social and cultural history of French medicine in the early modern period, which he is writing with Professor Colin Jones of Exeter University.

Johanna Geyer-Kordesch is Director of the Wellcome Unit for the History of Medicine, University of Glasgow. She has written a number of essays on medicine in the eighteenth century, in particular on Georg Ernst Stahl's holistic theory of medicine. She is now interested in medical case histories, their narrative structure, and their literary importance because it illuminates how medical science and illness experience structure the diverse tensions within such a seminal period as the Enlightenment.

Isobel Grundy formerly of Queen Mary and Westfield College, London University, is Henry Marshall Tory Professor at the University of Alberta. She is author of *Samuel Johnson and the Scale of Greatness* (Leicester and Georgia, 1986); co-author with Virginia Blain and Patricia Clements of *The Feminist Companion to Literature in English: Women writers from the Middle Ages* *to the present* (Batsford and Yale, 1990), and co-editor with Susan Wiseman of *Women, Writing, History 1640–1740* (Batsford and Georgia, 1992). She has produced a revised edition of Lady Mary Wortley Montagu, *Essays and Poems* (Oxford, 1993: first edited with Robert Halsband, 1977) and the first scholarly edition of Eliza Fenwick, *Secresy, or The Ruin on the Rock* (Broadview Press, 1994: first published 1795). She is at work on a new life of Lady Mary Wortley Montagu.

Mark Jackson is a research fellow at the Wellcome Unit for the History of Medicine at Manchester University. His Ph.D thesis (to be published in 1995 by Manchester University Press) was on cases of suspected new-born child murder in the eighteenth century. He is currently working on an intellectual and social history of what was originally referred to as 'mental deficiency'. From September 1994, he will take up a research post in Manchester developing a training and research programme in twentieth-century biomedical sciences, with a particular interest in immunology.

Ludmilla J. Jordanova is Professor of History at the University of York. She is author of *Lamarck* (1984) and *Sexual Visions* (1989) and has edited *Images of Earth* (1979, with Roy Porter), *Languages of Nature* (1986) and *The Enlightenment and its Shadows* (1990, with Peter Hulme). She is currently working on medicine in Britain and France between 1780 and 1820.

Mary Lindemann is Associate Professor of History at Carnegie Mellon University. She is author of *Patriots and Paupers: Hamburg, 1712–1830* (New York: Oxford University Press, 1990). She has just completed a monograph on health and healing in seventeenth- and eighteenth-century Germany.

Andreas-Holger Maehle is a Wellcome Research Fellow in the History of Medicine at the University of Durham and Privatdozent at the University of Göttingen. His publications include *Johann Jakob Wepfer (1620–1695) als Toxikologe* (Aarau: Saauerländer, 1987) and *Kritik und Verteidigung des Tierversuchs: Die Anfänge der Diskussion im 17. und 18. Jahrhundert* (Stuttgart: F. Steiner, 1992). He is currently working on a history of pharmacological and toxicological research in eighteenth-century Britain.

Roselyn Rey has written a thesis entitled 'Birth and growth of vitalism in France, from the second half of the eighteenth century to the end of the first empire' (forthcoming in *Studies on Voltaire and the eighteenth century*). She has published some papers on French natural history (Buffon, Cuvier) and has recently published a *History of Pain,* (Paris: La Dècouvat, 1993). She is a Research Fellow and teaches history of medicine and history of life sciences at the EHESS.

Andrea A. Rusnock is Assistant Professor of History at Rensselaer Polytechnic Institute. She is editor of *The Correspondence of James Jurin (1684–1750),* (forthcoming). She is currently working on a history of medical and political arithmetic in eighteenth-century Britain and France.

David E. Shuttleton is a lecturer in English Literature at the University of Wales, Aberystwyth. He is at present preparing his doctoral thesis, *'My own Crazy Carcase': The life and works of Dr George Cheyne (1672–1743)* (Edinburgh University, 1992), for publication, and is working on a study of Romanticism from a lesbian and gay perspective in collaboration with Dr Patricia Duncker.

Akihito Suzuki is a research fellow at the Wellcome Institute for the History of Medicine. His Ph.D thesis was on the history of medical and philosophical concepts of madness in the eighteenth century. He has published articles on the history of psychiatry, and is currently working on a history of psychiatric practice in early nineteenth-century England.

Philip K. Wilson is Assistant Professor in the History of Science at the University of Hawaii. He studied medical history at the Johns Hopkins University and the Wellcome Institute, receiving his Ph.D from University College London for his thesis on the career and writings of the London surgeon and physician, Daniel Turner (1667–1741). He is currently working on a history of surgeons and their practices in Enlightenment England.

Introduction

The paradoxes of medicine in the Enlightenment are legion. The earlier triumphs of the New Philosophy and the Scientific Revolution created great expectations for what Francis Bacon called 'the relief of man's estate', which undoubtedly included the relief of suffering, the overcoming of disease and the prolongation of life. Physicians and *philosophes* alike looked to a medical revolution that would complement and complete the Scientific Revolution, and (as Ludmilla Jordanova shows in her 'Reflections on Medical Reform: Cabanis' Coup d'Œuil') constructed mythic histories of medicine that trumpeted such a transformation.[1] Yet disease remained rampant throughout the *ancien régime* and morbidity and mortality rates stayed appallingly high. Only one disease's ravages were checked by medical action – smallpox – and then, as Andreas-Holger Maehle shows in his 'Conflicting Attitudes Towards Inoculation in Enlightenment Germany', such improvement was only partial and sporadic. So-called 'new diseases',[2] including rickets and tuberculosis, took larger tolls. And, more scandalously, many contemporaries believed that Enlightenment outlooks and lifestyles themselves – sedentariness, urbanity, the cult of politeness, the new obsession with *belles lettres* and fiction, a powerful if pernicious instrospective bent – were actually creating nervous, hysterical and hypochondriacal disorders and uncertainties about the principle of life.[3] This indeed is emphasized in two essays in this volume, David Shuttleton's 'Methodism and Dr George Cheyne's "More Enlightening Principles"' and Roselyne Rey's 'Vitalism, Disease and Society' – which, like several other contributions, emphasizes how biomedical formulations can be fully grasped only if set in their wider sociocultural contexts.[4]

Paradox was, to some degree, the stock-in-trade of Enlightenment criticism, and it should be no surprise that that the satirist physician Bernard Mandeville was to the fore in noting the contradictions for health of the march of mind, not least the spread of literacy and the reading habit. In 'Honeyed Words: Bernard Mandeville and Medical Discourse', Francis McKee surveys an Enlightenment physician writing medical works to demonstrate how reading medical works precipitates hypochondriacal indigestion![5]

Several of the contributors address another aspect of the Enlightenment paradox: the shadow side of *Aufklärung*, or, alternatively, the silver lining to be found in various clouds.[6] Enlightenment ambitions often yielded little direct fruit, yet in diverse ways progress was being made on the health front; and it is the historian's duty to discern nuance and to make balanced judgements on complex changing situations. In 'An Enlightenment Science? Surgery and the Royal Society', Philip Wilson adduces evidence to call into question the low regard traditional historians have had for Enlightenment surgery.[7] In her 'Sarah Stone: Enlightenment Midwife', Isobel Grundy shows that (despite the stereotypes advanced in traditional histories of obstetrics) eighteenth-century midwives were not all benighted – and (despite the rhetoric of more recent feminist historians) traditional women-centred childbirth was not entirely natural and safe.[8]

Three essays scrutinize the complexities of eighteenth-century attitudes towards mental illness. Treatment of the mad was neither a matter of happy (or barbaric) neglect nor the mobilization of what Michel Foucault dubbed the 'great confinement'.[9] Nor did the 'age of reason' succeed in establishing a Newtonian science of the mind, healthy or sick. Psychological theorizing and psychotherapeutics were alike complex. In 'Anti-Lockean Enlightenment? Mind and Body in Early Eighteenth-Century English Medicine', Akihito Suzuki reveals how historians have been mistaken in their widespread assumption that Locke's model of human understanding played a major part in shaping models of mental disorder in the early Enlightenment.[10] Jonathan Andrews' 'The Politics of Committal to Early Modern Bethlem' maintains that the question of the use of confinement in lunatic asylums in the eighteenth century for the purpose of social control is immensely difficult to evaluate. And Roy Porter argues in 'Shaping Psychiatric Knowledge: The Role of the Asylum' that small private mental institutions in late Enlightenment England, for all the undoubted horrors of the 'trade in lunacy', may well also have served as key sites in psychiatric innovation.[11]

Two essays that form a pair – Mary Lindemann's 'The Enlightenment Encountered: The German Physicus and His World, 1750–1820', and Andreas-Holger Maehle's 'Conflicting Attitudes Towards Inoculation in Enlightenment Germany' – explore the ambiguous implications of enlightened absolutism for medicine in German-speaking Europe. In their different ways, these two contributions relate how the centralizing and bureaucratic regimes of German princes gave medicine heightened official status. Nevertheless, German cameralism also subordinated medicine to administrative protocols – and often prejudices – and district physicians might be coopted to serve as minor functionaries. It remains a moot point whether the uptake of inoculation was ultimately helped or hindered by archducal dictates – variolation certainly spread faster and wider in free-market England, an issue assessed in Andrea A. Rusnock's 'The Weight of Evidence and the Burden of Authority: Case Histories, Medical Statistics and Smallpox Inoculation'.[12]

These dilemmas are mirrored by a further pair of papers that explore the diffusion and deployment of medical knowledge within the public and political domains. Lawrence Brockliss's 'Medical Reform, the Enlightenment and Physician-Power in Late Eighteenth-Century France' analyses the tensions underlying new trends in French medical education in the eighteenth century: idealistic reformers campaigned for a revised rational and scientific curriculum, whereas would-be practitioners sought a practical training that would win a large clientele and secure a good living.[13] The difficult passage undergone by Enlightened medical science in the real world is also laid bare by Johanna Geyer-Kordesch's 'Whose Enlightenment? Medicine, Witchcraft, Melancholia and Pathology', which shows, in a way comparable to Brockliss's paper, that the rational and progressive medical reasoning of the professors did not necessarily square with the practicalities of legal and administrative procedures in the chamber and the council, the court-room and the Court. Similar power struggles form the focus of Mark Jackson's 'Developing Medical Expertise: Medical Practitioners and the Suspected Murders of New-Born Children'. Examining infanticide trials in eighteenth-century England, Jackson demonstrates the unresolved battle between the authority of the law, the expertise of the medical profession, and the opinion of the public.

Two conclusions suggest themselves. First, no simple model of a medical Enlightenment – no idealized representation of it as a body of advances in theories and practices helping to transform society – remotely corresponds to reality. Second, it would be a mistake, for that reason alone, to dismiss the concept of a medical Enlightenment out of hand, and to revert to talk of a barren century of idle medical chatter. The eighteenth century produced extensive and innovative medical discourses. Medical images – diagnosis, therapy, regimen – were central to the socio-political visions of the *philosophes;* and integral to more secular and materialist images of the future, the improvement of health under the guidance of a wise medical profession became highly influential.[14] The Enlightenment no more resolved its medical than its cultural, social and political paradoxes. It is the aim of this volume to explore some of these intriguing contradictions.

Notes

1. Lester S. King, *The Medical World of the Eighteenth Century* (Chicago: University of Chicago Press, 1958); *idem, The Road to Medical Enlightenment, 1650–1695* (London: Macdonald, 1970); *idem, The Philosophy of Medicine: The Early Eighteenth Century* (Cambridge, Mass.: Harvard University Press, 1978); Roy Porter, 'Medicine in the Enlightenment', in Christopher Fox, Roy Porter and Robbey Wokler (eds), *Inventing Human Science: Eighteenth-Century Domains* (Berkeley: University of California Press, 1995); Andrew Cunningham and Roger French (eds), *The Medical Enlightenment of the Eighteenth Century* (Cambridge: Cambridge University Press, 1990).
2. L. Stevenson, '"New Diseases" in the Seventeenth Century', *Bulletin of the History of Medicine,* xxxix (1965), 1–21.
3. Roy Porter, 'Civilization and Disease: Medical Ideology in the Enlightenment', in J. Black and J. Gregory (eds), *Culture, Politics and Society in Britain 1660–1800* (Manchester: Manchester University Press, 1991), 154–83; many of the chapters in G. S. Rousseau (ed.), *The Languages of Psyche. Mind and Body in Enlightenment Thought* (Berkeley: University of California Press, 1990) are relevant; see also G. S. Rousseau, 'Psychology', in G. S. Rousseau and Roy Porter (eds), *The Ferment of Knowledge* (Cambridge: Cambridge University Press, 1980), 143–210.
4. See also David E. Shuttleton, '"My Own Crazy Carcase": The Life and Works of Dr George Cheyne, 1672–1743' (Ph.D. thesis, University of Edinburgh, 1992); George Cheyne, *The English Malady,* Roy Porter (ed.), (London: Routledge, 1990; 1st edn 1733); F. Duchesneau, 'Vitalism in Late Eighteenth-Century Physiology: The Cases of Barthez, Blumenbach and John Hunter', in W. F. Bynum and Roy Porter (eds), *William Hunter and the Eighteenth-Century Medical World* (Cambridge: Cambridge University Press, 1985), 259–95.
5. Francis McKee, 'The Earlier Works of Bernard Mandeville, 1685–1715' (Ph.D. thesis, Glasgow University, 1991).
6. See P. Hulme and L. Jordanova (eds), *Enlightenment and its Shadows* (London: Routledge, 1990).
7. Valuable is Christopher Lawrence (ed.), *Medical Theory, Surgical Practice: Studies in the History of Surgery* (London & New York: Routledge, 1992).
8. See David Harley, 'Ignorant Midwives - a Persistent Stereotype', *Bulletin of the Society for the Social History of Medicine,* xxviii (1981), 6–9; Valerie Fildes, Lara Marks and Hilary Marland (eds), *Women and Children First* (London and New York: Routledge, 1992).
9. Michel Foucault, *La Folie et la Déraison: Histoire de la Folie à l'Age Classique* (Paris: Librairie Plon, 1961); trans. and abridged as *Madness*

and Civilization: A History of Insanity in the Age of Reason, Richard Howard (trans.), (New York: Random House, 1965); Arthur Still and Irving Velody (eds), *Rewriting the History of Madness: Studies in Foucault's 'Histoire de la Folie'* (London/New York: Routledge, 1992).

10. Akihito Suzuki, 'Mind and its Disease in Enlightenment British Medicine' (Ph.D. thesis, University of London, 1992).
11. William Llewellyn Parry-Jones, *The Trade in Lunacy: A Study of Private Madhouses in England in the Eighteenth and Nineteenth Centuries* (London: Routledge & Kegan Paul, 1971).
12. J. R. Smith, *The Speckled Monster. Smallpox in England 1670–1970, with Particular Reference to Essex* (Chelmsford: Essex Record Office, 1987).
13. Compare, for a Scottish parallel, Lisa Rosner, *Medical Education in the Age of Improvement: Edinburgh Students and Apprentices, 1760–1826* (Edinburgh: Edinburgh University Press, 1991).
14. Dora B. Weiner, 'Le Droit de l'Homme à la Santé – une Belle Idée devant l'Assemblée Nationale, 1790–1791', *Clio Medica,* v (1970), 209–23.

1

The Politics of Committal to Early Modern Bethlem

Jonathan Andrews

Introduction

The scholarship of the past three decades on the treatment of the insane in early modern France has stressed (*inter alia*) the political dimensions of incarceration and the highly politicized nature of contemporary definitions of insanity. Writing in the 1960s Michel Foucault emphasized the mixed nature of the French institutions of 'the classical age', in which the insane were interred alongside other symbols of *deraison.* Vagrants, prostitutes, felons, dissenters, idiots and the mad were jumbled together quite indiscriminately in L'Hôpital Général, and at a host of other hospitals, *maisons de santé* and prisons. The situation seems to have been particularly acute at the Bicêtre, where not only was madness blended with little distinction from criminality, but political deviancy also found a place under folly's guise.[1] In 1975 Erwin Ackerknecht outlined with greater specificity how the Bicêtre, the Salpêtrière and other 'mixed' institutions were used to confine and silence political and social dissent in pre-revolutionary, revolutionary and Napoleonic France.[2] It is now generally accepted, as Jan Goldstein has expressed it, that 'it was standard Old Regime practice for one party who wanted another removed from the scene for whatever nefarious reason to obtain a *lettre de cachet* from the Crown authorizing incarceration on grounds of lunacy'.[3] Colin Jones' survey of treatment of the insane in eighteenth- and early nineteenth-century Montpellier has also underlined how often social and political motivations prevailed over medical reasons in dictating confinement.[4] It was not merely that the centrality of issues of 'public order' and 'moral danger' politicized lunacy, according to Jones, but the persistently lax nature of admission policies meant that individuals continued to be 'unjustly imprisoned for various nefarious reasons' throughout the century.[5] It was only during the later eighteenth century that French hospital administrators, magistrates and savants began actively to object to 'arbitrary or repressive imprisonment – even by *lettre de cachet*'.[6] Despite the campaign against *lettres de cachet* during the decades immediately after the Revolution, contends Jones (in agreement with Foucault), there is scant evidence that the scope for the false detention of individuals as insane was more limited.

It has, of course, been the work of Foucault and scholars with particular affinities for the 'social control school' of history,[7] that has fuelled this accentuated appreciation of the political and social elements underlying early modern definitions and labelling of deviancy. More recently, Goldstein has further demonstrated, for the post-revolutionary period, how closely intertwined emergent French psychiatry was with the central state bureaucracy, applying the term 'political medicine' to the policy making and legislation enacted in respect of lunacy administration. Goldstein was more preoccupied, however, with the formation of the French psychiatric profession and the prevailing of state medicine over corporate medicine, than he was with admission policies and patients themselves.

Most English scholarship has tended to maintain how different England was from France. Roy Porter and other scholars (baulking, in particular, at Foucault's paradigm of a great, state-sponsored moral '*renfermement*' of the insane during the eighteenth century) have rightly maintained that English institutions for the insane were largely 'voluntary' or private establishments, set up and run by private benefactors and subscribers, and removed from direct state supervision and intervention.[8] The eighteenth century was distinguished by its free 'trade in lunacy',[9] and its relative lack of legislation on the issue of the insane. Nor (despite their unregulated state), did madhouses, prisons and Bridewells in England, share to the same degree the agglomerating tendency so marked in contemporary French responses to the mad and other forms of deviancy. When the law *was* called upon to decide on the property, offences and custody of 'alleged fools and lunatics', proceedings in England, according to Porter and others, 'probably treated [them] ... more sympathetically than the equivalent arrangements in France'.[10] More recently, Akihito Suzuki has emphasized how little evidence there is in early modern Quarter Session records for the kinds of moralistic and politicized definitions of insanity evidently so common in contemporary France.[11] A major explanation for these differences was the radically different nature of the state bureaucracies in the two countries. English government has often been distinguished by scholars for its heterogeneous localism and its '*laissez faire*' response to lunacy. By contrast, lunacy administration in France has usually been characterized as part of a large, centralized bureaucracy, with closer links to the peripheries of local government, allowing for a more interventionist, state-directed policing of lunacy and deviancy.

Other recent English scholarship, however, has begun to look more closely at the political nature of native institutions. Craig Rose, in a study of the Royal Hospitals of London, has revealed how profoundly the hospitals and their personnel were affected by the political upheavals of the 1680s and 1690s.[12] Indeed, the Royal Hospitals clearly experienced something of a 'Glorious Revolution' in their own governments during that period. In fact, they spent the seventeenth century intermittently engaged in a struggle for autonomy, regularly frustrated in their desire for self-government and regularly locking horns with both the monarchy and the City over questions of income, patronage and appointments. Rose did not include, in his survey, the administration of the Hospitals of Bridewell and Bethlem, which underwent similar upheavals during the political crisis of that time. Nor was Rose much concerned with the patient population of these institutions, the political implications of their admission policies, or their governors' roles in such policies.

Other scholars, such as Mary Fissell and John Pickstone, however, *have* examined these aspects more fully, with relation to a wide range of institutions in early modern Britain. Fissell demonstrated for the Bristol region how much the character of charitable institutions was determined by divergent ideologies and 'factional interest[s]', and how definitions of those poor people 'worthy' for admission were the predicates of various 'sectarian and political alliances'. Her concentration on 'the recipients of charity as well as the givers', and the pathways by which the poor sought relief at and beyond the institution, led her not only to stress the active, voluntary ways in which individuals and families sought help, but also the importance of the sponsorship they procured from patrons and benefactors and its conditioning by the ideologies of these sponsors.[13] In Fissell's model, 'the structure of the admission process ... mimicked the politics of the great', in that the personal patronage exercised over admissions required the conformity of applicants, although she also emphasized the reciprocal nature of the obligations entailed on both sides.[14] Pickstone explored the intimate connection between the development of institutions in late eighteenth-century Manchester and its region, the rising prominence of issues of public health, and the transition of these concerns to a more central position on the political agenda. He showed how profoundly the evolution and regulation of hospitals and dispensaries reflected the struggles of different political, religious and social groupings for power and status. His work also underlined the responsiveness of admissions to these institutions to political forces.[15] Like Fissell, Pickstone pointed to the attractiveness of the powers of patronage open to subscribers through their rights of nominating patients. Work on Scottish institutions too, like Guenter Risse's study of the Edinburgh Royal Infirmary, has stressed the political, social and economic advantages that attracted subscribers. Risse pointed to the letters of recommendation required for the admission of patients and their more sympathetic evaluation when 'coming from the most generous benefactors'.[16] Studies of early modern Italian hospitals, such as Sandra Cavallo's work on Turin,[17] have also highlighted the political motivations of benefactors, and the political nature of admission policies which (for example) granted a privileged status to 'citizens'. Cavallo demonstrated how strategies for the institutional relief and accommodation of the poor might reflect 'the needs of political consolidation and conflict', although, like her colleagues, she acknowledged the multiform explanatory elements behind 'the development of forms of poor relief'. All of this scholarship has, to varying degrees, affirmed the importance of understanding what Pickstone has called the 'political ecology' of hospitals: that is, 'the complex interrelations between hospitals and the communities they were built to serve'.[18]

The majority of recent scholarship on institutions, nevertheless, has been about administrations and benefactors rather than patients, about networks of patronage and relationships between élites, rather than how patients were actually received into an institution (not to say that these issues are unconnected). Furthermore, most scholars have concentrated on general hospitals and other specialist and non-specialist institutions for the ordinary sick and poor, rather than on early modern asylums. Recent studies of nineteenth-century asylums have addressed these questions more comprehensively. To name just a few: John Walton's study of the 'casting out and bringing back' of the insane has been particularly influential, and much cited in subsequent historical studies.[19] Walton made provocative comments about the political dimensions to this process. Taking his lead from Foucault and Scull, he asked questions about 'how working-class people come to be defined or labelled as insane and as fit candidates for asylum admission'.[20] Yet Walton found only 'a handful of ... cases' admitted to Lancaster County Asylum where 'political dissent' was a significant constituent of their malady, or in their committal.[21] Indeed, his conclusion that most committals arose from 'domestic' rather than political troubles has been confirmed by other recent studies of nineteenth-century asylums. The surveys of Anne Digby and Charlotte Mackenzie (considerably more comprehensive than Walton's) have convincingly shown that it was family problems which were predominant in determining the reasons and processes whereby patients were admitted to asylums.[22] Current research on the history of people with learning difficulties[23] has also endorsed this view of the family as primary arbiter in the identification and institutionalization of mental deficiency or handicap. Since the 1960s, then, much of the bite seems to have been taken out of the social control approach to the history of mental health, although the various debates are far from resolved.

For the early modern English madhouse, questions about the political and social nature of confinement have still received comparatively little attention. As far as the Hospital of Bethlem is concerned, historians like Michael Donnelly and Peter Rushton have candidly confessed that we know little about how patients were admitted.[24] This neglect is partly explained by historians' over-reliance on literary accounts of Bethlem, or at best on O'Donoghue's antiquated history,[25] texts which largely ignore the process of committal to the Hospital. It is also to be explained by the fact that the focus of recent historical endeavour has been to deny the applicability of the French-Foucauldian analysis to the English context. My work on early modern Bethlem, however, suggests that admission to the Hospital was considerably more politicized than the emphatic nature of this denial would sustain.

It is not my intention, here, to advocate any kind of return to the social control model, which most historians now recognize and utilize merely as a flawed, but useful, point of common reference, rather than as a legitimate theoretical foundation for an analysis. Yet, despite and because of the provocation of the social control school, questions about the extent to which lunacy was politicized in England, have only partially been confronted. In distinguishing which offenders were appropriate for Bethlem, which for other institutions, and which might be pardoned, authorities were plainly imposing, marshalling and developing limits within which (it was felt) lunacy required to be contained. In order to assess how far lunacy and deviancy were intertwined, it is these limits which need to be understood more thoroughly. When was it that lunacy, to quote Chistopher Hill, 'overstepped the bounds of the politically endurable'?[26] More importantly, what or where were those bounds, and how much, in drawing up and policing those bounds, was lunacy itself being politicized?

Bethlem as an Arm of State

What soon becomes clear when studying Bethlem is that it was very much a city institution, and also a royal institution, owing allegiance to both arms of government. The Hospital had been given to the City by Henry VIII in 1547, but only in custody, and its history during the seventeenth century was punctuated by wrangles with and between the Crown and the City over patronage rights to appointments at Bethlem. After a suit between these two authorities over rights to the Hospital in the 1620s and 1630s, for example, Charles I reconfirmed 'the house and soyle of Bethlem' in 1638, but the Lords also felt free to instruct the Governors (the same who also governed Bridewell Hospital, London's archetypal house of correction) that they had no right to prejudice the rents and leases of either hospital, or to give away the money of the poor.[27] Indeed, Bridewell and Bethlem and the other royal hospitals continued to be considerably dependent on royal sanction when it came to leasing or selling lands and properties.[28] Bethlem's governors were dominated by city tradesmen and politicians, On Bethlem's governing board sat the leading potentates of the City's central administration – the Lord Mayor, Recorder of London, Aldermen, members of the Court of Common Council, and representatives of the major guilds and trades houses – including, by the 1670s and 80s, men like Sir Thomas Player, City MP and Chamberlain of London, and the radical 'republican' Whigs Slingsby Bethell, Henry Cornish and Thomas Pilkington. Yet at the same time, if less prominent, amongst the Hospital's governors were some of the leading supporters of the royal prerogative, men like James Butler, the Duke of Ormonde, Sir Richard Mason and Sir William Wiseman (also a London Chamberlain). Some were rather hybrid figures, on the one hand representing the City, but on the other hand cultivating royal patronage. On the Building Committee which supervised Bethlem's rebuilding at Moorfields, for example, were figures like Sir William Bolton, onetime Lord Mayor of London and a major player in City politics, but also a man who, when censured by the Bethlem Court of Governors in 1674–5, was able to call on royal support for his reinstatement.[29]

Part and parcel of this dual allegiance owed by Bethlem was a virtual obligation to receive patients sent to it by both the royal and the city authorities. In some respects, Bethlem *was*, in fact, a state institution, and it was due to its traditional relationship with the State that, during the late eighteenth and early nineteenth centuries, it was Bethlem (rather than St Luke's or any other hospital) which took into custody attempted regicides, assassins and their accomplices, such as Margaret Nicholson, James Hadfield and Bannister Truelock. Throughout the period Bethlem received numerous cases committed with the personal stamp of royal authority, from the Secretary of State and from other notables within the royal administration. During the seventeenth century Bethlem admitted patients committed by the House of Lords, by the Privy Council, and by the High Commission. From the late seventeenth century it also became the main receptacle for mad and disorderly individuals who came under the provenance of that new overseer of the royal household, the Board of Green Cloth (a branch of the Lord Steward's Department), as well as for those deemed mentally unfit for service in the army and navy. Particularly large numbers of patients were sent by the Sick and Wounded Seaman's Office and by the War Office. In addition, throughout the period, Bethlem regularly received patients committed by the Lord Mayor, the Court of Aldermen, the Court of Common Council and the London and Middlesex Sessions. The Lord Mayor, in his capacity as chief city magistrate, head of the Court of Aldermen and frequent chair at the meetings to conduct the business of the royal hospitals, had a particularly important role in the committal of lunatics to Bethlem. It is in these cases, sent by the major outside authorities, rather than by private individuals, or by poor families and parishes, that the political implications of confinement are most apparent. It is with such cases, and especially with Board of Green Cloth cases, that I shall be largely concerned here. The nature of the Hospital's records and other available data means that the most eloquent and detailed information on state committals to Bethlem is to be derived from seventeenth- rather than eighteenth-century sources. My analysis will inevitably be biased accordingly.

'Lewde wordes in tyme of frensey': Early Political Limits to Speaking One's Mind

Christopher Hill has emphasized the apparent tolerance for the mad in political circles in England during the first half of the seventeenth century.[30] He cited cases like Arise Evans and Lady Eleanor Davies who were permitted considerable immunity, despite the political sensitivity of their self-appointed roles as prophets – until, at least, 'they overstepped the bounds of the politically endurable'.[31] State papers, Privy Council records and the Minutes of the Bridewell and Bethlem Court of Governors confirm that this tradition of immunity for the mad was a long and resilient one, and underline the frequency with which madness was actually conceived of as an excuse and absolution for offences, even if of a highly political nature. The options of punishment or confinement open to authorities were often waived as merely aggravatory to the condition of the insane. For example, on John Watson's complaints against the Bishop of London in 1579 being declared groundless and Watson found '*non compos mentis*', the Star Chamber decided that imprisoning him 'might further distracte him'. Instead, they enjoined him 'to repaire unto his Lordship, and ... acknowledge his faulte', leaving Watson's future care to the Bishop's discretion.[32] Even when an individual *was* 'committed to Bethlem for certeyne lewde wordes in tyme of frensey spoken agaynst the Kinges Majeste', as was one typical offender on the Privy Council's orders in 1546, he was often discharged soon after, once it 'appered' that 'there [was] ... no malice in him'.[33] In other cases guardianship was preferred over confinement. When William Williams of Newport, Monmouth, was found 'franticke' in 1580, having made 'certen unduetifull speaches uttered againste her Majestie' (for which he had been 'committed to the common gaole of Glocester'), the Council ordered his release into the custody of a guardian, requiring only that 'restitucion' be made of 'the gelding & c.' he had stolen.[34] If madness, however, tended to excuse slandering the magistrates, theft and other serious offences, this was only in so far as it appeared that the threat posed by madness could be contained and negated, and that the type of offence and the condition of the lunatic concerned permitted adequate amends to be made. The discharge of such cases depended on evincing the innocuous nature of their madness (the absence of a malicious or dangerous intent towards the lieges), on obtaining sufficient restitution for the offence committed, and on ensuring the future safe-keeping of the lunatic. When it came to this latter condition, in the absence of large-scale institutional provision, the family and the parish, or the guardian, served as the first and second rank guarantors, and the established authorities were generally happy for them to do so.

Clearly it was not always easy *per se* for the authorities to determine whether an offender was mad or not. In addition, there was no standard, or legally enshrined, procedure for certification, and this contributed to a considerable and widely recognized confusion in official policies towards the insane and to some individuals being falsely confined. Contemporary tests for lunacy, whether conducted by medical men or laymen, were primitive and deficient, and were figures of fun as depicted in the literature of the time. The political authorities plainly strove to make the right decision, however, and occasionally conducted their own independent examinations on doubtful cases. In 1575, the Privy Council were informed by the

Mayor of Leicester, that:

> Richard Sheffield had utterid certein sedicious wordes and speeches, clamying him self to be sonne to King Henry the Eight, and by sume was thought madde as he had ben many times before, and by others it was dowbted whether he were so or no.[35]

Seeking a 'better understanding of the trothe', the Privy Council ordered that he be examined, and that, if found insane, he was 'to be used as a man of that sorte' and his wife (who had been imprisoned by the Mayor) was to be released. While Sheffield had in fact been confined in Bridewell despite being found 'a lunatike', he was soon discharged, once his sister petitioned 'their Lordships' and offered 'to take the charge of him'.[36] In other cases, the ascription of madness served to commute a sentence from jail to the madhouse. William Ellis, locked up in the Gatehouse and examined before the Privy Council in 1617, having previously been arraigned before the Bishop of Bath and Wells for being a 'a wyked anabaptist', guilty of 'desperate speeches' and 'much ill affection by lewde and scandulous wordes against his Majestie's sacred person', was committed to Bethlem upon being found insane.[37] The evident lack of intervention from families and friends in Ellis' case, by contrast with Sheffield's, reveals the importance of social connections at this time. The implication, however, that confinement was preferred for Ellis because his disaffection to the monarchy and his anabaptism were adjudged graver offences than Sheffield's rather more obviously fallacious pretension to the throne, suggests one political determinant of the bounds of confinement, and how important politics were in discriminating one case from another.

Hill has emphasized how much scope there was for folly and playing the fool in the writings of the political and religious radicals of the period. Furthermore, Hill has demonstrated how aping madness was one way for political and religious dissenters to gain an exculpatory license for their unorthodoxies. The Erasmian tradition of praising folly, as Screech has argued particularly well,[38] was a very durable one. There was clearly a sense in which radicals were adopting a pragmatic strategy when calling themselves fools and mad, while denouncing establishment figures and orthodox beliefs. Popular caricatures of visiting Bethlem during the early modern period indulged in depictions of the Hospital as a welcome asylum for political and religious dissidents. Ned Ward turning the common mirror of madness on the outside world, in his *London Spy* of 1699, presents us with a prime example. Depicting one Bedlamite he had rebuked for ranting 'against Kingly government', Ward had the patient respond by calling *him* a fool and extolling the benefits of being free to speak his mind in Bethlem, whereas his visitor and those outside were required to guard their tongues:

> I can tell great men such bold truths as they don't love to hear, without the danger of a whipping post.[39]

This exculpatory side to madness, furthermore, helps to explain why so many individuals were brought before the Bridewell and Bethlem Court of Governors deemed to be 'counterfeits' and 'impostors', posing as insane.[40] Bethlem was anyway too small to take nearly all the deranged individuals who came before the authorities, and there were few other alternative lock-ups available, apart from houses of correction, or prisons. Neither Bethlem, with a capacity of only 20 at the beginning of the seventeenth century, and no more than 50 before 1677, nor Bridewell, could accommodate large numbers of the mad or bad, for whatever reason. Indeed, the tolerance for the insane spoken of by Hill was partially a product of lack of institutional provision (although the apparent failure to perceive a need for such further suggests that tolerance was the general rule).

Nevertheless, many individuals *were* sent to Bethlem by the Government upon slandering or questioning the established authorities. There was quite another side to the caricatures of Ward *et alia*, which implied that political or religious deviance alone could suffice to land one in Bethlem, and that, far from simple exculpation, identifying and confining individuals as mad might be one way for hierarchy to suppress or contain deviancy. 'Persecuted' throughout the land, said Ward's fictional madman, truth flew to Bethlem 'for sanctuary'.

Bethlem had long, in fact, been used as a receptacle for unruliness by the central and municipal government, and had long (especially since being gifted to the City in 1547 and joined with Bridewell in 1557), been associated with the repression of political and religious deviancy. It is often difficult to know what to make of accounts of confinements at Bethlem for political motives, especially those of the florid kind which spoke of riots being provoked amongst the local populace. One Elizabethan journal, described how on 5 June, 1595:

> a certain citizen, being a silkweaver, came to the Lord Mayor's house, using some hard speeches concerning him and in dispraise of his government. The Lord Mayor said he was mad and so committed him to Bedlam as a madman, but not having his officers about him sent him thither by some of his own servants; but without Bishopsgate he was rescued by prentices and divers other to the number of two or three hundred persons.[41]

We know that weavers were, and continued to be, for much of the seventeenth century, something of a mainstay of popular dissent. Weavers were also conspicuous inmates in both Bethlem and Bridewell, while slandering the magistrates ranked highly amongst the offences of State committals to both institutions. We also know that riotous behaviour was commonly associated with both apprentices and Bethlem, and remained peculiarly definitive of the Hospital's environment. None the less, it is very difficult to separate fact from fiction in such representations, to know where hyperbole and polemic ends and fair reconstruction begins.

One limit to tolerance for lunacy, as Hill has pointed out so well, was clearly breached when lunacy transcended the individual and the private, and entered the public sphere. It was when unorthodox ideologues and prophets gained active adherents that they became most dangerous to the established order. A typical example is that of Bartholmew Helston, who, according to one diarist, went about town in 1607 (like Richard Sheffield before him) 'giving himself forth to be Queen Mary's son', and (unlike Sheffield) was 'oftentimes gathering people about him'. When apprehended, Helston was adjudged of 'a seditious disposition' rather than lunatic, and was sent to Bridewell (despite his rather odd comment 'that he was stolen from Hampton Court where he was born'). The choice subsequently left to Lord Salisbury, however, was simply 'whether he remain in Bridewell or be sent to Bedlam' (the governors of Bridewell having evidently found his behaviour incongruous with the orderliness of their house).[42]

This highlights the emphatically political use to which Bethlem could be put as an alternative place for the incarceration and correction of individuals whose fundamental transgression had been against the established order. Bethlem was often spoken of by its own governors, as well as by outsiders, in the early seventeenth century, as a 'prison', and its inmates as 'prisoners', being conceived of in a way scarcely distinguishable from Bridewell. Indeed, that as late as 1672, Privy Council ministers could still refer to Bethlem's inmates as 'prisoners'[43] (when most other, lesser authorities had abandoned this terminology), suggests the inveteracy in the highest circles of conceptions of the Hospital as primarily a detention centre.

The apprehension of those, like Helston, who 'went abroad' and caused public tumults was an aspect of social policing. Many such individuals had also infringed the vagrancy laws, and were a threat in that they were 'at large', free of any familial or seigniorial supervision, and their disorderly conduct was thus apt to impinge upon sane society. As Beier's and many other studies of the social and political threat of vagrancy have pointed out, such waywardness was dangerous in itself, because it was unpredictable, and because it was 'masterless' or irresponsible, in that it severed all customary links between the individual and his household, place of work and settlement.[44] Vagrancy appeared at its most capricious when it involved the insane, who were not only particularly prone to wander, but whose wandering, apparently without rhyme or reason, appeared particularly rootless, arbitrary and volatile. In their attempts to impose limits on such wandering, central authorities issued directives repeatedly to magistrates and local officials, and the mad were occasionally explicitly singled out for apprehension. In 1630, for example, the Privy Council issued a warrant to the Westminster JPs for the arrest and committal to Bethlem of:

> certaine persons who run up and downe the streetes and doe much harme, being either distracted or els counterfeictes, and therefore not to be suffered to have their liberties to range

specifically naming a 'King Robert', 'Doctor Owen' and 'Mistris Vaughan'.[45] Just how closely bound up the threat of insanity (especially pauper insanity) was with the threat of vagrancy, or the fact of the insane being on the loose, is implied by the failure to separate insanity as a problem from vagrancy within the poor law until 1714. It is also manifested by the frequency with which individuals wound up in Bethlem because they had strayed from their lodgings, and had no one at home to provide for their future safeguard, or else were discharged by the Governors once guarantees, or security, had been given for their custody, or keeping within doors. Confining the insane, then, was often synonymous with containing their vagrancy. For example, Mary Davies wound up in Bethlem in 1676, because she had 'frequented' Whitehall Palace' 'for some space of time' and was 'much distracted', but also because 'she hath noe certaine abode'.[46] Therefore, she was cut off from the parochial or familial support that might have offered another option in her case, or vouchsafed that she would no longer constitute a threat at large to royalty. The vagrancy of the insane was especially dangerous when it impinged directly on the ruling classes. It was not just because Tobias Hume was 'distracted' and his 'words & Accons' were 'disorderly blasphemous and distemp[er]ed', that he was committed to Bethlem in 1642. He was also 'daingerous in goinge abroad of doeinge hurt', and 'by pressinge uppon sev[er]all ho[ora]ble Parsonnages', namely the five •.rls who signed the petition and warrant for his committal.[47] The Charterhouse, where Hume was a pensioner, had clearly been unable to contain his unruliness, not just within the bounds of what was permissible, but within its own physical or territorial limits.

While there was a clear recognition that Bethlem was for 'real' lunatics and Bridewell for rogues, these two institutions were often interchangeable and boundaries between them often blurred in this early period. Cases were sent back and forth from one house to the other. That Bethlem was regularly full only encouraged this symbiosis. The mad, and (more especially) dubious cases of madness, were often sent to Bridewell prior to their transfer to Bethlem, while awaiting either a vacancy or further assessment. It seems to have mattered little to some authorities whether an individual was confined in Bethlem or Bridewell. In 1638, for example, Henry Wayne's fellow parishioners succeeded in obtaining a written order from the Privy Council for his committal to Bethlem, but 'acknowledged ... in Courte that he is more a knave than a Madman'. There being, anyway, 'noe roome in Bethlem', the Governors agreed to set him to work at Bridewell, 'untill tryall may be made whether he be madd'.[48] The carpenter, George Goodwyn, hauled before the Bridewell Court on Sir Nicholas Rainton's warrant in the same year, and accused of having 'spoken seditious words against the king and blasphemous words against God', was set at work at Bridewell despite being conceived 'crackbrayned' and his mother's corroborating testimony that he was 'weak headed' and had not worked in his trade for months.[49] Sometimes, the fluidity of distinctions between the mad and the bad, and the use of Bridewell to punish and deter offenders who may have been insane, and more appropriate for Bethlem, was even more explicit. This confusion seems to have been particularly manifest in cases involving politico-religious dissent. Although 'suspected' to be 'madd', Richard Whetstone, for example, was committed to Bridewell by the Privy Council in 1615, because of 'a certaine lewde and wicked paper written by him'. At Bridewell, he was 'to bee ... corrected with the whipp' and not allowed 'at any time to goe abroade', and only 'if ... hereafter' he appeared to be mad, was Whetstone to be 'conveyed into Bedlem'.[50] Little seems to have distinguished Whetstone's case from that of others, before and after him, who merely received summary punishments at Bridewell. Typically, Luce Marten was sent to Bridewell in 1626, having 'writ and presented to his Majestie many foolish and idle lynes, some of them being scandelous against the Queene's Majestie', and was simply ordered to be 'well corrected with the whipp and then ... sett ... at libertie'.[51]

'Great Men' Policing the Boundaries of 'Bold Truths': State Committals, the Board of Green Cloth and Other Central Authorities

It is in the Board of Green Cloth's dealings with Bethlem that the political nature of confinement appears at its most emphatic. This Board sent over 40 patients to Bethlem during the period 1670–1750. With authority over that sacral territory known as 'the verge of the Court' – that is over any disorder occurring on royal property within 12 miles of wherever the Court was sitting – the Board's dealings with offenders inevitably had political implications. There were few more highly sensitive political arenas, and offences committed within the bounds of the verge were immediately, *per natura,* invested with political threat. Here, it is as important to see the arena of the verge as a semantic arena, invested with its own symbols and meanings, as it is to see it as a real location, where physical acts took place. In *The Politics and Poetics of Transgression,* Peter Stallybrass and Allon White emphasized how much ideology is defined by its particular 'domains' or 'places of production', and by the traffic and controls operating between and through these domains.[52] Whether it be the court, or the market place, every arena produces 'its own rules governing interaction, the body and language'.[53] One can see this very clearly in the discursive domain of the verge.

Merely intruding on to royal property carried an element of danger to the lieges. *Table 1* shows how highly the mere act of 'intrusion' into the royal domain figured in the reasons for patients' committal to Bethlem by the Board. In at least 17 (or 41 per cent) of the 41 cases 'intrusion' was specified as one of the offences. There was naturally an accentuated sense of trespass where royalty was concerned. Yet royal palaces, royal parks and other areas frequented by the royal family were strikingly permeable and insecure places, very open to the public. Though owned by the Crown, the royal parks were used by a large, heterogeneous throng of the general populace. Entrances and passages through park and palace walls also allowed limited freedom of public access, while ancient rights of immunity attached to the special jurisdiction of the verge had long made it a hideaway for debtors and other offenders. Board of Green Cloth proceedings are replete with problems over public concourse through royal property. In fact, an increasing propensity is perceptible on the Board's part from the later seventeenth century to restrict the formerly wide license for indiscriminate access – to brick up doorways and entrances, to block passageways and to apprehend and prosecute the motley crowds of 'thieves, Robbers,

Vagabonds, Vagrants, Begg[ar]s, Masterless men, boys','pick pockets and lewd women', who loitered about royal property.[54]

Table 1

Reasons for Admission of Patients Committed to Bethlem by the Board of Green Cloth, 1670–1750[1]

Reasons	Men	Women	Totals
Attempted suicide and wife's complaint	1	0	1
Treasonable words/writings and troublesome within verge	3	0	3
Counterfeiting a minister and troublesome etc.	1	0	1
Intrusion and troublesome etc.	8	8	16
Intrusion and troublesome etc. and house of correction unable to cope	1	0	1
Threatened violence (drawing sword/suspicion of malice/threat to throw stone)	2	1	3
Actual physical assault (wounding/ throwing fruit at King)	3	0	3
Disorders within royal household	0	1	1
Soldiers and sailors	5	0	5
Unknown	6	1	7
Totals	30	11	41

1. Derived from Bethlem's Admission Registers and Board of Green Cloth Minutes and Letter Books

The visibility of royalty and nobility was particularly marked during this period, and was a powerful source of attraction for the ordinary citizen, let alone the alienated or psychotic. This may all sound rather familiar, given the present-day furore about press access to, and the visibility and security of the royal family. Yet, in early modern times the power and person of the Monarch were peculiarly immanent within the public sphere. Royalty not only visited Bethlem, but presided in Council over the committal of apparently crazy individuals to Bethlem and elsewhere. Self-appointed correctors of the public morals, like the one-time Bedlamite Alexander Cruden, might even gain an audience with, and kiss the hand of, the Monarch.[55] A touch from the monarch was held to cure scrofula ('the King's Evil'), while petitioning the monarch or the royal ministers was an accepted form of obtaining redress. The royal palaces and parks were commonly beset by throngs of people waving petitions, or waiting for a sight or a touch of royalty. Contemporaries felt their relation to monarchy and hierarchy even more acutely, and individuals were perhaps more prone to referring the confused riddle of their identities and their out-of-focus grievances to the ultimate authorities. They were certainly more liable to be incarcerated for so doing. Indeed, these considerations may help to explain why so many were sent to Bethlem believing themselves emperors, kings or queens, or for infractions within the verge, or why the mad king or queen had such a prominent place in representations of the population of Bedlam. No doubt, this is more intimately connected with the strong association of madness with pride during this period, a subject that has already been examined by numerous scholars,[56] while the pervasiveness of such images in literary caricatures of madness may encourage a tendency to exaggerate the importance of the phenomenon. I am far from wanting to suggest that the psychotic do not still commonly identify with potentates and celebrities.

Quite apart from bothersome intrusions into the verge, violence, or the threat of violence, also seems to have featured prominently in Board of Green Cloth committals to Bethlem. Six or nearly 15 per cent of all cases in *Table 1* were accused of threatening violence, or actual physical assault inside the verge. In a significant number of cases, furthermore, the vague description 'troublesome' is used in the Board's minutes and warrants, terminology which may conceal rather more serious offences. When Deborah Lydall was committed to Bethlem in 1677, it was not her frequent trespassing and 'severall disorders' in St James's Park that seem to have provoked the Board to act. More 'p[ar]ticularly' it was her having 'tooke a Stone offering to throw it at the Queene' and the distracted nature of 'her whole Carriage and deportment'.[57] Similarly, Richard Harris, had been a 'frequent' intruder and 'committed several disorders' in St James's Park, and had 'long ... shewed himselfe ... distracted', before the 'p[ar]ticular' act of 'throwing an Orange at the King', in 1678, provoked his incarceration in Bethlem.[58] His act may have had some more meaningful motive (or was, at the very least, full of irony!), in that the Board's Entry Books during the same year record a great want of oranges and lemons in the town and the difficulties of the grocer getting 'fitting' samples even for the King.[59] Edward Price wound up in Bethlem in 1715, having 'lately become Lunatick ... been troublesome and offensive' to the Court at St

James's, and moreover for having 'wounded one of the Soldiers of the Guard with another's Bayonett'.[60] These cases suggest that committal often followed an extreme type of misdemeanour, and was far from the first resort for dealing with the incursions of mad individuals.

The context in which violent offences took place, and the individuals against whom violence was directed was plainly vital in such cases. Matthew Pugh, whose conveyance to Bethlem, in 1745, by order of the Board of Green Cloth and in the Company of one of the King's Provost Marshalls, created a minor stir in the press, had made the mistake of drawing his sword in St James's Chapel – much too close to royalty and nobility for comfort.[61] Captain White, sent to Bethlem in 1691, had not merely intruded into Windsor Castle and Palaces, but 'in a Violent Manner did Assault one George Buthwaite one of the Poore Knights', had 'Committed severall high Misdemeanours' and had previously 'wounded Captaine Hull the Governour of the Poor Knights'.[62] There was also the apprehension that such offenders 'may do other Mischiefes', against which incarceration offered some guarantee of 'prevention'. In White's, as in most other cases, however, it was not the political threat entailed in such violence that identified them as insane and appropriate for confinement in Bethlem. Rather, it was that the assaults by White and others had been made 'without any Provocation' (or at least without any provocation considered legitimate, or rational), which, primarily, seem to have shown them to be 'much discomposed & disordered in ... Braine'. This may help to explain why the authorities so rarely actually discussed the motivations for such acts (although this, itself, must qualify my conclusions about their meaning with some reservations). Motivations were generally held to be non-existent amongst the insane, or else deluded and therefore irrelevant.

The Board of Green Cloth also dealt with disorders and verbal indiscretions within, or close by, the royal household. While often taking the form of essentially inter-personal disputes, mutinous words from a royal footman, or a violent altercation between an inferior servant and a lieutenant of the Tower might also have worrying political ramifications. If Voltaire worried about being too candid with Enlightenment ideas in front of servants, then how much more must the Board have worried about seditious utterances or actions inside the royal household. Catherine Edwards, servant to the Duchess of Richmond and living in Whitehall Palace with her husband, John (servant to the Duke), was admitted to Bethlem in 1679 having 'been guilty of many disorders contrary to the good Government of his Ma[jes]ties Household'.[63] Two years earlier, Nicholas Valiant, one of the King's Footmen in Ordinary, had also been admitted to Bethlem at the King's 'express com[m]and', having 'been guilty of many disorders' and having 'for a long time shewed himselfe to be a p[er]son distracted & voyd of right understanding'.[64] More especially, Valiant had 'of late uttered treasonable words saying he had rather kill the King then my Lord of Pembrook'. It was emphatically a preventative and security-conscious concern about such a dangerous presence in the royal household (or, to quote verbatim from the warrant, 'for ye prevention of any danger or mischeife that may ensue'), that Valiant was passed into Bethlem's 'safe custody'. Concern for Valiant's cure was conspicuous by its absence from the warrant.

Many social historians have emphasized the importance of the household in this period in defining the limits of acceptable behaviour. Quite apart from the royal household, preserving the peace of the household was a significant concern in many admissions to Bethlem. Moreover, there was clearly a relation between the threat to hierarchy entailed in disorderly conduct within, or nearby, the royal household, and the threat to familial hierarchy and harmony entailed by domestic strife. Unruly apprentices and servants, and disobedient wives, threatened not only the ability of the household to subsist, but also the established scales of authority on which the stability of the household (often conceived as a microcosm for the state) was held to rely. When committal orders from the Green Cloth and the Sick and Wounded Board stressed subjecting patients (like Catherine Edwards and Thomas Gallop) to 'the order and discipline' (or 'Government') of the 'house' of Bethlem, it was clearly intended that the Hospital's regime would supplant and re-instil an alternative (and, often, harsher) internal regime to that adjudged to have failed within the individual's original household.[65]

Far beyond the verge, hostility to the powers that be voiced without sufficient circumspection frequently invoked the force of the law and was seldom safe from informers eager for rewards. As a recent study of the language of madness by Allan Ingram has underscored,[66] madness, in this period, was very much identified by words and the language people spoke. While the blasphemy laws were rather laxly enforced in England by comparison with other European countries, imprudent or passionate words, whether blasphemous or disrespectful of royalty, were still readily deemed treasonable or threatening to the established order. Individuals 'speakeing daingerous words', or cursing the names of the King or one of his ministers were regularly informed on and arraigned before justices. Such individuals appear quite regularly in the minutes of the Bridewell and Bethlem Governors, and in the proceedings of the Privy Council, the Board of Green Cloth and other courts. They were not always people who had come into contact with the major authorities, but were often apprehended for simple civil disorders and vagrancy, as part of the ordinary policing of the streets. The extrovert and the insane, furthermore, were apt to do their cause no favours by speaking disrespectfully and out of turn once brought before their elders and betters. Indeed, if telling 'great men bold truths' risked being stigmatized as insane in this period, the mad were themselves peculiarly liable to speak their minds recklessly, to disregard the strictures of etiquette and decorum, and to outrage the bounds of hierarchy and propriety. James Williams, for example, admitted to Bethlem in 1662, had been apprehended 'for being a disorderly p[er]son & causeing tumults in the streetes', but went on to compound his situation before the Bridewell Court by 'uttering here this day wicked & seditious words concerning the Kings Ma[jes]tye'.[67] When Anne Bassett was found 'distracted' and sent to Bethlem, after appearing before the Bethlem and Bridewell Court of Governors, in 1647, accused of being an 'idle disorderly p[er]son', her crime and condition seem to have been no worse than that of many other women who were simply sent home. That her warrant had been signed by Sir John Wollaston, the Hospitals' President, and that Bassett 'abused the court', however, may have made the difference between confinement and deliverance in her case, and others like it.[68] Military authorities were, not surprisingly, particularly intolerant of insubordination and disaffected words against any superior, let alone the monarchy. Slandering royalty, even in jest, was liable to land men on a charge, and might be the cause of an expulsion from a military hospital and from the support of a military pension. Greenwich Hospital's Governors, for example, dealt most stringently with Thomas Wynn, drumming him out in 1733 for his insolence towards the royal family (he had called the children 'whelps' and wished them back in their 'own Country'). Wynn had originally tried to excuse himself by putting his remarks down to 'mirth', which cut little ice with the Greenwich Board, who were more concerned about the 'dangerous consequence' such might have 'for the rest of the Pensioners, & People of the House'. The Board also rejected Wynn's subsequent claim, when petitioning the Admiralty for reinstatement, that his indiscretions had been the consequence of 'Frenzy', asserting that on the contrary they arose from 'Disaffection'.[69]

Of course, expressions of disaffection to the established authorities were far from sufficient on their own to suggest insanity or irrationality. Apparently sane individuals sent to the Bridewell and Bethlem Governors by the Green Cloth and other authorities for scandalous words (or, like Edward Smith in 1638, for 'having noe dep[end]encie upon any p[er]son in the Courte' and 'resorteth hither and pestereth and annoyeth the same'), more often received a whipping and/or a brief period of custody at Bridewell, before their deliverance. (Both institutions were still, however, more or less bound to await a warrant from such authorities before they could release a prisoner).[70] While it was often, as in the case of Edward Harris in the 1730s, 'Treasonable Expressions', uttered in the wrong places, which first brought individuals to the attention of the authorities, it was, normally, only when other evidences from an individual's language, demeanour, behaviour or deportment, suggested insanity, that committal to Bethlem was deemed appropriate. Harris was originally committed to Newgate, and was only subsequently found 'disordered in his Senses' and transferred by order of the Secretary of State to Bethlem. It was the nature of Mary Coglan's 'whole Carriage & deportm[en]t' that identified her as insane when examined before the Board in 1677 (rather than merely her making as if to hurl a stone at the Queen). Coglan had originally been conceived to be simply 'rude & disorderly', 'a Disturb[er] of the Peace of his Maj[es]t[y']s House', and 'a Counterfeit', rather than a real lunatic, and had been sent to a house of correction. When, *vice versa*, seeking to defend himself against the imputation of insanity that had landed him in Bedlam in the 1690s, the Jacobite 'Scribe of Christ', Richard Stafford, had emphasised the absence of 'Extravagancy' in his 'Deportment', and the gentleness and composure of his 'voice' and 'manner'.[71] In 1692, a year after Stafford's confinement, another individual was identified as 'a madman' and sent to Bethlem, having 'came into the House [of Commons], up to the very Table with his hat on, and bid the Speaker come out of the Chair'.[72] Likewise, it was the lack of any signs of insanity in Richard Farnham's 'words or gestures' which were to signify his sanity in 1637, just as they had signified him as insane a year earlier. The power of mere gestures and deportment in conveying clear socio-political messages, outraging established norms of etiquette and hierarchy, and identifying individuals as irrational should not be underestimated. Plainly the authorities sought to distinguish political deviancy from actual lunacy and to respond differently in accordance. On the explicit grounds that the aforementioned disturber of the House of Commons was mad, the House had decided initially to mitigate its outrage, merely expelling him and forgoing the usual custodial sentence with 'the Serjeant at Arms' (although it took just another two days before the President of Bethlem was ordered to 'take care of' him and 'put him in Bedlam'). Yet such cases still suggest how easily the distinction between irrationality and affronting hierarchy, or between madness and badness, was liable to blur.

Keeping the Insane Close: Special Instructions for State Committals

For most individuals discussed so far, committal was politicized merely, or primarily because their transgressions took place in a political arena, or touched upon establishment figures. Yet it is necessary to strive to distinguish these cases from others confined emphatically for political reasons, whose offences actually altered and politicized the normative character of confinement, or whose committals suggest that the content of lunacy itself was being politicized. Individuals who merely trespassed on royal property, or threw things at the royal family, and who were committed to Bethlem without any special arrangements made, appear plainly to be of the former sort. Others, however, whose committal orders stipulated peculiarly stringent requirements for their custody, or who, like Richard Farnham and Richard Stafford (discussed below), landed themselves in Bethlem chiefly on account of actions and words in contradiction of established norms, belong to the latter.

It was not just that bodies like the Board of Green Cloth and the Privy Council sent persistent and vociferous nuisances to Bethlem. They also occasionally issued special instructions to impose an extra degree of confinement upon such patients, or to deprive them quite emphatically of any voice, or audience for their words. The Privy Council warrant committing William Ellis (who had 'expressed ... scandulous wordes against his Majestie's person') to Bethlem in 1617, ordered that he be kept 'safe their in chaynes until farther order'.[73] A rather more explicit warrant from the Council committing Richard Day to Bethlem in 1639, ordered that no-one be permitted 'to have Access unto him or to speake w[i]th him, but in the presence of his keeper' – although Day was to spend but a fortnight in Bethlem.[74] In 1673, a warrant from the Secretary of State, Henry Coventry, ordered the Bethlem porter not only 'to lock up Dun ... a Person in his Custody', but:

> not to Suffer him to be seen or spoken to by any person in his room. And when it should be thought fit to suffer him to walk out, that no body be permitted to talk with him.[75]

The objectives of securing and silencing individuals were clearly paramount in such committals. Any aim of curing Ellis, Day and Dunn was not even mentioned. Of course, this does not mean that cure was not an implicit concern. Cure (as I argue more fully below) *was* stipulated in other state committals, while the government was making some sort of distinction about the peculiar function of Bethlem merely in choosing it for the insane over penal institutions like the Tower, or the Marshalsea. Indeed, one should beware taking the rather formulaic language of warrants too literally. Just as differentiations were being made in the choice of custody for the mad and bad, those choices presumed and predicated differences in the way cases were to be treated. Yet, when it came to actually specifying terms and provisions for custody and treatment in Bethlem (in such cases as Day and Dunn), the government sometimes made very little distinction between the insane and the felonious. Indeed, the orders it issued for the detention of dangerous felons in its prisons were sometimes almost identical to those issued for committals to Bethlem.

Questions of security were clearly important in most committals to Bethlem, but loomed particularly large in state committals. In the later seventeenth century, even when warrants from the Board of Green Cloth instructed that patients be treated 'in the usual manner', it was also assumed and specified that this entailed patients being 'secured'.[76] Confinement, furthermore, did not only tend to be more severe for state committals – its length and character might depend more explicitly on the individual's capacity for moral reformation. When, three years before Richard Day, Richard Farnham had wound up in Bethlem at the command of Laud and the High Commission, he had been ordered to be kept in similarly close confinement. Farnham was only granted 'the Liberty usually afforded to others in that house' once the Hospital's officers had themselves sued for it and testified that he 'did not appear either by words or gestures to be madd or Lunatiq[ue]'.[77] This was, in addition, only on the Privy Council's condition that Farnham continue to 'behave himselfe well and soberly, and lives Orderly' – language in which the moral and the mental merge quite overtly. There seems little doubt that such language was strongly informed by judgements about Farnham's moral culpability as an alleged bigamist and blasphemer. Confinement, in such cases, had a deterrent aspect to it. One might compare the terminology used in Farnham's case with that used 40 years later, in the case of John or Jean Stafford. Stafford was ordered discharged from Bethlem in 1688 on the Physician's certificate to the Green Cloth that he was 'not distracted' and 'has behaved himself very civilly and orderly since he hath bin in the Hospitall'.[78] Of course, assessing patients in terms of their civility and orderliness was a conventional means of judging sanity/insanity during this period, and not peculiar to patients confined by the State. Yet, the especial emphasis placed on the civility and orderliness of lunatics and alleged lunatics has obvious wider implications about the authoritarian and hierarchical nature of society. In state committals, furthermore, this emphasis appears to have been particularly marked and to have invested insanity, and its associated rudeness and unruliness, with particularly heavy social and political overtones.

Farnham was still in Bethlem a year and a half after being declared sane, when the Hospital petitioned Archbishop Laud directly, pleading lack of space for other lunatics and that Farnham was 'not ... soe Lunatiq[ue] as still to [need to] continue there'.[79] Even then, Farnham was not to gain his liberation. After the passing of one more year saw his acquittal on the charge of bigamy, in July 1639, Farnham was sent to Bridewell (another example of the two institutions' alternating relationship). The Court of Session's verdict on this occasion that he had been shamming lunacy – in so far as 'he is not so distracted as he woulde make himselfe, but is able to worke and gett his living' – may reinforce Hill's point about the advantages of counterfeiting madness. Yet it also suggests how closely madness was bound up with social and economic gauges, such as ability to work and financial means of support, and how hazy and value laden were the criteria for determining mental disorder.

Madman or Politico-Religious Dissenter? The Case of Richard Stafford

Perhaps the most explicit example of how Bethlem was used to silence politico-religious dissent, is the case of Richard Stafford. Indeed, his case is eloquent enough to merit a somewhat more detailed analysis.

Richard Stafford (1663–1703) was the second son of John Stafford (d.1705) of Thornbury, Gloucester, the grandson of William Stafford (1593–1684), a moderate parliamentarian pamphleteer, and the nephew of Sir John Stafford, Constable of Bristol Castle. He clearly came from respectable and wealthy stock. His family were prominent amongst the local Gloucestershire gentry. They owned the estate of Marlwood Park in Thornbury, and Richard was able to dispose of land and property in Cloestone parish on his death mortgaged to the value of £500. Embarking on an education to the bar, Stafford soon found himself paying more attention to divinity, of which he became a voracious, largely self-instructed student, taking the precepts of the Old Testament in particular to his heart. Richard's upbringing and inclinations led him increasingly to the more radical side of Protestant dissenting religion, in a parish that was something of a nonconformist heartland. He may have attended the Quaker meeting house established at Thornbury in 1690, although, a decade later, he was on closer terms with the parish vicar, Ralph Grove, whom he made an overseer of his will.[80] His first entry into print, a tract entitled *Of Happiness* (1689), reads like a personal creed of faith, with plain, ingenuous instructions on how happiness was to be achieved by following God's commandments. Yet Stafford was also a devout constitutional monarchist, firmly convinced of the divine right of kings. By the time his first publication appeared, the Glorious Revolution had seen the Catholic James II exiled in favour of his daughter, Mary II, and his Dutch son-in-law, William III, and Stafford launched himself into much more dangerous and contentious waters. Convinced not only that William's accession was unconstitutional and against God's law, but of his own divinely appointed mission to bring the government to its senses, Stafford was to publish tract after tract saying just that and declaring himself a Scribe of Jesus Christ. His stand and his writings struck loud chords with dissenters and gained the active support of Jacobite publicists. Bold from the start in distributing his pamphlets at the very doorways of government, Stafford was to find himself twice arrested (on both of which occasions he was dealt with as a sane offender), before he was finally declared insane and sent to Bethlem. Delivering the first of his anti-government pamphlets to the sitting parliament, on 4 January, 1690,[81] Stafford had been indicted under the common law and was confined in Newgate for a week. On publishing another two pamphlets and delivering them to Commons members at the beginning of the following April (having already left two letters on the back stairs at Whitehall),[82] his punishment was more severe. (It is unlikely that Stafford helped his case by issuing a further petition and remonstrance whilst in custody).[83] He suffered another four weeks' detention in the custody of the Sergeant-at-Arms, had his chamber searched and was handed over to his father's safe-keeping in Gloucester. It was a year and a half later, once Stafford had published several more tracts and had returned to London to distribute them around the Queen's Court, that he was sent to Bethlem.

Stafford was committed to Bethlem in November 1691, where he was to remain for nearly eight months. The reasons for his committal specified in the warrant were being 'distracted' and moreover 'very troublesome to their Ma[jes]ties at Kensington By Dispersing Books & Pamphlets full of Enthusiasme and Sedition'.[84] His case is of particular interest, because it is one of the clearest and best documented examples we have of the political uses of confinement. Indeed, there can be few other cases where the political motivations for incarcerating an individual as insane in this period appear more paramount, or where the stigma of insanity serves so effectively and designedly to discredit and silence dissent. Not to say that Stafford's is an open and shut case of psychiatric abuse, or that Stafford failed to provide signs of mental instability sufficient to sanction a charge of insanity. Yet the primary motivations behind his confinement were undoubtedly political.

Regrettably, it is rare that the historical record is sufficiently explicit to be sure exactly what was said by such individuals, and what made their words appear so dangerous, or so insane. Sometimes, as in the case of Charles Burroughs, a confectioner who, in 1716, uttered (amongst a host of 'treasonable words') 'indecent expressions concerning the King & Madam Kilmarnock', the censorship of language 'not fitt to be incerted' was openly admitted by the authorities.[85] Fortunately, however, many of Stafford's pamphlets were printed and are still extant. Reading these writings, it is soon apparent that they contain, at the very least, signs of mental peculiarity, being deeply self-referential, obsessive, and (increasingly, as time goes on) full of delusive hubris and contradiction. Yet Stafford's writings, particularly his early productions, are not merely the 'violent and incoherent tirades' that O'Donoghue once dismissed them as.[86] Indeed, by contrast with the tracts of Lady Eleanor Davies (where the Biblical quotations are often the most coherent features), there was nothing incoherent about Stafford's writing. Complaining bitterly about the illegality and unconstitutional nature of William's accession to the throne, Stafford gave quite lucid and potent expression to a widely felt outrage at the 'Glorious Revolution'.

> In the late Revolution of putting down one King, and setting up another ... they have actually departed from that Established and fixed Order of Things he [God] hath set up,

declared Stafford in his 1690 pamphlet *A Supplemental Tract of Government ... referred to the Consideration of the Lords and Government.*[87] Deposing 'a King' to whom, Stafford went on:

> those of the pure Reformed Religion had Sworn a Solemn Oath of Allegiance and Supremacy ... [knowing him] to be a Papist ... makes *Protestantism* stink, and be evil spoken of throughout the World.

It was his *Tract of Government* that landed Stafford in Newgate, which is hardly surprising given his claim that 'the late Revolution' departed from God's law, and given the very personal affronts and admonitions he hurled at William, Mary and the Clergy. Yet the pamphlet contains few obvious signs of insanity, and neither do Stafford's two subsequent productions, both of which repeated condemnations of 'Popery and

Arbitrary Government' and warnings to the monarchy and clergy, merely adding brief comments about other dangers to the nation, such as the very real threat of a French and Irish invasion.[88] Stafford's writings also encapsulated much of the dilemma felt by the Protestant dissenters, who had only been permitted the right to worship in 1689, but had continued to be debarred from office in Church and State by what Stafford and his co-religionists regarded as 'contradictory Oaths'. Stafford's deep conviction of the need for purification and reform in the established Church, and his profound concern about the popish tendencies of Church and State,[89] was a typical dissenting standpoint. In order, no doubt, to mitigate his culpability in the eyes of the authorities, Stafford sought to portray himself as on the moderate, rather than the extreme, side of nonconformity. In his *A Clear Apology and Just Defence* of 1690, while complaining about the severity of the legal penalties that had been imposed upon dissenters, he defended himself as a mild dissenter, who had been loyal and regular in his observation of Church of England services, taking communion thrice a year and continuing to attend 'sometimes', even after the Toleration Act of 1689.[90] This strategy of 'occasional conformity' was common to most dissenters before and after 1689, but Stafford seems to have followed it with less cynicism than most. Nevertheless, Stafford's total intolerance for Catholicism undoubtedly set him on the more extreme side of dissent. Indeed, he would probably have been one of those nonconformists, who, rather than see Catholics in office, would have opposed moves to repeal the same Test Acts which excluded Protestant dissenters from office too. Much more than this, it was Stafford's inability to accept the legitimacy of the new Government, the vociferous and uncompromising way he condemned it, the insistence of his claims to be speaking directly from the mouth of God, and the determined persistence with which he attempted to force these views down the throat of the Government, which identified him as no ordinary dissenter, but a dangerous and crazy radical.

In his *Apology*, which was published soon after his second period of confinement and the year before his committal to Bethlem, Stafford was already aware of a campaign to identify him as a lunatic, which he conceived as merely an attempt to discredit his views. The comments he made on this subject cannot simply be attributed to growing paranoia or a persecution complex. 'A malicious and false imputation may be cast and endeavoured to be fastened on anyone', declared Stafford, six months prior to being sent to Bethlem:

> And also, what is a little new or unusual, or doth somewhat exceed common apprehension, may seem to the vulgar sort, yea, and be

> called by them madness; but this is so trivial, that it is sufficient answer only to take notice of such an Ignorant Calumny.

His remarks on how insanity had been used in this way, and the devices he deployed to turn the mirror on his accusers, show Stafford to have been capable of considerable insight and composure. In fact, he was developing an old theme, adumbrated in his very first publication, *Of Happiness* (1689), and very much at the heart of dissenting religious tradition. 'Distraction and Restlessness of mind', said Stafford, in a long digression on melancholy,[91]

> ... do pass in the World for pure Melancholy. It is an Aspersion cast upon sincere Religion [that] ... All Thoughts of God ... are by the Ignorant and Ungodly thus esteemed.[92]

Stafford emphasized the positive, scriptural definition of melancholy as synonymous with sorrow, and how giving way to melancholy could be a means for the Holy Spirit to act on the conscience. On the one hand, Stafford championed melancholy as a natural and legitimate way of knowing God, of entering into his commandments and experiencing the 'regrets of Conscience'. On the other hand, he condemned the medical, materialist explanation of melancholy, which 'would impute [it] to the blackness of blood, and heavy flegmatick Constitution', and warned how 'inward Religion is in danger to be destroyed' by the tendency to mistake 'all regrets of Conscience ... for Melancholy, and the Workings of God's Spirit for Enthusiasm or Fancy'.[93] Stafford stood most firmly, here, within a rich religious heritage of praising folly and cults of melancholy, spanning Erasmus and Burton to nonconformists like Richard Baxter and Timothy Rodgers.

Apparently, then, Stafford was already feeling the brunt of the vigorous campaign against 'enthusiasm' in politics and religion that Michael MacDonald and others have shown to be so distinctive of post-Restoration orthodoxy.[94] Extremists on either side of the religio-political divide were increasingly denigrated in the literature of the age as irrational bigots, and their ferocious temperaments represented as mirrored in the animalistic distortion of their faces and in their deformed and distempered minds.[95] 'How stark mad beyond Moorfields or Hellebore', declared one of Stafford's contemporaries in a publication narrated under the guise of modesty and moderation, 'the Red Hot Bigotts of both sides have lately bin'.[96] Indeed, it was the declared agenda of this publication (and many others of the same ilk), to expose the madness at the heart of religious and political passion:

> to represent the great Furioso's on either hand in their own Colours, to dress em in their own distorted Faces ... to shew the madness and unreasonableness as well as danger in any such desperate Heats.

To return to specifics, Daniel Finch, 2nd Earl of Nottingham, the Secretary of State who ordered Stafford's confinement and whom Stafford was most hostile to amongst the King's Ministers, is unlikely to have been receptive to Stafford's opinions, especially given his own politico-religious views. A stout Anglican and leader of the High Church Tories, Nottingham was, despite his sponsorship of the Toleration Act, extremely hostile to any radical form of religious dissent. He was neither friend to nonconformists' ambitions for office, nor to the legitimacy of occasional conformity.[97] Stafford embarked on his preaching career in the same year as Nottingham became Secretary. If it is tempting to see Stafford's periods of confinement as, in a significant sense, explained by particular political events, and particular political prejudices, nevertheless, bias tends to cut both ways. It seems rather more persuasive to see Stafford's (and a number of other state committals) as partial consequences of an increasing tendency to anathematize dissent, to stigmatize ideological or spiritual ardour and individual claims of inspiration as intemperate or mad. There was much more, however, to the cases of Stafford *et alia* than simple repression.

Stafford was one of a small minority of individuals sent to Bethlem whose transgressions took their most explicit form in politico-religious dissent, while it was evidently not this dissent alone which signified Stafford as mad. It was only gradually, after a number of confirmatory evidences from Stafford's writings and conduct, that the government seems to have determined that he was mad. Stafford's *Apology*, moreover, does present some perceptible signals of deterioration in his mental processes. His assertion 'I speak nothing of my self, but from his Word only', and its preface by a detailed account of his own education and attainment of credentials 'at the School of Prophets', was but one of a number of somewhat extravagant contradictions. This, and other assertions, such as his claim to have given away a hundred copies of his petition to parliament, and to have ordered a thousand, 'more then sufficient for all the Representatives of the whole Nation', do seem to suggest that his delusions of grandeur were reaching new heights. By claiming to be a divine messenger, Stafford may well have been compensating somewhat for the 'personal Deformity and Lameness' which he blamed in the *Apology*, amongst other things, for his being called mad.[98] (Arise Evans also seems to have suffered from physical deformities.)

Stafford was treated seriously enough, however, to be responded to quite candidly and without any slur of insanity by the government publicist, Edward Stephens. Replying in his own *Apology*, Stephens devoted an entire pamphlet to the self-elected scribe. Although a firm Whig who welcomed the Revolution and attacked the Quakers, Stephens was also a supporter of tolerance in religious affairs and of rapprochement with Protestant dissenters. Adopting a rather gentle, admonishing tone to Stafford, Stephens referred to him and others like him as simply 'honest mistaken People'.[99] Stephens used his response to Stafford to rebuke other, less honest dissenters within the Government itself, who had gained office through insincere oaths of allegiance. There is nothing, however, to suggest that Stephens thought Stafford mad. Indeed, he saw sufficient cause in Stafford's stand to ask whether:

> we do not give occasion to Mr. Stafford, and other very honest People, to suspect, and plainly signify to the World abroad ... that we our selves are not well satisfied in what we have done.

Significantly, it was not Stafford's opinions themselves which Stephens deemed so 'extraordinary and rare' (indeed, it was the very popularity of Stafford's opinions that was most worrying to Stephens and the government). What was exceptional was 'the Zeal ... he ... shewed ... for what he thought to be true', so much so that it could be dismissed as bizarre, or, as Stephens put it: 'it could not deserve to be taken notice of in print'. Both Stephens' and the government's attitude to Stafford and how to deal with him was soon to change, however, as the increasingly aggrieved tone of Stafford's writings was itself to signify.[100]

One should not expect to find categorical signs of insanity in Stafford's early works, perhaps, when it was three more of his publications that apparently altered the government's attitude towards him and provoked his committal to Bethlem. There is, however, little difference in either the tone, or the subject matter, of the pamphlets of 1690 and those of 1691. In the first of his 1691 pamphlets, *The Truth Which God hath shewn to his Servant Richard Stafford* (March 1691), Stafford declared, with little change in his emphasis:

> They count it an odious or invidious thing, to speak or preach against the *Government* that now is, for according to their wanted manner of *turning things upside down,* they call that the Government, which is only an unnatural and unjust Usurpation.[101]

Stafford's last production before his committal was merely a few additions to his previous book *Things Plain and weighty*, and contributed nothing that was noticeably any madder than his previous works. Yet Stafford's awareness was even more acute, in these works, that his ambition (God willing) to 'blow the unjust Possessors out of the Throne' with his words, 'might be lookt upon', not only as 'forward and vain', and savouring 'of high Self-conceit or rank Enthusiasm', but even as 'like the ... droppings forth of Mad Men'.[102] It was not just his words, his egoism and his presumption, however, which seem to have convinced the government that he was mad. It was also his very persistence, his going beyond all normal, reasonable avenues to get himself heard, his disregard for all warnings and all natural instincts of self-preservation, the brazenness of his dissension, the unbridled nature of his zeal. Stafford, himself, had recognized the dangers of succumbing to 'a furious unwarranted Zeal' when writing *Of Happiness.* After being accused by Edward Stephens of displaying a zeal quite 'extraordinary and rare to be met with',[103] it was but a few more short steps beyond the pale for Stafford's zeal to be dismissed as simply madness. At no stage did Stafford attempt to conceal his activities or identity. If he was clearly, therefore, no ordinary, surreptitious plotter, what else could he have been but a fool, or a madman? It seems to have been knowingly that Stafford contravened the strictures of 'Custom and Usage' by handing his petitions to Commons members.[104] Yet to have transgressed a third time and handed another letter personally to Kensington Palace on 3 November, 1691, after repeated warnings and punishments, argued Stafford to be not just a stubborn transgressor, but a senseless one. Showing a modicum of self-restraint after his release from Bethlem, Stafford resolved to leave his latest book with the Clerk of Parliament, rather than attend the sessions 'in Person almost every day'. He noted the important lesson he had learned:

> that my coming and appearing so often in Person, would seem somewhat like a Mad-man, which mine enemies have falsly reproached me to be.[105]

On the day of his arrest at Kensington, Stafford had, in fact, already been refused permission to 'deliver my Books in Person' and 'turned ... out of Doors' by the King's servants, when he chose to drop them on the ground outside the doors.

The mention of royal servants raises another issue about the politics of confinement. The angry reaction of these particular servants, who proceeded to burn Stafford's book and throw him into a coal cellar, indicates just how important were the lower ranks of the hierarchy in the process of committal. It was beadles, marshallsmen, sergeants and other members of the royal household, or else the constables and petty officials of local parishes (like, St James's Westminster), who were monarchy's first line of defence against transgressors. It was offences committed within the reach or hearing of these lesser authorities which tended to cause individuals to be apprehended and arraigned before the Board of Green Cloth. Bothering royalty or the government was, in some cases, less significant than bothering beadles. It is an obvious over-simplification to say that such committals merely reflected the circumscriptions endorsed by the political élite. Indeed, while these lesser officials were certainly representatives of the established order, being royal or civic employees, and dealing with offenders very much according to the guide-lines laid down by the Green Cloth and other higher authorities, they were also autonomous individuals, with their own peculiar antipathies, and their own particular ways of imposing the boundaries of transgression. Power is not necessarily less politicized, however, because it is devolved. In fact, while it is quite often that one finds these lesser royal officials being hauled before their superiors for failing to arrest vagrants, beggars and other disorderly intruders, laziness and corruption, rather than any scrupling at the overarching ideology is more often the root cause. Explicit evidence of inferior officials acting according to their own, divergent prejudices, by either arresting or pardoning an insane transgressor in contradiction of their briefs, is somewhat exceptional.

Stafford had continued to publish even during his confinement at Bethlem, and it is the strategy adopted by the government towards him during this time which most of all underlines how thoroughly the Hospital could be used for purposes of political repression. Just a week after Stafford's committal, the Green Cloth were informed that 'many persons do frequently resort to him'. Fearing that he would resume 'his former evill practices, and be incouraged to write and publish more of his treasonable Books and Papers', they instructed the Governors to withhold all writing materials from him, unless he was writing to his father or close friends, and the letter had been perused by the Governors or a trusty servant.[106] The government's main concern, then, in keeping Stafford in Bethlem was silencing his troublesome dissent. Never in its communications with the Hospital did the Green Cloth express any concern about Stafford's recovery. What was plainly more important to the government was the 'seditious', 'treasonable' and 'scandalous' nature of Stafford's writings. It mattered little whether or not they came from the pen of a madman.

Five months later, the Board was informed 'that a great Concourse of people' was still seeing Stafford, and hearing him 'preach and Scandalously reflect on ye Governm[en]t'. Moreover, these people were providing him with writing materials, were receiving his productions through his cell window, and were carrying them to the printing press. Furthermore, claimed the Green Cloth, these 'Pamphletts & Libells' were 'more full of Treason & Sedition then those for which we Sent him to yo[u]r Hospitall'. In his pamphlet entitled *The Truth Which God hath shewn unto his Servant Richard Stafford*, printed just before his confinement in Bethlem, Stafford was already defiantly declaring that he 'would speak in the Ears of the People that are by the Prison Walls', and may well have done just that when in Newgate.[107] As a result of the irregularities of Stafford's confinement at Bethlem, the Board ordered (recalling the above-mentioned cases of Day and Dunn) that he 'be more closely Confined' and barred from any visitor 'except in the presence of a keeper', while no 'suspected Person' was to be 'Suffered to come to him'. From Stafford's own writings we may surmise that he was subsequently removed to a more secure and rather less salubrious cell at Bethlem.[108]

There can be few more conclusive proofs than this of how the government attempted to use Bethlem for political quarantine, or of the muzzling potentials of madness. Stafford's words were dangerous and needed to be quelled, not because they were insane, but because they expressed a radical disaffection to government that was coherent enough, and was shared widely enough, to win adherents, to be dispersed and to inflame popular dissent. Ultimately, it mattered less whether the government believed Stafford really was mad or not, than that he could be (and, indeed, was being) taken seriously by others. While the members of the Green Cloth recognized that they depended on Bethlem's Governors to enforce their orders, their comment that 'we must leave the further Care of suppressing these infamous Practices, to you who are ye Governours of ye Place' was a clear rebuke and allowed the Governors little space for objection. On the other hand, it was ultimately impossible to use Bethlem like the Bicêtre, to silence political dissidence, given the Hospital's identity as a public resort and the unregulated and open nature of its environment (a conclusion that agrees with the findings of studies on other English carceral institutions). Devotees of Daniel, Cromwell's canting porter, in Bethlem during the 1640s, also seem to have been allowed such indiscriminate access to him, by means of his cell window, that they were able to follow his Bible readings. There was no such thing as the Goffmanesque 'total institution'[109] during this period.

It is by no means sure, of course, that all of Stafford's advocates thought him entirely sane, and there may have been an element of cynicism in the way Stafford was exploited by Jacobite publicists. Furthermore, Stafford's tracts plainly took on a rather more acute and aggrieved sense of persecution during and immediately after his confinement in Bethlem, a development reflected, perhaps, in the Green Cloth's statement that his libels out of Bethlem were even more extreme than those that had got him there. Stafford's *Mystery of Iniquity* and his *Last and concluding Testimony* are particularly poisonous texts. Here, Stafford not only condemns William's 'Malice' and the 'Satanical Subtlety' that had got him into Bethlem, but also suggests that the King is 'possessed' and prophesies that William's dead body will 'be thrown into devouring Fire and everlasting Burnings'.[110] Stafford's subject matter became more and more self-referential, his protests about his sanity more and more insistent, agonised and elaborate, and his need to bolster his own ego more and more pronounced and out of touch with reality. Stafford even offered himself as a hostage for William's safe conduct if the King would agree to abdicate and 'return into Holland'.[111] Stafford may also have been losing the faith of many of his old allies, for it was no longer just the slurs the government had placed on his character from which he felt the need to defend himself. His madness was increasingly 'the false Reproach of the Multitude' (although it is questionable how literally *we* should take such Biblical quotations), while, ironically, 'many People' were subsequently to accuse Stafford himself of breaking his word.[112]

It is difficult to be sure how much Stafford was not only deluding himself, but was experiencing pathological delusions, when one has little but his own versions of events to go by. At times he admitted interpolating passages into his accounts. When publishing the undertaking he claimed to have given to Nottingham to obtain his release from Bethlem, he owned that certain words 'were not expressed, yet they were intended in my Mind'. And yet these words, he went on to assert, were the very basis 'upon which my solemn Promise was founded'.[113] Indeed, Stafford's attempts to reconcile his own contradictions, and to wriggle out of having broken his 'promise before God' – by, for example, dismissing parts of his petition as pure oratory, to which he had no intent to be held – became increasingly desperate and irrational. Of course, when examining states of contemporary consciousness, like Stafford's, that were so attuned to the disembodied word of God, the inner promptings of conscience, and the gauge of the spirit, it is no simple matter deciding where spiritual and psychological truth ends and delusion and madness begins. When, however, it came to spiritual inspiration being used as an endorsement for challenging the established worldly authorities, in a context where personal, 'untutored' claims of access to divine truth were regarded with increasing suspicion, the situation was bound to be judged somewhat differently. It is such judgements that would seem to indicate how profoundly madness was being politicized at this time, or, in other words, set outside the boundaries of orthodoxy and authority.

It may be easy to see Stafford's identification whilst in confinement with other persecuted figures, such as John the Baptist, the prophet Jeremiah, Judge Jenkins, *et alia*, as delusions of grandeur. One can also see them, however, as obvious and profound points of reference for anyone who experienced the Bible as the living word, and as strategies of self-preservation against what Stafford plainly conceived of as much more than 'the slings and arrows of outrageous fortune'. While he thought of himself as divinely chosen, Stafford never mistook himself for Jeremiah, nor, indeed, for anyone but Richard Stafford. Prior to his confinement, unlike Lady Eleanor Davies, Stafford made no *explicit* temporal prophesies (either of joy or of doom) directed at any individual, beyond vague and general references to punishments awaiting and the Day of Judgement being nigh for the King and his government. (Granted, of course, the legitimacy of prophesy within the politico-religious context of the 1690s was less established than it had been 50 years earlier.) Stafford, moreover, seems to have resisted the more grandiose and delusional notions of conspiracy theory developed by such Bedlamites as James Tilly Matthews (whose case has been well documented by Williams, Howard and Porter).[114] If his claims of persecution and that he was discharged only after a recantation had been 'forced and extorted' out of him – by 'Grievous foregoing Bondage and Oppression', and by 'putting me down into a low, dark, narrow, and stinking Room for seven Weeks and three days'[115] – seem biased, overblown and a little paranoid, they are not without legitimacy. Bethlem was clearly not a very salubrious place, and Stafford was far from the only one to express disgust for its standards of accommodation. Before his liberation into the safe-keeping of his father, in June 1692, Stafford had indeed been required to issue a written recantation to the Secretary of State, to 'beg Their Majesties Pardon, for [his] ... Offence', and to vow 'never .. more to come within the Gates of Whitehall or Kensington Court', nor to 'Write and Publish any thing more against the Government'.[116] Indeed, the Queen's order for his release arrived the very day after Nottingham had received Stafford's submission.[117]

On the other hand, it may be argued that Stafford was still treated with remarkable lenience under the circumstances. The 'madman' mentioned earlier, who, in 1692, just six months after Stafford's release, disrupted proceedings at the House of Commons, 'would [likewise] have been taken into custody of the Serjeant at Arms', 'if he had not been [judged] a madman'. Unlike Stafford, however, it took just two more days for this individual to be ordered taken care of at Bethlem. Stafford, on the other hand, was an indomitable offender, having had a number of tussles with, and warnings from, the authorities before being sent to Bethlem. The government could not easily have ignored Stafford's tirades, which were repeatedly delivered right under their very noses at Westminster, Whitehall and Kensington, and in an extremely insecure political climate. Despite a forced recantation and his subsequent banishment to his father's care in Gloucester, and even if the government ordered certain printers not to publish his works in future (as Stafford alleged), Stafford continued to publish dissension in contradiction of his former promise and continued to escape further punishment for the remainder of his life.[118] Indeed, within a month of his release, Stafford wrote to Nottingham expressing regret for his petition and threatening Nottingham's damnation if he should be imprisoned again.[119] Subsequent criticism from some that Stafford had perjured himself by his publications since his release from Bethlem provoked the over-sensitive scribe to respond with a further vindicating pamphlet *c.* 1693.[120]

According to Dr Richard Kingston, writing after the issue of yet another of Stafford's pamphlets *c.* 1695, Stafford may have only 'escaped' more 'trouble' because he had 'a father in Government and persons of quality his relations in both Houses'.[121] Indeed, claimed Kingston, Stafford's family had actively 'represented him as a madman' in order 'to save his life'. This reinforces the arguments of Hill, Screech and Porter about the exculpatory cloak of madness. Yet it also suggests how effectively the taint of madness had negated Stafford's discourse, which could mean little if everyone that mattered believed him mad. Stafford's popularity as a persecuted Jacobite in Bethlem may have taught the government that (as contemporary medical treatises often counselled) ignoring the discourse of the mad was a more effective disempowering ploy than paying it the attention it craved. That of course, and the fact that the government's position seemed safer as the 1690s progressed. Stafford, too, no doubt, contributed to his own vilification by the vanity, obsessiveness and lack of circumspection in his outpourings. By 1696, furthermore, although still calling for James's restitution, Stafford had somewhat cooled in his attitude to the deposed King, and his rather more critical accounts of James and his intriguing to regain the throne must anyway have appeared less threatening.[122]

The importance of friends or family in high places was clearly critical in cases like Richard Stafford's throughout the period, although the less formalized nature of committals at seventeenth-century Bethlem seems to have allowed extra scope for such influences. The significance of family connections as an element in the evaluation of committals to Bethlem itself underlines the political side of the familial. It also indicates how dependent were the definitions and implications of mental disorder on domestic, as well as political and social, variables. When, in 1687, Chichester Trelawney was freed from the King's Bench prison and remitted the fine of 500 livre originally imposed upon him, he too was preserved from a worse fate by his breeding (as well as by the financial means at his disposal). Writing to Trelawney's brother, the Bishop of Bristol, Henry Guy explained that the King was willing to accept two alternatives: either 'he be sent to Bedlam or otherwise he be kept in custody and provided for out of his own estate by his relations'.[123] As Trelawney fails to appear in the Hospital's admission registers, his family evidently preferred the latter option. Trelawney's case can be compared to that of many others with powerful friends. When, over a century earlier (in 1579), for example, Richard Brotherton appeared 'to be distempered in his wittes', the Privy Council asked the Dean of 'Poules' whether 'either by counsell or phisicke he maie be reduced to order; or otherwise bestowed with some of his friendes that maie take ... care of him', all the more especially 'bicause it seemeth that he hath a good opinion in the said Deane'.[124] The right connections, then, might tend both to preserve the insane from confinement, and also to encourage more attention to the curative side of their care.

Outvoting People as Insane? Power, Authority and Confinement

Cases like the above provoke real questions about the nature of power when it came to defining insanity. How much can madness be seen in this (or, indeed, any other) period as 'just a scapegoating stigma, which power uses to patrol its own boundaries and validate itself'.[125] The words of the dramatist, Nat Lee, who, after being sent to Bethlem by his family and supported there by the Green Cloth, declared 'They said I was mad; and I said they were mad; damn them they outvoted me', as Porter has observed, 'put the politics of this view in a nutshell'.[126] Richard Stafford was saying something very similar when he described the way in which 'the multitude' labelled the unusual and the zealous mad, and when he told Nottingham and his government, after his release:

> what ye lately did to me, was ... only Gotten Power, and the Will of

> Men. It was so done meerly because ye were stronger; and it could be so done.[127]

It was not just about the minority view against the majority, it was about where exactly authority resided in society. For Stafford, Lee and others who took the Bible quite literally to their hearts, the ultimate authority was God's word, as freely interpreted by men and women of conscience. Likewise for many Puritans and Quakers, it was the sanction of their own religious customs and beliefs that encouraged and justified them in interrupting church services, and criticizing Church and State. Here, perhaps, it is Foucault's analysis of power that is most helpful, where confinement is seen essentially as the 'articulation of social difference'. While the establishment allied itself firmly with law and reason, and increasingly with Anglicanism and Whiggism, stigmatizing its enemies as the forces of anarchy and unreason, those identified and incarcerated as mad might, like Stafford, protest that, what 'is called the Government of Reasonable ... Men', is 'rather' a 'Government of unreasonable Men'.[128] Yet power, as Foucault emphasized, has positive as well as negative aspects. In some cases, as we have seen, where it was enshrined in the family connections of an offender, power might be exercised to prevent, or mitigate, punishment and incarceration.

Going beyond a Foucauldian notion of institutionalization as the drawing up boundaries of propriety by the arbiters of rational, polite culture, or the consolidation of the power of various élite groups, Fissell and other scholars have rightly asserted how negotiated were the institutional entities of early modern Britain. Much more than 'reflecting', in any rigid sense, 'the definition of social boundaries', 'charities were ... an arena in which such boundaries were made, tested, and reinforced'. While negotiation and reciprocation were important forces at work in admissions to all institutions, however, this was not so much the case when it came to admitting the insane. Volitional seeking of relief and direct returns for such relief were more easily expected from the ordinary sick poor – who tended to petition for their own admissions, who were required to express their gratitude to the hospital on their discharge, and whose continuance in hospital was dependant on their observance of codes of conduct, partially enshrined in particular institutional regulations. Such negotiation was rarely expected from patients admitted to Bethlem, however. On the contrary, lunatics were supposed to remain in Bethlem so long as they continued radically to depart from those codes of conduct endorsed by their custodians and by sane society. It was not the insane, but their friends and parishes who negotiated for their admission, while, for patients sent to Bethlem by the State, this negotiation was carried out between, rather than with, authorities and élites.

Ordering the Care and Cure of the Insane: Political Tolerance for Persistent Nuisances?

Stafford's case is unusual in that comparatively few of Bethlem's patients *were* committed or discharged with special instructions for their closer detention from outside authorities. Such special instructions were more common in seventeenth-century committal orders than in those of subsequent times, when Bethlem's administration and medical officers seem to have been more successful in asserting their autonomous and professional authority over admissions. Yet even in the seventeenth century, the Board of Green Cloth, the Privy Council and other bodies generally left it to the Hospital to 'take care of [patients] in the same manner as is usual' or 'customary ... in such cases'. Nor were these authorities only concerned with the detention of the mad, or the allegedly mad. Occasionally, the Board and other authorities even stipulated that individuals had been sent to be 'cured' at Bethlem, or that the Hospital should 'have Care of' their 'Lunacy'. Even when committing recidivists like Mary Coglan to Bethlem, the Board of Green Cloth might specifically request that she 'be put into a way of recovery'. Sometimes special requests for good treatment were made. In the case of the Mariner, Thomas Dunn, committed to Bethlem in 1667, for example, the Privy Council asked that he be 'treated as well as that Place will affoard'.[129] In other cases, like that of the above-mentioned Catherine Edwards, servant to the Dutchess of Richmond, there is evidence of a period of grace, and even of former efforts to obtain a recovery, before committal to Bethlem was deemed necessary. Edwards was said to be 'at certaine times very much distracted ... not withstanding all the endeav[our]s & means us[e]d by her ... Husband'. Even after Edwards had perpetrated 'many [further] disorders', and the Green Cloth ordered her readmission and that she be 'treated' in Bethlem 'according to the order and discipline of yo[ur] house', the Board may be seen to be bearing the curative efficacy of the Hospital firmly in mind – for this was seen as located essentially in the order and discipline of Bethlem's regime.[130]

Furthermore, many of those individuals committed to Bethlem by outside authorities carried a long record of incursions and disorders, whether in connection with city property or notables, or with royal property. Again, I would emphasize, there was no simple transition in this period from toleration to intolerance. Board of Green Cloth warrants for admission to Bethlem conventionally declared that individuals had 'been *frequently*' or '*for some time* [my italics] very Troublesome to their Maiesties' or to 'ye Court'.[131] William Landy, for instance, was in and out of the verge, despite being given fair warning, 'banished [from] the Court & charged not to come againe ... upon paine of his Maj[es]t[y]'s displeasure'. He was also in and out of Bethlem, in a series of 'short, sharp, shock' type, admissions which failed to have much impact on him.[132] Mary Coglan had likewise been frequently admonished to avoid the Royal Court, been 'turn'd out of [various palace] Gates', and been 'for some space of time much distracted', before being sent to Bethlem.[133] Prior to this she had merely served a brief spell in Tuthill Fields Bridewell (where, she had already been warned she would be sent if found at Court again).[134] It is worth stressing, here, the inadequacies of the legal machinery available to deal with cases of persistent lunatic offenders. The authorities plainly had few convenient options open to them. Confinement was often the last of these. In this light, it may seem less surprising that confinement was meted out in a language often suffused with the ideology of deterrence. In so far as incarceration served as a last-ditch response to recidivists, however, it is more difficult to sustain the argument that the authorities were placing lunacy on the other side of very stringently defined and enforced boundaries.

That trespassers on royal property and other politically charged detainees who wound up in Bethlem were often guilty of numerous transgressions suggests a modicum of tolerance, even in the most sensitive of places. Far from all those people committing disorders within the verge were sent to Bethlem. Those who were, were clearly a rather incorrigible minority. Persistence, as well as a quality of irrationality, incomprehensibility, wantonness, or aimlessness to their actions or behaviour, distinguishing them from ordinary offenders, was usually required before the Board saw Bethlem as the appropriate answer. Cases like William Bodyman, found to be 'Lunatick' and to 'infest & disturb' St James's Palace in 1711, might simply be delivered to their Churchwarden and Overseers (or else to their families), 'to be by them taken Care off according to Law & usuall Custome'. Others bound for Bethlem, like John Pomfrett, who was to be committed in 1731 on the normal charge of being 'troublesome and offensive to his Ma[jes]t[ie]s Court', might even be 'discharged out of Custody and not sent to Bethlem' on their 'Madness going of[f]'. Cases like Pomfrett's indicate that an individual's madness might be conceptualized quite distinctly from, and was generally more important than, the nature of his, or her, actual offence. As Peter Linebaugh has emphasized in his study, *The London Hanged*,[135] one must ask why some individuals were not apprehended, incarcerated or executed, as well as why some were. In other words, the nature of confinement and punishment is also defined by what has rather inelegantly been called 'excarceration', or by those who managed to avoid it and the reasons for their avoidance. Thomas Whittmore, Yeoman of the King's Pantry, who was ordered admitted to Bethlem in 1680, on his wife, Mary's, complaint to the Board that he was distracted and had attempted suicide, was 'released' on the subsequent discovery that he was 'not Lunatick'. The exclusively male Board's explanation that he was rather 'only discontented & melancholy by reason of his said Wife's disorderly course of life', could be taken at face value. It might also be interpreted as a reflection of how social and gender prejudices exerted a compromising influence on official sympathies and distinctions.[136] Indeed, this may help to explain why not the slightest suggestion of insanity was made in the case of Richard Shee, an Irish Catholic resident within the verge, who flew into a 'great Passion' out of jealousy and 'rage' over his wife's conduct and disdain of his authority, was guilty of 'rudness and affronts' to Green Cloth officers, and 'drew his sword', threatening to fight them and then 'kill himself'. Shee seems only to have landed himself in the Marshalsea, after a brief spell in the Porter's Lodge, because he refused 'to give security for his future good behaviour'.[137]

That the mad were, however, as I have argued above, quite often confused with the bad, and *vice versa*, manifests considerable ambiguities in government policies towards offenders. It suggests that, while irrationality might itself explain and exonerate offences, merely troubling and offending the highest authorities could be perceived as innately irrational. Nevertheless, the majority of individuals guilty of such offences were dealt with quite differently by authorities like the Green Cloth. Most would not even have become part of the written record, having been dealt with on the spot and turfed out of prohibited areas by petty officials. Those who were arrested, were mostly arrested on civil charges by marshallsmen, beadles, etc., according to the authority invested in their offices, or according to the general warrants issued by the Board for the apprehension of vagrants, those who disturbed the peace and others who had trespassed, or infringed the law, on various royal properties. And it was on these civil charges that detainees tended to remain. In very few cases is there evidence that any suspicion of madness was attached to the nature of the crime itself. If confinement was imposed, the sentence tended to be a brief spell in a

Bridewell, or in prison. Cases like William Glaseborough, sent to Tuthill Fields Bridewell 'to be punished' after apprehension by the marshallsmen as 'a Sturdy Beggar & Vagabond', and Elizabeth Gibbs, who spent 16 days there for 'often' intruding into the King's palace, 'though forbid', after which she was discharged to her parish,[138] are much more typical of the government's policing activities, than those cases sent to Bethlem I have been focusing on here.

Rare Objections to Political Committals

Bethlem had little option but to admit patients sent to it by authorities like the Privy Council and Board of Green Cloth – a fact well illustrated by the customary wording of some warrants: 'not doubting of yo[ur] compliance', 'will be acceptable service to the King'.[139] On the other hand, the Hospital had its own criteria of suitability for admission, criteria which became increasingly sophisticated as the period progressed and which the Governors were not averse to citing when rejecting or discharging patients who did not qualify. Indeed, most public bodies, even the Board of Green Cloth, acknowledged at times that admission depended on whether 'upon Examination he/she appear a fit Object', as in the case of the Reverend Joseph Ward in 1741.[140] After the Restoration, and especially at times when the royal prerogative was less assured, royal authorities had to be rather more deferential to both the City and the Hospital authorities when seeking an individual's admission. Writing to the Lord Mayor in 1683 to express his Majesty's wish that one such individual 'might be sent to Bedlam', for instance, Secretary Jenkins supposed that 'none ... is received there but by allowance of yourself and the Governors'.[141] The man in question was apparently not regarded as politically dangerous, but the Secretary's evident pique that he had 'pretended to give me informations relating to dangerous persons, but all his discourse was of having been poisoned and bewitched by his enemies, etc,' may suggest a different bias in this committal.

On some rare occasions, the Governors objected in quite categorical terms to the billeting of unsuitable cases at the Hospital by other authorities. Just as, indeed, despite letters from royal ministers recommending the appointment of royal nominees to offices in Bethlem and Bridewell and 'not doubting of' the Governors' 'ready Complyance', the Governors went ahead and appointed their own independently chosen officers, they might also reject or discharge patients comitted by the State.[142] In 1675, John Taylor, 'conceived to be distracted', was sent to Bethlem from by the House of Lords.[143] Taylor had originally been sent to Guildford Gaol 'for uttering

Blasphemous Words' or 'Speeches' (said by the Lords to 'tend immediately to the Destruction of all Religion & Government'). He was subsequently tried in person at the House of Lords, after the Lords had perused the Surrey Justices' examination. Just a few days after his committal to Bethlem, however, Taylor was declared quite sane by the Bethlem Physician, Thomas Allen. Allen was ordered by the Court of Governors to acquaint the Clerk of Parliament with this fact in no uncertain terms. Indeed, Allen was to inform the Clerk not only 'what hee conceiveth [Taylor's] ... Disposition to be' (i.e. highly culpable), but moreover 'that there is noe punishment for any kept in Bethlem'. The Governors had taken severe umbrage at the tone of the Lords' warrant to them, which had ordered 'the Master or Keeper of ... Bedlem', not only to take custody of Taylor but to see that he was 'kept there with bread and water and such due bodily Correccon as may conduce to his Recovery from the Madnes wherewith hee seemes to be possessed'. Plainly, even the Lords had not been convinced that Taylor was insane, having also stipulated that if he 'shall not prove to be mad but persist in the said blasphemyes', he was 'to be delivered to be proceeded against according to the Law' in such cases. Yet, the implication that Taylor was committed to be cured of his blaspheming suggests that lunacy was being considerably politicized. That merely persisting in such blasphemies might be seen as evidence of simple perversity, rather than insanity, manifests the ambivalence at the heart of official policies. Furthermore, it suggests that the currency of conceptions of insanity as a transient mental aberration, or curable disorder of cognition, allowed ample space for confusion and for more punitive responses to manifestations of both mental and political deviance. In this instance, as in most instances, Parliament was clearly recognizing that Bethlem was primarily a place for the cure of the insane, but it was also attempting to ensure that Taylor received correction and punishment for his blasphemy. While Bethlem refused (at least overtly) to perform the latter role, the Hospital also assisted Parliament and served to endorse Taylor's conviction and punishment for felony, by identifying him as bad rather than mad. Indeed, the Governors even offered suggestions to Parliament as to how Taylor should be dealt with, asking whether he should either be sent 'to Newgate' to await prosecution 'for blasphemy', or 'to Bridewell to be kept att hard Labo[ur]'. Furthermore, Taylor was not actually released from Bethlem to be prosecuted in the courts for another five months. In the meantime, Taylor himself addressed his own humble appeal for 'Liberty' to Charles II [see *Figure 1*], by way of a petition in verse form, the first letters of each line spelling the name 'Charles Stuart'. If Taylor's blasphemy was incurable, then Parliament was clearly content to use Bethlem as a convenient holding place, and (as far as his immediate liberty was concerned) Taylor's petition fell on deaf ears.

Figure 1
The humble ptic[i]on of J[oh]n Taylor a Prisoner in Bethlem
To y[e]Kings most Excellent Ma[jes]ty

C hrist thy Crowne his kingdome is divine
H e is thy Soveraigne Prince as thou art mine
A power into thy hands is freely lent
R elease a Prisoner yt is Inocent
L ove softer is then Downe on Angells wings
E ternall love is the great King of Kings
S ubjects are Children Princes Parents are
S ent down from heaven w[i]th Gentle love & care
T o save the tender Lamb and harmles dove
V ictorious mercy Reaps Triumphant Love
A noynted king thou art of Brittons Land
R uler of Nations Sway'd from thy right hand
T ender thy Lambs and heale them in destresse
E ndless will be thy peace and hapynesse

Yo[ur] Pet[icione]r assuredly knowing the tendernesse of yo[ur] princly nature whose mercy like the Beams of the Sunne hath shined upon many humbly Supplicates yo[ur] Ma[jes]ty to p[re]sent my Cause to ye hon[ora]ble ye house of Peeres by whom I was com[m]itted that by yo[ur] clemency I may enjoy my Lib[er]ty
And I shall daly pray for your Eternall peace &hapynesse
J[oh]n Taylor

Reproduced from *House of Lords RO. Braye MS. 3*, fol. 96, 1675.

The Green Cloth's committal of the previously mentioned John or Jean Stafford, in 1688, was evidently another case of dubious confinement where Bethlem's authorities acted promptly and independently to liberate the offender. Stafford had spent just ten days in Bethlem on the usual charge of being 'distracted ... apt to do mischiefe' and 'troublesome' within the verge, when the Bethlem Physician certified that he was 'not distracted', and 'has behaved himself very civilly & orderly since he hath bin in the Hospitall', and Stafford was ordered discharged by the Green Cloth.[144] Yet such cases were highly exceptional. Rarely, in practice, did the Bethlem Governors object to state committals, even if, in principle, it was mutually accepted that these individuals might be 'improper objects of the Charity'. While, during the first three decades of the eighteenth century, about four applicants for admission a year were being rejected by the Bethlem Governors, not a single one of these cases appears to have been committed under the warrant of the Green Cloth, or any other state authority.[145]

While Bethlem was clearly not a 'mixed' institution in the sense of French hospitals like the Bicêtre, there were evidently times when its boundaries were rather hazy. Other institutions too, patently not specializing in the custody or cure of the insane, such as houses of correction, might occasionally be used by the state authorities for both these purposes. Having 'Com[m]itted greate disorders' in Whitehall Palace, Richard Hutton, for example, was quite consciously sent to Tuthill Fields Bridewell in 1670, despite being recognized as 'a person distemp[ere]d in his braine'. What is unusual in Hutton's case, however, is that this was explicitly with the objective 'that he might be there reclaimed & Cured of his distemp[er]'. Only subsequently, when it was acknowledged that Hutton had got worse in Bridewell, where he had been left 'in want of those ordinary meanes & helps that might Contribute to his Cure', was he ordered transferred to Bethlem. Bridewells and workhouses were quite frequently employed in this period, of course (particularly in the eighteenth century), to house small numbers of the insane. Such provision was normally confined, however, to the putatively 'harmless' and 'incurable' insane (and the mentally handicapped), and to simple custody, rather than cure. Indeed, it was quite customary for such institutions to refuse to take dangerous cases, or to dismiss or transfer cases to Bethlem once they became violent or destructive. Thus, when Hutton was found to have 'growne to so high a distemp[er] of braine & disorder that' Tuthill Fields had no means 'to secure the lives of other p[er]sons now in the said house', his transfer to Bethlem was to be expected. While the Board of Green Cloth were clearly concerned that he 'should be put into the way of Cure' at Bethlem, they were also looking to the Hospital simply to act as a holding place for somebody who was politically a danger, as there was no other way '(if he should have Liberty) to keepe him out of his Ma[jes]t[y']s Pallace'.[146]

Continuities and Discontinuities

The treatment of cases like Richard Stafford in the seventeenth century may be compared and contrasted to that of other political deviants a century later, for whom there seems to have been rather less tolerance. Egbert Lamborn's committal to Bethlem by the Green Cloth in 1761, like Stafford's, stipulated that he be kept 'in close confinement he appearing to us a Desperate Lunatick'. There is little evidence, however, of persistent abuses by Lamborn, who had merely 'delivered ... Letters', 'within the Verge of the Court' in 1761, even if the Board considered them 'of a most heinous Nature', while Lamborn was to spend not eight months, but the remaining 35 years of his life in confinement as a lunatic.[147] Alexander Hatton, apprehended the year after Lamborn 'in the Apartments of His Majesty's Palace at St James's ... behaving in such a manner as to give suspicion that he had some ill Design', and ordered 'into Confinement' by the Board of Green Cloth, likewise remained in Bethlem until his death in 1765.[148] Thomas Stone, too, sent to Bethlem in 1787 by the Secretary of State, died there in 1805, having had his fate sealed not only by the Bethlem Physician's examination, but also by the King personally perusing the letters he had continued to write whilst in confinement.[149] The case of James Tilly Matthews, who was locked away for nearly 20 years in Bethlem, after some deranged and ill-chosen remarks in the gallery of the House of Commons, is, perhaps more than any other, the best illustration of how times had changed. That Matthews continued to be perceived as dangerous to the government, despite numerous and medically-endorsed attempts to free him, and no evidence at all of any violent propensities, suggests how difficult it was now becoming for such individuals to obtain their liberty. Matthews' writings, too, had been exploited as evidence to justify his continued incarceration. All four of these last mentioned individuals had been transferred to the incurables wards, the provision of which after 1728 had clearly furthered the tendency of patients to remain for life.[150] My examination of those cases sent to Bethlem by the Green Cloth after 1700 suggests that comparatively few qualify as incorrigible nuisances to the Court, rarely being recorded as 'frequent' transgressors, while many had only 'lately become a Lunatick'.[151] On the other hand, of course, the formal nature of the language of such warrants makes it rather difficult to assess with confidence exactly how often these individuals had offended, let alone exactly what types of behaviour were meant by standard formulae like 'hath committed severall disorders', 'apt to do mischiefe', or 'troublesome and offensive'. Warrants are often all one has to go on when evaluating the dynamics of state committals, and, constituting merely the final judgment on a case, rarely convey much information about the processes by which that judgment was determined.

Of course, there are still many significant signs of continuity between seventeenth and eighteenth century treatment of insane offenders, who often continued to be dealt with leniently and to receive exculpation for their crimes, even if of a highly political nature. There is obvious continuity in the treatment of cases like Richard Harris (introduced above) and Deborah Lydall, who were sent to Bethlem for throwing (or threatening to throw) objects at royalty, and cases 100 years later, like that of John Frith. Although arraigned and confined in Newgate for throwing a stone at the royal coach in 1790, Frith was subsequently declared 'unfit to plead by reason of insanity' and was freed from gaol on condition of security being given 'that he should be confined in some proper place as a lunatic, or in some other manner taken care of '.[152] Throughout the period, there was an effort discernible in state committals to communicate a sense of the graciousness, sympathy and forgiving nature of monarchy in dealing with the insane, reinforced by the stress placed on the personal role of royalty in such cases. Significantly, for example, Frith's treatment was 'to answer his Majesty's most gracious intentions'. It is perhaps not surprising that Margaret Nicholson, given the seriousness of her crime in attempting to assassinate George III, was confined in Bethlem for life where she spent the first year in chains at the Government's command. The air of punishment in her committal would have been no less marked (if anything, it would have been more so) in the previous century. Subsequently, moreover, she seems to have been treated quite leniently. She was personally enquired after by the King, was permitted to have the same freedom as ordinary patients after a year in confinement, and was allowed to receive numerous, respectable visitors.

Conclusions

The extent to which lunacy was politicized in early modern England has been underestimated. A significant number of individuals were plainly incarcerated as lunatics first and foremost by reason of the political threat they were deemed to pose. Bethlem clearly operated rather more than some historians have appreciated as a state institution, not only receiving politically dangerous individuals, but actually subjecting them to a more extreme form of confinement and silencing than was customary for ordinary patients, at the express behest of the royal and civic authorities. In other words, Bethlem was used in a way that, in some senses, was not so different as might have been supposed from Bicêtre, L'Hôtel Dieu and other French institutions. There was plainly a considerable element of ambivalence in distinguishing between those fit for Bethlem and those fit for prison, or the house of correction, a conclusion well illustrated by the relationship between Bridewell and Bethlem. This ambiguity seems to have been particularly marked in the seventeenth century, before admission policies at Bethlem had been subjected to more thorough regulation. By in large, nevertheless, unlike the mixed institutions of late eighteenth century France, internment in Bethlem did, by definition, imply insanity. Political motivations can only be said to have predominated in a minority (if still a significant minority) of cases. Even when politics did figure in patients' committal, this was seldom sufficient alone to get a patient admitted to Bethlem. Outside authorities tended to respect the peculiar competence of the Hospital for the insane, and do seem to have striven to reserve committals to it to those they conceived to be truly mad. Walton has observed: 'why bother to use the complicated and controversial machinery of certification for insanity when ... straightforward physical and legal coercion could also do the job'.[153] On the other hand, while no less controversial, in procedural terms certification was certainly less complicated in the seventeenth and eighteenth centuries, than it was in the next century. Furthermore, as I have shown, more customary forms of coercion were not always deemed adequate, while certification seems to have been a rather more ambivalent and politically-loaded procedure than has commonly been acknowledged.

Ultimately, however, I would pick few bones with Walton's and others' assertion that it was domestic strife and more mundane social and economic realties, rather than politics, which tended to instigate, and prevail in, the processes by which patients were committed to (and discharged from) Bethlem.

Notes

1. Michel Foucault, *Madness and Civilisation: A History of Insanity in the Age of Reason* (London: Tavistock, 1967), originally published as *Histoire de la Folie* (Paris: Librairie Plon, 1961), especially ch. viii, 224–5, 234–40.
2. Erwin H. Ackerknecht, 'Political Prisoners in French Mental Institutions before 1789, during the Revolution, and under Napoleon I', *Medical History*, 19 (1975), 250–5.
3. Jan Goldstein, *Console and Classify. The French Psychiatric Profession in the Nineteenth Century* (Cambridge: CUP, 1987), 107.
4. Colin Jones, 'The Treatment of the Insane in Eighteenth- and Early Nineteenth-century Montpellier. A Contribution to the Prehistory of the Lunatic Asylum in Provincial France', *Medical History*, 24 (1980), 371–90.
5. *Ibid.*, 381–2.
6. *Ibid.*, 377.
7. See, for example, George Rosen, *Madness in Society. Chapters in the Historical Sociology of Mental Illness* (London: Routledge & Kegan Paul, 1968); *idem*, 'Social Attitudes to Irrationality and Madness in Seventeenth and Eighteenth Century Europe', *Journal of the*

History of Medicine and Allied Sciences, xviii (1963), 220–40; *idem,* 'Enthusiasm', *Bulletin of the History of Medicine,* xlii (1968), 393–421; David Rothman, *The Discovery of the Asylum* (Boston: Little Brown, 1971); Robert Castel, *L'ordre Psychiatrique. L'âge d'or de l'aliénisme* (Paris: Les Editions de Minuit, 1976), republished in English as *The Regulation of Madness. The Origins of Incarceration in France* (Berkeley; Los Angeles: University of California Press, 1988); Andrew T. Scull, *Museums of Madness* (London: Allen Lane, 1987); *idem,* 'A Convenient Place to Get Rid of Inconvenient People: the Victorian Lunatic Asylum', in A. D. King (ed.), *Buildings and Society* (London: Routledge & Kegan Paul, 1980), 37–60; D. Ingleby, (ed.), *Critical Psychiatry: The Politics of Mental Health* (Harmondsworth: Penguin , 1981), and *idem, The Problem of Medical Knowledge: Towards a Social Constructivist View of Medicine* (Edinburgh: EUP, 1982).

8. Foucault, *Histoire de la Folie* (note 1), ch. ii, 'Le grand renfermement', 56–91; Roy Porter, *Mind-Forg'd Manacles. A History of Madness in England from the Restoration to the Regency* (London: The Athlone Press, 1987), especially 113–14; and *idem,* 'Foucault's Great Confinement', *History of the Human Sciences,* 3, 1 (1991), 47–54.
9. William Llewellyn Parry-Jones, *The Trade in Lunacy. A Study of Private Madhouses in England in the Eighteenth and Nineteenth Centuries* (London: Routledge & Kegan Paul, 1971).
10. Porter, *Manacles (note 8),* 114, and especially ch. 3, 110–68.
11. Akihito Suzuki, 'Lunacy in Seventeenth and Eighteenth-Century England: Analysis of Quarter Sessions Records. Parts I and II, *History of Psychiatry,* ii (1991), 437–56, and iii (1992), 29–44; *idem,* 'Family, Community and Lunacy in Early Modern England: An Analysis of Quarter-Session Records', paper given at SSHM Annual Summer Conference, 'Communities, "Caring" and Institutions' (July, 1992). See also, A. Fessler, 'The Management of Lunacy in Seventeenth Century England: an Investigation of Quarter-Sessions Records', *Proceedings of the Royal Society of Medicine,* xlix (1956), 901–7; Peter Rushton, 'Lunatics and Idiots: Mental Disability, the Community and the Poor Law in North-east England 1600–1800', *Medical History,* 32 (1988), 34–50, and *idem,* ' "Idiocy", the Family and the Community in the Early Modern Period', paper given at SSHM Day Conference, 'From "Idiocy" to "Mental Deficiency": Historical Perspectives on People with Learning Disabilities' (October 1992).
12. Craig M. Rose, 'Politics at the London Royal Hospitals, 1683–92', in L. Granshaw and Roy Porter (eds), *The Hospital in History* (London; New York: Routledge, 1989), 123–48; *idem,* 'Politics, Religion and Charity in Augustan London, 1680–1720' (Cambridge: Ph.D thesis, 1989).
13. In this connection, see also Roy Porter, 'The Gift Relation:

Philanthropy and Provincial Hospitals in Eighteenth-century England', *ibid*, 149–78.

14. Mary E. Fissell, *Patients, Power, and the Poor in Eighteenth-Century Bristol* (Cambridge: CUP, 1991), especially 6-7, 86–93, 113–17, 122–5, 198–9, and 'The "Sick and Drooping Poor" in Eighteenth-century Bristol and its Region', *Social History of Medicine*, 2 (April, 1989), 1, 35–58.
15. John V. Pickstone, *Medicine and Industrial Society. A History of Hospital Development in Manchester and its Region, 1752–1946* (Manchester: Manchester University Press, 1985), especially 2, 11, 17–20, 24–9, 63–75; *idem* and Stella V. F. Butler, 'The Politics of Medicine in the Early Industrial City; a Study of Hospital Reform and Medical Relief in Late Eighteenth-century Manchester', *Medical History*, 28 (1984), 227–49.
16. Guenter B. Risse, *Hospital Life in Enlightenment Scotland. Care and Teaching at the Royal Infirmary of Edinburgh* (Cambridge: CUP, 1986), 11, 19, 28, 82–3.
17. Sandra Cavallo, 'Charity, Power and Patronage in Eighteenth-century Italian Hospitals: the Case of Turin', in Granshaw and Porter, *op. cit.* (note 12), 93–122; *idem*, 'The Motivations of Benefactors. An Overview of Approaches to the Study of Charity', in Barry and Jones (eds), *Medicine and Charity*, 46–62; *idem*, 'Hospitality, Civic Ideals and Pre-industrial Charity in Sixteenth- and Seventeenth-century Turin', paper given at SSHM Conference, 'Communities, "Caring" and Institutions' (1992).
18. Pickstone, *op. cit.* (note 15), 2.
19. John K. Walton, 'The Treatment of Pauper Lunatics in Victorian England: The Case of Lancaster Asylum, 1816–70', in Andrew T. Scull (ed.), *Madhouses, Mad-Doctors and Madmen* (London: Athlone Press, 1981), 166–200; *idem*, 'Casting Out and Bringing Back in Victorian England', in W. F. Bynum, Roy Porter and Michael Shepherd (eds), *The Anatomy of Madness. Essays in the History of Psychiatry*, 3 vols (London: Tavistock, 1985–8), ii, 132–46.
20. 'Casting out', *ibid.*, 135.
21. *Ibid.*, 139.
22. Ann Digby, *Madness, Morality and Medicine. A Study of the York Retreat, 1796–1914* (Cambridge: CUP, 1987); Charlotte Mackenzie, *Psychiatry for the Rich. A History of Ticehurst Private Asylum 1792–1917* (London; New York: Routledge, 1992), and *idem*, 'Social Factors in the Admission, Discharge and Continuing Stay of Patients at Ticehurst Asylum, 1845–1917, in Bynum, *et al., op. cit.* (note 19), iii (1988), 147–74.
23. See especially Matthew Thomson, 'The Problem of Mental Deficiency in England and Wales, *c.* 1913–1946' (D.Phil., University of Oxford, 1992); *idem*, 'Community Care and Control of Mental Defectives in Inter-war Britain', paper given at SSHM Conference, 'Communities,

"Caring" and Institutions' (1992); David Wright, 'The Role of Family and "Community" in the Institutionalisation of Mentally Handicapped Children in Nineteenth-century England', paper given at same conference, and *idem*, ' "Childlike in his Innocence": lay attitudes to "Idiots" and"'Imbeciles" in Victorian England', paper given at SSHM Day Conference, 'From "Idiocy" to "Mental Deficiency"...' (October 1992). In much of his work, however, Thomson explores and emphasizes the ideological rationales for solutions to the problem of mental deficiency. For example, Thomson, 'Sterilization, Segregation and Community Care: Ideology and Solutions to the Problem of Mental Deficiency in Inter-war Britain', *History of Psychiatry*, 3 (December, 1992), 473–98.

24. Michael Donnelly, *Managing the Mind. A Study of Medical Psychology in Early Nineteenth-Century Britain* (London: Tavistock, 1983), 6; Peter Rushton, 'Lunatics and Idiots', *Medical History*, 32 (1988), 34–50.
25. Edward G. O'Donoghue, *The Story of Bethlehem Hospital from its Foundation in 1247* (London, Fisher & Unwin, 1914).
26. Christopher Hill, *The World Upside-Down: Radical Ideas During the English Revolution* (Harmondsworth: Penguin, 1978), 223–4.
27. *Bridewell and Bethlem Court of Governors Minutes* (henceforth, *BCGM*), 2 April, 1638, fol. 173.
28. See, for example, *State Papers Domestic* (henceforth, *SP)*, Entry Book, lxxi (8 December, 1684), 364.
29. Bolton was dismissed as a governor of Bethlem in 1676, but was reinstated by the King's command. See Jonathan Andrews, 'Bedlam Revisited: A History of Bethlem Hospital, *c.* 1634–1770' (Ph.D thesis: University of London, 1991), 161 and note 120.
30. Hill, *op. cit.* (note 26), 223-4; *idem, Change and Continuity in Seventeenth-Century England*, revised edition (New Haven and London: Yale University Press, 1991), especially 48–77, 270–1, 316–19; *idem* and Michael Shepherd, 'The Case of Arise Evans: a Historico-psychiatric Study', *Psychological Medicine*, 6 (1976), 351–8.
31. Hill, *op. cit.* (note 19), 223–4.
32. *Acts of the Privy Council*, xi (1578–80), 284.
33. *Acts of the Privy Council*, i (1542–47), 388, 481. Both references seem to refer to the same man, namely Richard Cheeseman, of the parish of Lye in Surrey, who had originally been brought before the Privy Council 'for lewde wordes' on the warrant of Sir Matthew Browne.
34. *Acts of the Privy Council*, xii (1580–1), 15 February, 1580, 328.
35. *Acts of the Privy Council*, ix (1575–7), 23.
36. *Ibid.*, 299.
37. *Acts of the Privy Council* (1616–17), 25 and 29 November, 1616, and 21 December, 1617, 387–9 and 392–3.
38. M. A. Screech, *Erasmus: Ecstasy and the Praise of Folly* (London: Penguin/Peregrine, 1988; orig. Duckworth, 1980); *idem*, 'Good Madness in Christendom', in Bynum *et al., op. cit.* (note 19), i

(1985), 25–39.

39. Edward Ward, *The London Spy* (London: 1699), K. Fenwick (ed.), (London: Folio Society, 1955), 50.
40. A particular type of counterfeit, who used the pretence of being patients, or ex-patients, as a license for begging, was so worrying to the Hospital's Governors during the 1670s and again in the 1780s that they issued a public repudiation in the London press. *BCGM* 13 August, 1674 and 18 June, 1675, ff. 29 and 138; *The London Gazette*, 17–21 June, 21–4 June, 24–8 June, 28 June –1 July; 5–12 July, 1675. For an individual case of a 'Tom of Bedlam', see e.g. *BCGM* 23 April, 1673, ff. 501, case of William Scavenger. Madness was, of course, just one amongst a large wardrobe of disguises.
41. G. B. Harrison, *The Elizabethan Journals. Being a Record of the Things Most Talked of During the Years 1591–1603* (London: Routledge, 1939; revised edn of 1928 edn), 27.
42. See G. B. Harrison (ed.), *A Second Jacobean Journal. Being a Record of Those Things Most Talked of during the Years 1607 to 1610* (London: Routledge & Kegan Paul, 1958), 41, 9 July, 1607.
43. *PRO SP44/31*, 28 March, 1672, fo. 86.
44. A. L. Beier, *Masterless Men: The Vagrancy Problem in England 1560–1640* (London: Methuen, 1987).
45. *Acts of the Privy Council* (*PRO PC2/40*), 10 November 1630, 108.
46. *PRO LS13/104*, fo. 79; *BCGM* 1 July, 1676, fo. 277.
47. *BCGM* 27 May, 1642, fo. 385.
48. *BCGM* 22 August, 1638, fo. 193.
49. *BCGM*, 20 December, 1638, fo. 217. See similar case of Thomas Stevenson, sent to work at Bridewell for begging, despite being found 'somewhat crackt brayned': *ibid*, 21 November 1638, fo. 211.
50. *Acts of the Privy Council*, 1615–16, 23 September, 1615, 285.
51. *Ibid.*, 1625–6, 15 April, 1626, 432.
52. Peter Stallybrass and Allon White, *The Politics and Poetics of Transgression* (London: Methuen, 1986).
53. *Ibid.*, 195.
54. See, for example, *PRO LS13/86*, fo. 51; *LS13/105*, ff. 66, 68; *LS13/115*, fo. 116; 13/172, fo. 91; *LS13/173*, ff. 106–7. Recent social historians from Peter Burke and Robert Malcolmson to Roy Porter have stressed how much the masses rubbed shoulders with the élite in early modern society, and what a volatile brew this could be, socially and politically. They have also suggested that the divide between popular and élite culture and recreations was actually increased during the course of the period. See Peter Burke, *Popular Culture in Early Modern Europe* (reprint, Aldershot: Wildwood House Ltd, 1988); Robert W. Malcolmson, *Popular Recreations in English Society 1700–1850* (Cambridge: CUP, 1973); Roy Porter, *English Society in the Eighteenth Century* (Harmondsworth: Penguin, 1982). The multiplying regulation of rights of passage to royalty and royal

property, and the penalizing of individuals guilty of infringement, may be seen as another aspect of this growing demarcation.

55. See *Bethlem Admission Registers*, fo. 184, 17 December, 1743; *The Adventures of Alexander the Corrector* (London: 1754); *The Gentleman's Magazine*, 24 (1761), 601.
56. See, for example, Max Byrd, *Visits to Bedlam* (Columbia: University of South Carolina Press, 1974); Michael V. Deporte, *Nightmares and Hobbyhorses: Swift, Sterne, and Augustan Ideas of Madness* (San Marino, California: Huntingdon Library, 1974); L. Feder, *Madness in Literature* (Princeton: Princeton University Press, 1980).
57. *PRO LS13/104*, 16 August, 1677, fo. 89.
58. *PRO LS13/104*, 12 January, 1678, fo. 94.
59. *PRO LS13/172*, 16 December, 1678, fo. 18.
60. *PRO LS13/176*, 18 April, 1715, fo. 27.
61. *London Evening Post*, Nos 2804 and 2805, 23–6 October and 26–9 October, 1745; *Bethlem Admission Registers* (henceforth, *BARs*), 28 October, 1745 and 18 October, 1748, ff. 255 and 223.
62. *BARs*, letter dated 18 August, 1684.
63. *PRO LS13/104*, ff. 98 and 105, 8 July, 1678 and 17 April, 1679. See, also, cases of Anthony Boad, an Italian servant to the Queen, admitted on 13 May, 1685, Elizabeth Jelly, presumably a maid in the Queen's Kitchen, who was sent to Bethlem *c*3 March, 1688, on a warrant from William Yardley, Clerk to the Queen's Kitchen, and Edward Macklew, 'one of his Majesty's Household Servants ... deprived of his Reason by a violent Fever' and ordered into Bethlem's 'safe custody' in 1775. *PRO LS13/105*, ff. 4, 6, 48; *LS13/179*, fo. 223; *BARs*, letters dated 13 May, 1685 and 3 March, 1688.
64. *PRO LS13/104*, 4 December, 1677, fo. 90.
65. *PRO LS13/104*, 8 January, 1678 and 17 April, 1679, ff. 98 and 105; *BARs*, 29 January, 1706, fo. 73; *PRO Kew ADM96/6*, 29 January, 1706.
66. Allan Ingram, *The Madhouse of Language. Writing and Reading Madness in the Eighteenth Century* (London; New York: Routledge, 1992).
67. *BCGM*, fo. 17, 22 October, 1662.
68. *Ibid.*, fo. 301, 16 April, 1647.
69. *PRO Kew ADM67/124*, 14 and 17 December, 1733, ff. 86–88; *ADM67/125*, 7 November 1737, ff. 59–60. See, also, the case of John Welch, a Roman Catholic, expelled for abuses of the same nature in 1738 and 1744; *ADM 67/126*, 7 December, 1744, fo 252.
70. *BCGM*, fo. 174, 11 April, 1638. See, also, case of Fulwood, who 'used certaine scandelous and seditious speeches against his Majestie and the State', and, although claiming to have been drunk, was ordered by the Privy Council to be punished with the whip in Bridewell as an 'example' to others: *Acts of the Privy Council* (1613–14), 12. And see cases of Thomas E[a]den alias Sampson, John Coates and Elizabeth

Briton, sent to Bridewell for, variously, 'scandalous words against his Ma[jes]tie', 'daingerous words against Parliament', etc., and whose discharges depended on warrants being issued by some outside authority: *ibid.*, ff. 202, 393 and 40, 17 October, 1638, 15 July and 15 September, 1642.

71. Richard Stafford, *The Mystery of Iniquity Somewhat Laid Open. In a Letter to the Present Governour; Wherein is also Contained an History and Recital and Proposal of Sundry Things to be Made Known and Remembred, and to be done Accordingly. In that Letter which I Carried to Thine House at Kensington on November 3 1691 which was there Burnt (as Near as I Can Remember) the Words Contained Therein was to this Following Effect* (7 January, 1693), (London: 1693), 3.
72. Henry Horwitz (ed.), *The Parliamentary Diary of Narcissus Luttrell 1691–1693* (Oxford: Clarendon Press, 1972), 10 December, 1692, 307–8.
73. *Acts of the Privy Council* (1616–17), 21 December, 1617, 392–3; Ellis was also mentioned *supra.*
74. *PRO PC2/50*, 28 July and 12 August, 1639, ff. 546 and 594.
75. *PRO SP44/28*, 7 October, 1673, fo. 92; *Calendar of State Papers Domestic* (henceforth, *CSPD*), Car. II, 1673, 571.
76. For example, cases of Peter Massey, Deborah Lyddall and Nicholas Valiant, *PRO LS13/104*, 29 September, 1675, 16 August and 4 December, 1677, ff. 73 and 89–90.
77. *PRO PCR, II*, 26 January, 1637, fo. 537.
78. *PRO LS13/105*, 17 January, 1688, fo. 54.
79. *BCGM*, 20 June, 1638, fo. 186.
80. Biographical information about Stafford, and the chronology of his writings and periods of confinement, may be pieced together from his extant publications (although this is not without risk of bias). See, especially, Stafford, *A Clear Apology* (London: 1691). See, also, the wills of Richard Stafford and John Stafford, Gloucs. RO; Anthony A. Wood, *Athenae Oxonienses* (New York; London: Johnson Reprint Corporation, 1967), iv, 781–2; Joseph Foster, *Alumni Oxonienses* (Oxford; London: Parker and Co., 1891), 1405; *DNB*, liii, 459. For Thornbury, see Ralph Bigland, *History, Monuments and Genealogical Collections relative to the County of Gloucester* (London: 1792; facsimile edn, Stroud: Bristol & Gloucester Archaeological Society, 1992), 3 vols, iii, 295–314. Ralph Grove (b.1673) was appointed vicar of Thornbury in 1701, a year after receiving his MA from Christ Church, Oxford, and was to officiate there until his death in 1728. See, Foster, *op. cit.*, (above), i, 616.
81. *A Supplemental Tract of Government, to be Annexed unto the Book of Happiness and c, Chapter 3 Circa page 147. Which may be Applied to all Nations; But is now Particularly Referred to the Consideration of the Lords and Commons assembled in the Present Parliament at Westminster, 4 January, 1690* (London: 1690). See also his *Of Happiness: Wherein it*

is Fully and Particularly Manifested, that the greatest Happiness of this Life consisteth in the Fear of God and keeping his Commandments in Opposition to the Pleasures of Sin, or the pretended conveniency of Disobedience (London: 1689).

82. *Things Plain and Weighty, Referred Unto the Consideration of both Houses of Parliament, 25 March, 1690* (reprinted, with additions, London: 1691); *A Copy of Two Letters left on the Back-Stairs at Whitehall, Jan. 26, 1690* (London: 1690), and *The Case of Richard Stafford Humbly Offered to Both Houses of Parliament* (London: 1690).
83. *A Short Printed Petition to the Knights, Citizens and Burgesses in Parliament Assembled. Delivered to them whilst I was their Prisoner under the Custody of the Seargeant at Arms* (London: 1691), and *A short Remonstrance of Richard Stafford unto the Parliament of England, upon their not Receiving and Hearing of his Testimony, but Shutting Him up in Prison for the same* (London: 1691).
84. *PRO LS13//105*, fo. 69; *BARs*, letter dated 4 November, 1691, fo. 140.
85. *PRO LS13/86*, 31 August, 1716, ff. 57–8; *LS13/115*, fo. 51.
86. O'Donoghue, *op. cit.* (note 25), 241–2, 406. The *DNB* also dismissed Stafford's tracts as 'more or less incoherent', while Wood judged Stafford 'little better than craz'd or rather bigotted with religion' (*op. cit.* (note 80), iv, 781).
87. Stafford, *op. cit.* (note 81), *A Supplemental Tract*, 1; *Things Plain and Weighty*, 9.
88. Stafford, *op. cit.* (note 81), *Things Plain and Weighty*, 11–12.
89. See, for example, Stafford, *op. cit.* (note 80), 25.
90. For background on Protestant dissenters during this period, see, for example, Hill, *op. cit.* (note 26), Douglas R. Lacey, *Dissent and Parliamentary Politics in England, 1661–1689: A Study in the Perpetuation and Tempering of Parliamentarianism* (New Brunswick, Rutgers University Press, 1969); Richard L. Greaves, *Enemies Under His Feet. Radicals and Nonconformists in Britain, 1664–1677* (Stanford: Stanford University Press, 1990); Geoffrey Holmes, *Politics, Religion and Society in England, 1679–1742* (London and Ronceverte: The Hambledon Press, 1986).
91. Stafford, *op. cit.* (note 81), *Of Happiness*, 657–65.
92. *Ibid.*, 657.
93. *Ibid.*, 657, 662–3.
94. Michael MacDonald, '*Mystical Bedlam: Madness, Anxiety and Healing in Seventeenth Century England* (Cambridge: CUP, 1981); *idem*, 'Popular Beliefs About Mental Disorder in Early Modern England', in Wolfgang Eckhart and Johanna Geyer-Kordesch (eds), *Münstersche Beiträge zur Geschichte und Theorie der Medizin* (Münster: Burgverlag, 1982), 148–73; *idem*, 'Lunatics and the State in Georgian England', in *Social History of Medicine*, 2, 3 (December, 1989), 299–314; *idem*, 'Insanity and the Realities of History in Early Modern England', in R. M. Murray and T. H. Turner (eds), *Lectures on the History of*

Psychiatry. The Squibb Series (London: Gaskell/The Royal College of Psychiatrists, 1990), 60–77.

95. For early examples of the pathologizing of religious fervour, see Meric Casaubon, *Treatise Concerning Enthusiasme, as it is an Effect of Nature: but is Mistaken by Many for Either Divine Inspiration, or Diabolical Possession* (London: 1655); Henry More, *Enthusiasmus Triumphatus, or, a Discourse of the Nature, Causes, Kinds, and Cure, of Enthusiasme; Written by Philophilus Parresiastes* (London, 1656). For later attacks, see George Lavington, *The Enthusiasm of Methodists and Papists Compared* (London: 1757); Thomas Evans, *The History of Modern Enthusiasm* (2nd edn; London: 1757).
96. *A Modest Attempt for healing the Present Animosities in England. Occasion'd by a late Book Entitled, A Modest Enquiry, and c. In a Dialogue between* ***Testimony,*** *a Zealous Dissenter; and* ***Hot-head,*** *a Chollerick Bigot;* ***Trimmer,*** *Moderator* (London: 1690).
97. On Nottingham, see e.g. Henry Horwitz, *Revolution Politicks: The Career of Daniel Finch Second Earl of Nottingham, 1647–1730* (Cambridge: Cambridge University Press, 1968); Lacey, *op. cit.* (note 90), 232, 234–7, 240–1; Stafford, *op. cit.* (note 80); Holmes, *op. cit.* (note 90) especially 132, 155, 187, 192, 199.
98. *Apology*, 15–16.
99. Edward Stephens, *An Apology for Mr. Richard Stafford, with an Admonition to Him and Other Honest Mistaken People* (London: 1690).
100. Following his discharge from Bethlem, and clearly bearing a whole host of grudges against his persecutors, Stafford was to blame a Mr. Robert Stephens (presumably, the same man) for the refusal of 'several Printers' to publish his works (claiming that Stephens was acting under the Secretary of State, Nottingham's, orders); Stafford, *Because that to Many People, I have Seemed to Falsify my Word and Promise, which I Made on Being Discharged out of Bethlehem Hospital* ... (n.d., *c.* 1693), 3.
101. *The Truth which God hath Shewn*, 42.
102. *Ibid.*, Preface.
103. Stafford, *op. cit.* (note 81), 660; Stephens, *op. cit.* (note 99), 1.
104. See, his *Apology*, (note 80), 13, where Stafford describes ordering his petition to be printed and given to Commons members, 'though I knew before this was contrary to Custom and Usage'.
105. Richard Stafford, *To the Lords Spiritual and Temporal, and to the Commons of England assembled at Westminster; at their Sessions begun on November 7 1693* (1693).
106. *PRO LS13/105*, fo. 70, 11 November, 1691. According to the diary of Narcissus Luttrell, within another fortnight, Stafford had managed to get some more of his productions as far as the Speaker of the House of Commons. On the Speaker taking notice in the House of 'a packet of seditious papers', asserts Luttrell, it was recommended that the President of Bridewell and Bethlem, Sir William Turner, be asked to

ensure that Stafford be deprived of pen, ink and paper 'to prevent his writing such scandalous papers'. The proximity and similarity of these two episodes, and the lack of any reference to the latter in the Bethlem archives, however, may suggest that they both refer to one and the same event. Horwitz (ed.), *Diary of Narcissus Luttrell*, 25 November, 1691, 38; Wood, *op. cit.* (note 80), iv, 782.

107. Wood, *op. cit.*, 40–1.
108. See Stafford, *op. cit.* (note 100), 2, where Stafford speaks of being conveyed into an oppressive cell at Bethlem 'for seven Weeks and three days'. While the chronology does not exactly tally, as Stafford was ordered kept more closely confined by the Green Cloth on 11 April, 1692, exactly ten weeks and a day before he was ordered discharged, it is not unlikely that there was some delay in implementing the Green Cloth's orders. *PRO LS13/105*, 11 April, 1692, fo. 73; *SP44/98*, 21 June, 1692, fo. 488.
109. Irving Goffman, *Asylums* (New York: Anchor Books, 1961).
110. *Richard Stafford A Scribe instructed in the Law of God, his Last and Concluding Testimony unto the Princes, the Priests, and the People Inhabiting the Island of Great Britain. Concerning the Great Sin which they Committed in the Year 1688, by Putting Down one King, and Setting Up Another; With his Final Exhortation unto Them (who at this Day Continue in the same Transgression) to come into Repentance and Restitution* (n.d., *c.*1693), 6; *The Mystery of Iniquity*, 1–3, 7. In the latter, written largely whilst Stafford was in Bethlem, Stafford emphasises fires which occurred at Kensington and Whitehall, and a cannon shot that had narrowly missed William when he was at the Hague.
111. *Stafford, op. cit.* (note 71), 9.
112. *Ibid.*, 11; and *op. cit.* (note 100).
113. *Ibid.*, 2.
114. David Williams, 'The Missions of David Williams and James Tilly Matthews to England (1793)', *English Historical Review*, liii (1938), 651–68; Robert Howard, 'James Tilly Matthews in London and Paris 1793; his First Peace Mission – in his Own Words', *History of Psychiatry*, 2 (March, 1991), 53–70; Roy Porter (ed.), *Illustrations of Madness* (1810), by John Haslam (London: Routledge, 1988), introduction.
115. *Stafford, op. cit.* (note 100), 2.
116. *Ibid.*
117. Stafford's account is verified by the fact that his own version of this order is almost verbatim with that amongst State Papers Domestic and that in the Hospital's own records. *PRO SP44/98*, 21 June, 1692, fo. 488, and *BAR*s, 21 June, 1692.
118. Amongst Stafford's publications subsequent to his discharge, were: *To the Right Honourable Daniel Earl of Nottingham Principal Secretary of State, and To the Other Members of the Privy Council Richard Stafford,*

a Scribe of Jesus Christ, Sendeth Greeting (n.d., *c.*1692); *Some Thoughts Concerning The Life to Come: With a Brief Account Of the State of Religion, As it is Now in the World* (London: 1693); *Because that to Many People ...* (n.d., *c.*1693), and *Richard Stafford A Scribe ...* (n.d., *c.*1693). In his *The Mystery of Iniquity Somewhat Laid Open ...* (1692), Stafford spoke of being imprisoned 'four times' (p.10), while in his *last ... Testimony* (p.1), Stafford claimed to have been 'imprisoned ... five times'. I have been unable, however, to find any other evidence of Stafford being confined more than three times, or subsequent to his discharge from Bethlem.

119. See, *To the Right Honourable Daniel ...*, reproduced in *Because that to Many People* (note 100), 2–4.
120. *Ibid.*
121. *HMC Report of the MSS of the Marquess of Downshire* (London: HMSO, 1924), i, ii, 601; *HMC Downshire MSS*, xxx, 94.
122. Stafford, *To the Representatives of the People and Nation of England, Assembled at Westminster at their Session, begun October 20 1696* (London: 1696).
123. *SP, Out Letters (General)*, xi, 28 July, 1687, 151; *CSPD, Treasury Books* (1685–9), viii, iii, 1494.
124. *Acts of the Privy Council* (1578–80), xi, 14 April, 1579, 100–1.
125. Porter, *Manacles* (note 8), 2.
126. *Ibid.* Although Lee was not a state committal, once his independent means of support had been exhausted, he was subsequently supported in Bethlem by the Green Cloth, presumably because as writer to the King's Players, he was counted as a quasi-member of the Royal Household.
127. Stafford, *To the Right Honourable Daniel, op. cit.* (note 118), 3.
128. *Ibid.*, 3.
129. *PRO PC2/58*, 8 February, 1665, fo. 36; *PC2/59*, 16 January, 1666, fo. 271. For another case where special treatment was requested, see, for example, *BARs*, 7 March, 1688, case of Thomas Palden.
130. *PRO LS13/104*, ff. 98 and 105.
131. *PRO LS13/104*, ff. 79, 89, 90, 94; *LS13/105*, fols 34, 79, 87; cases of Mary Davies, Deborah Lyddall, Nicholas Valiant, Richard Harris, William Wenham, Thomas Brookes and Mary Gammon, all admitted during the 1670s.
132. *PRO LS13/172*, fo. 37.
133. *PRO LS13/86*; *LS13/104*, fo. 95; *LS13/171*, fo. 356.
134. *PRO LS13/104*, fo. 73; *BCGM* 29 September, 1675, fo. 186. See also the case of Peter Massey, *PRO LS13/175*, fo. 85.
135. Peter Linebaugh, *The London Hanged: Crime and Civil Society in the Eighteenth Century* (London: Allen Lane/Penguin, 1991).
136. *PRO LS13/104*, fo. 111.
137. *PRO LS13/88*, 21 March, 1694.
138. *PRO LS13/87*, discharge warrants dated 10 June and 6 November,

1687. See also case of George Bells, discharged on 23 March, 1688.

139. For example, *PRO LS13/105*, fo. 134; *BCGM*, 10/18 July, 1686, 25 August, 1688, 13 February, 1690, cases of the soldiers John Greene, James Walker and Eric Prenson.
140. *PRO LS13/177*, fo. 98.
141. *SP, Entry Book 64*, 137.
142. See, for example, *PRO SP44/31*, fo. 86, *SP29/361*, No. 94 and *SP44/31*, fo. 132, re. the appointments of the Bethlem Apothecary in 1672 and the Bridewell Minister in 1674.
143. For Taylor's case, see *BCGM*, 19 May, 1675, fol. 129, and warrant dated 14 May, 1675 at end of same Court Book; *House of Lords Journals*, xii, 691, 700–1; xiii, 18–19, 26; *House of Lords RO, Braye MS. 3*, fo. 396.
144. *PRO LS13/105*, 17 January, 1688, fo. 54.
145. *Bethlem Sub-Committee Minutes*, 1709–17, 1717–27, 1727–35.
146. *PRO LS13/104*, fo. 46.
147. *PRO LS13/179*, fo. 12; *BSCM*, 12 September, 1761; *Bethlem Incurables Admission Register* (*BIAR*), fo. 46.
148. *PRO LS13/179*, fo. 17; *BSCM*, 3 August, 1762; *BARs* and *BIARs*.
149. *BSCM*, 27 September, 1788.
150. Andrews, *op. cit.* (note 29).
151. See, for example, cases of Dorothy Jones, William Robinson, Jacob Widdekeller and Revd Jospeph Ward, in *BARs*, ff. 26, 100, 210; *PRO LS13/176*, ff. 70, 183; *LS13/177*, ff. 20 and 98.
152. Ida Macalpine and Richard Hunter, *George III and the Mad-Business* (London: Pimlico, 1991; orig. Allen Lane, The Penguin Press, 1969), 313; G. D. Collinson, *A Treatise on the Law Concerning Idiots, Lunatics, and Other Persons Considered Non Compotes Mentis* (London: 1812), Vol. i, 502–3.
153. Walton, 'Casting out', (note 19), 139.

2

Medical Reform, the Enlightenment and Physician-Power in Late Eighteenth-Century France

L. W. B. Brockliss

The Ancien-Régime Medical System

In eighteenth-century France medical practice was the domain of a complex web of licensed and unlicensed healers.[1] The official network of physicians, surgeons and apothecaries primarily served the social élite and was predominantly based in towns of over 2,000 inhabitants. The 80 per cent of the population that lived in villages, on the other hand, primarily relied on the services of unlicensed practitioners, clergy, local wise-women, bonesetters, itinerant quacks and so on. The distinction between town and country, licensed and unlicensed, however, should not be too tightly drawn. In the first place, unlicensed healers, particularly itinerants boasting a surgical expertise such as cupping for cataract, continually invaded the urban space and lured well-to-do clients from the clutches of official practitioners. Secondly, the most successful unlicensed healers who found their way to the court were frequently granted the *ad hominem* privilege of plying their trade, irrespective of royal edicts which emphasized that in urban France at least medical practice was to be monopolized by the qualified. Thirdly, the official medical profession, as in neighbouring countries, was plagued by too many internal rivalries and questioned distinctions to present a clear-cut contrast with the community of unlicensed healers.

Traditionally, in France as elsewhere, the official profession was supposedly hierarchically organized. At the top were the physicians, faculty graduates, who by dint of their university education belonged to the liberal professions and who alone had the legal right to practise physic (i.e. diagnose a disease and prescribe for its cure) in French towns.[2] Beneath them, acting as their subordinates, were the surgeons and apothecaries, who performed the surgical operations and prepared and administered the drugs that their superiors thought necessary.

The inferior, artisanal status of the surgeons and apothecaries was emphasized by the fact that they had to serve an apprenticeship, gained experience by going on a *tour de France*, then became qualified by being admitted to the *maîtrise.* By the eighteenth century, however, this theoretical structure had begun to break down and only existed in its pristine state in the minds of conservative physicians. In reality, there were always many surgeons and apothecaries who perforce had had to perform the role of physicians, because graduate practitioners tended only to be found in the large towns.[3] The distinction between licensed and unlicensed healers, therefore, was a blurred one, to say the least. As the eighteenth century progressed, moreover, the number of surgeons breaking bounds increased, for surgeons in the big cities in particular rejected their subordinate position, and began to neglect to consult with a physician in major surgical cases and even to prescribe for internal diseases. This reflected the fact that the century witnessed a rapid rise in their status. Through crown encouragement there emerged an élite corps of city surgeons, whose members had been educated in classics and philosophy,[4] had trained in the newly founded independent surgical colleges,[5] and were entitled by law to professional rather than artisanal status.[6]

At the same time, furthermore, members of the official medical community could find themselves practising illegally even when they kept to their professional last. This reflected the fact that the official medical community had no legal identity but consisted of two distinctive groups: those who belonged to medical corporations and those who did not. In towns where there was a legally recognized corporation of physicians, surgeons, or apothecaries only the incorporated could practise legally. Outsiders, however well qualified, were as much unlicensed healers as itinerant charlatans. For graduate physicians, therefore, a degree brought no licence to practise in the 40 largest cities of France; the right to practise in the most lucrative locations was dependent on leaping a variety of financial, social and practical hurdles which controlled admittance to the local medical corporation.[7] Restrictions on the activities of master surgeons and apothecaries were different but just as keen. The 3–400 corporations[8] of surgeons and apothecaries were also the bodies which granted the *maîtrise;* there was no separate accrediting body. Becoming qualified, therefore, meant at best gaining admittance to a local corps and gaining the right to practise within its legal *ressort.* But even this was not guaranteed, for the larger surgical corporations were empowered to grant different types of *maîtrise:* one which did bring admittance to the company, and others which only allowed the holder to practice in the local bourgs and villages where there was no corporation.[9] Not surprisingly, the monopoly of the corporations was a bone of contention. The bright and ambitious who had lacked the family means to enter a prestigious or lucrative corps were understandably frustrated, and many (their number was certainly growing in the economically buoyant eighteenth century) moved to the town of their choice to practise illegally. Paris, a rich city of 6–700,000 souls particularly attracted the qualified interloper, especially as a post at court, although not necessarily lucrative, brought the right to practise in the capital regardless of the privileges of the city's medical corporations.[10]

The extent to which boundary-breaking was a commonplace in pre-Revolutionary medical practice is evident from the frequency with which entrenched 'insiders' felt compelled to have recourse to the law to defend their monopoly position. Indeed, in some cases interlopers would be called before the courts, even when they apparently had the law on their side, so anxious were established practitioners to prevent unwelcome competition. In 1786, the physicians of Auxerre, for instance, who had no right of incorporation, tried to put an end to the medical practice of a recently arrived graduate physician called Guinault Descréaux. The *arriviste*, it was maintained, was an ertstwhile lawyer and medical charlatan, who had regularized his postion by taking a degree *à la hâte* at the 'foreign' university of Avignon.[11] Understandably, the tension between 'insiders' and 'outsiders' was most acute in Paris, where the incorporated physicians tried in vain to maintain their traditional monopoly and frustrate the attempt of the capital's surgeons to justify boundary-breaking by raising their status. In Paris, moreover, the quarrel between 'insiders' and 'outsiders' was not confined to the privacy of the courts, but placed firmly in the public domain as both sides defended their position at length in print.[12]

This great debate was at its height in the second quarter of the eighteenth century. What is interesting is that both sides were conservative in that neither really questioned the value of the existing official medical system. Paris physicians, like Philippe Hecquet (1661–1737), treated the surgeons as ignorant, unlearned sons of Adam, fired by greed to invade the privileged domain of their superiors. Their behaviour was immoral (the three-fold division was God-ordained), illegal and harmful to the Parisian public, since the surgeon–physician had an inadequate understanding of the science of medicine and employed dangerous drugs in a cavalier manner. Surgeon–physicians then were no better than empirical doctors, and their medical practice had to be stopped and the legal distinctions between physicians and surgeons confirmed in the capital for the benefit of the commonweal.[13] The surgeons and their supporters naturally jibbed at the aspersions cast on their morality and knowledge – indeed they repaid the compliment in kind.[14] But they essentially accepted Hecquet's insistence that the profession of physic should be monopolized by the academically trained, and accepted that most contemporary surgeons (outside the capital) were not fit to exercise the art. They argued not for the blurring of traditional boundaries, but that Paris surgeons in the second quarter of the eighteenth century represented a special case.

The most significant propagandist to defend the boundary-breakers was the erstwhile Mantes *accoucheur*, professor at the Paris *école de chirurgie* and future physiocrat, François Quesnay (1694–1774),[15] who published an extremely detailed and lengthy historical defence of the surgeons' independence in 1744. According to Quesnay Paris surgeons had been traditionally highly learned, so much so that in 1579 the pope had incorporated the Parisian company in the university as a separate faculty with the right to give lectures and give degrees in surgery. The physicians and the faculty of medicine had always resented the presence of learned surgeons, and had encouraged the city's barbers to set up as a rival company. Their machinations had come to fruition in 1660 when the crown had ordered the two companies to merge and the new company had been forbidden to teach or graduate students. Subsequently, until the turn of the eighteenth century, Paris surgery had languished. By the second quarter of the century, however, a group of surgeons had emerged anxious to restore the company to its pristine glory, and this, thanks to the aid of Louis XV, had been achieved, with the result that from 1743 the surgeons had once again been separated from the barbers. The rising status of the Paris surgeons, therefore, was not a radical departure, but a restoration of the traditional order of things.[16]

Quesnay, admittedly, did not always argue in such historical terms, but he was always careful not to rock the corporate boat too violently. Witness a pamphlet that he published in 1748.[17] Here again Quesnay acknowledged that Paris surgeons in the recent past had been ignorant barbers, and admitted that this being the case it was logical for the physicians to wish to supervise their activities closely. On the other hand, he insisted that *legally* surgeons had the right to treat external diseases independently. Although it was a nonsense to differentiate between internal and external diseases for the treatment of both required a knowledge of medical science, nevertheless it was the law, and the physicians were guilty of inventing novel rights for themselves in claiming the power to police the treatment of surgical cases. Fortunately, there was no need for the Parisian physicians to flout the law, for there was now a new generation of surgeons who were more than competent to treat external diseases without summoning a physician. These surgeons were just as learned as the physicians. Indeed, had this not been the case, then surgical knowledge would not have improved by leaps and bounds, as it had, in the first decades of the eighteenth century. Surgical advance depended not on manual dexterity but reading books and understanding Latin and philosophy. In fact, surgical *élèves* got very little practical training in operative techniques during their apprenticeship and attendance at the Paris college, for there were probably only 100 operations performed each year outside the Paris hospitals and the college course on surgical operations only lasted three months. Yet junior surgeons could perform lithotomies as well as their seniors:

> Ce n'est donc pas uniquement l'exercice continuel des mains qui apprend à opérer, comme le pense ceux qui n'ont aucune idée de l'Art de Chirurgie, & qui pour s'en former une, le comparent aux professions des Artisans, dans lesquelles on ne devient habile que par la seule habitude des mains, acquis par un exercice journellement répété.[18]

Surgery, then, was a science not an art, and because the modern Paris surgeon was learned, he was also perfectly equipped to treat internal diseases. This did not mean that the traditional monopoly of the physicians over internal diseases was thereby threatened, for Paris surgeons would limit their activities to the diseases of the poor. As the surgeons were forbidden by law from charging for consulting on internal diseases, they had no incentive to search out rich clients. The poor, on the other hand, could not afford to approach a physician, so the learned surgeons were filling a gap in medical provision, otherwise filled by barbers and charlatans. Moreover, much of this medical practice could be left to the surgeons' *élèves*, thus killing two birds with one stone. The *élèves* would be kept occupied and the pittance they received from the grateful poor would help to pay for their upkeep.[19] By emphasizing their independence, therefore, the Paris surgeons were not breaking boundaries at all, but in fact keeping the traditional medical system in good repair.

Quesnay's argument, of course, was tailor-made to strike a chord with the wider noble and professional Paris constituency at whom his pamphlets were presumably aimed. On the other hand, there can be little doubt that the surgical community at large would have been appalled, had critics accused them of really wishing to create an open medical market-place.[20] Indeed, it is quite clear that the Paris surgeons (learned or otherwise) were just as eager as the physicians to defend their monopoly rights. Thus, on the very eve of the Revolution the Paris surgeons were locked in a legal quarrel with their peers at court who claimed the right to practise in the capital by virtue of their royal office. The number of Paris surgeons in 1789 was relatively small (some 190). There were 120 surgeons of one kind and another attached to the royal household, so understandably, the Parisians feared the competition if all at court had the licence to practise in the capital. In fact, it was argued, less than 70 had the right to do so, for a significant proportion of the court contingent were actually surgical specialists, such as oculists and dentists, who could not be considered surgeons in the learned sense by any stretch of the imagination.[21]

Medical Reform

From what has been said, it is clear that the large majority of practitioners who belonged to the official medical system in eighteenth-century France were perfectly satisfied with its basic structure. Many might have been anxious to expand the scope of their corporate competence, but they were equally anxious that none should challenge their traditional monopoly rights. This conclusion is confirmed by the information provided in the *cahiers des doléances* that the medical corps drew up in 1789 to present to the Estates-General. Published examples of the surviving *cahiers* suggest that the corps was primarily interested in safeguarding its traditional rights against interlopers. In particular, hostility was directed against the custom of licensing the sale of secret remedies by alternative practitioners and their agents. The corps, on the eve of the Revolution, was not, it seems, interested in redrawing the medical map.[22]

However, in the final decade of the Ancien Régime there were signs that reform of the official medical system would soon be firmly placed on the political agenda. For the first time a handful of licensed and learned medical practitioners rose above the moralistic and historico-legalistic debate over the rights and wrongs of boundary-breaking, and viewed the existing medical system with a critical eye.[23] Significantly, given the current orthodoxy that the surgeons in eighteenth-century France represented the forces of modernity, the initiative came from a group of physicians.[24] Furthermore, these reformist physicians were either associated with or chose to address their reform proposals to the *Société Royale de Médecine*. This was a Paris-based institution of physicians, founded by the Crown in 1776, dedicated to medical progress through the collection of meteorological and epidemiological data.[25] Although theoretically not a threat to the existing medical system, it definitely helped to erode corporate solidarity among the community of physicians in that its permanent Parisian membership and provincial correspondents were generally drawn from existing corps. As association with the Society was supposedly a reward for making some positive contribution to medical science, its members were encouraged to consider themselves the cream of the country's physicians, medical pioneers whose focus of loyalty was the Society as much as, if not more than, their local corps. For this reason, the Society was particularly disliked by the old guard in the Paris college of physicians, all the more that the crown gave the new institution certain powers of medical police, such as licensing the sale of secret remedies, which the college coveted or felt were its own preserve.[26] Not surprisingly, in consequence, the Society was quickly identified as the institutional locus around which this small group of reform-minded physicians could gather.

The coming of the Revolution revealed that the reformers of the 1780s, while always a minority, spoke for a definite constituency within the official medical system. The establishment of the National Assembly in the summer of 1789 spawned a number of specialist committees whose brief was to investigate the ways in which existing social, cultural and professional institutions could be reformed to promote the general good. When the secretary of the *Société Royale*, Félix Vicq d'Azyr (1748–94), engineered the foundation of a separate *comité de salubrité* in September 1790, the floodgates were opened, and the committee received an avalanche of plans for medical reform from all over the country.[27] Reformers (as had been the case in the 1780s) offered a variety of solutions as to how the tensions in the existing medical system could best be resolved for the benefit of the people's health. Most of these again were the work of physicians, not surgeons. The most exhaustive and thorough of the reform proposals was the one drawn up by Vicq d'Azyr on behalf of the *Société Royale* and presented to the National Assembly only seven days after the foundation of the *comité de salubrité*.[28] A committee of the Society had been working on a new medical 'constitution' for France, and the *Plan* submitted by Vicq was clearly intended to be the basis for the report that the *comité de salubrité* would eventually draw up.[29] The *Plan*, it must be stressed, was not entirely Vicq's work, and therein lies its interest, for it was a document that drew heavily on other reform proposals, notably one submitted to the Society's committee by the Paris physician, Nicolas Chambon de Montaux (1748–1828), in October 1789. It was, then, a submission that was representative of the reform movement as well as its most detailed and carefully developed expression.[30]

The *Plan* promoted the introduction of a completely new medical system. In the first place, it took up a demand which had been voiced *sotto voce* by Quesnay in the pamphlet of 1748,[31] put more stridently in a pamphlet by the Rouennais surgeon Claude Nicolas Le Cat in 1766, [32] and had emerged as a central plank of the reform movement in the 1780s: the unification of the professions of surgery and medicine. Before the Revolution reformers had viewed such a development as a vain dream. Indeed, the Paris physician Antoine Petit (1718–94), writing in 1787 saw little chance of change in the imminent future: '... le temps où nos idées doivent germer n'est pas encore venu, je ne le crois pas prêt d'arriver'.[33] In the heady days of the Revolution, in contrast, Vicq d'Azyr felt that such a fundamental reform was quite within the realm of the possible, and was to be achieved by establishing a common form of institutional education for surgeons and physicians, and, more importantly, a common form of certification. The union of the two professions, it was believed, would put an end to the 'vicious' division between internal and external diseases, would regularize the status of medical practitioners (i.e. surgeons) who were encouraged by the public to practise both physic and surgery, and would end the quarrels between the two communities. Unification of the two professions, it was suggested, would restore the situation to what it had been in classical antiquity. The division of the two professions had been the result of the Church gaining control of all learning after the age of Justinian.[34] Pharmacy, however, according to the *Plan* was to remain a separate profession, even if apothecaries (now called pharmacists) were to be trained in future alongside prospective medical doctors. They would be examined for a separate diploma and, although their monopoly over the preparation of drugs was to be secured, they would be forbidden to practise medicine.[35] The reason for maintaining a separate pharmaceutical profession was not given, but on one level the decision to retain the *status quo* must have reflected the belief that the preparation of drugs was a specialist, complex, and time-consuming business. It must also have reflected the suspicion, shared by many reformers in an age when physicians all over Europe were singing the praises of expectant medicine, that apothecaries were the natural defenders of polypharmacy.[36]

In the second place, the *Plan* sought to dismantle completely the existing corporate medical system and end the monopoly privileges enjoyed by individual corps. Henceforth doctors and pharmacists would be divided into two groups. The first group would be given a certificate or diploma by one of the five medical schools that the programme envisaged erecting, and would be allowed to practise where they wished.[37] The second group would be trained in local *écoles pratiques* at the state's expense and would only be allowed to practise in their home *département* (the new administrative unit of the Revolution). This group would be expected in return for a state stipend to treat the poor in town and country for nothing, thereby ensuring that the whole population was able to consult with trained medical practitioners and (so it was hoped) putting an end to the army of charlatans and empirics. Vicq d'Azyr anticipated the establishment of some 6,000 rural cantonal doctors and an unspecified number of urban parish doctors, who would be based on a parish hospice. Except during epidemics Vicq believed that the number of indigent sick would be small, so that the departmental doctors would still be able to maintain a private practice.[38] Ideally, the cantonal doctors would also be in charge of delivering babies in the locality, but Vicq felt that such was the popular prejudice in favour of midwives that it would be a long time before they gained a monopoly. Thus it would be necessary for the *écoles pratiques* also to train midwives, again at the state's expense, at the rate of two per rural canton.[39]

An interest in extending the official medical system to the whole of the population was widely shared among the reformers. Indeed, the Montpellier-trained Swiss physician Samuel Tissot (1728–97), who practised outside France at Lausanne, seems to have been interested in training village doctors from the 1760s,[40] while one of the chief aims of the *Société Royale* was to learn more about popular epidemics in the hope that the sufferings of the poor could be eventually relieved.[41] Vicq, however, was not interested just in providing the human population of the countryside with trained medical personnel, for his programme also promoted the establishment of a veterinary department within the proposed Paris school of medicine and the foundation of a number of provincial schools where locals could be taught veterinary medicine.[42] There were already two veterinary schools in France at Alfort and Lyons, founded in the 1760s, but they tended to be research institutions. As a result care of animals remained the province of the blacksmith and the farrier, 'unqualified' healers who were not unknown to treat human ailments too.[43] Vicq clearly intended to establish a veterinary profession and extend the medical system to the whole animal realm. His personal interest in animal care was scarcely surprising, for he was an expert in comparative anatomy, he had been sent by the government to investigate the rinderpest epidemic of the mid-1770s, and had held a professorship at Alfort in the 1780s. Nevertheless, the programme's proposals were also the expression of a wider and novel interest a number of physicians had evinced in the care of livestock in the last years of the Ancien Régime. Indeed, the *Société Royale* itself had emerged out of a commission set up by the government to gather information about animal epidemics.[44]

In the third place, the *Plan* followed earlier proposals in placing great emphasis on completely restructuring the medical curriculum, so that the new integrated medical profession would be properly qualified for its herculean task of maintaining the health of the nation. Vicq said nothing about the quality of teaching provided by the new surgical colleges, but he was scathing at the expense of the 18 or so traditional medical faculties.[45] In his view the contemporary institutionalized medical education provided for aspirant physicians was useless as a training for medical practitioners. It merely produced an ignorant doctor, a virtual charlatan, who was left to 's'instruire par ses propres fautes'.

> Que peut-on attendre, en effet de quelques années d'étude, qui se passent à dicter ou à lire des Prolégomènes de Médecine, unique-ment formés de définitions & de divisions stériles? Que peut-on attendre d'Ecoles dans la plupart desquelles on n'enseigne ni l'Anatomie complette de l'homme, ni l'art de Botanique, ni la Chimie médicale dans toute son étendue, ni la Pharmacie, ni l'art de formuler, ni la Nosologie, ni l'histoire de la Médecine, ni la Traité des maladies; où l'on ne dit pas un mot des fonctions publiques du Médecin, où nul encore n'a professé son Art près du lit des malades, & d'où l'on sort enfin sans avoir rien appris de ce qu'un Médecin praticien doit savoir?[46]

Besides removing the bevy of minor medical schools in France and establishing five medical colleges with a complement of seven to ten professors, the solution to the problem of practitioner training was deemed to be twofold: to revolutionize the curriculum and institute a new system of examination.

The traditional core of the faculty curriculum, the study of theoretical medicine in the form of physiology, pathology, semiotics and therapeutics, was to remain important, but the professors would be required to keep their imaginations on a tight rein. Physiology would be closely tied to comparative anatomy, while the professor of pathology was warned 'à ne dire ce qu'il saura bien, à ne parler que d'après le souvenir des faits, [et] à ne jamais sortir de la route qu'il se sera tracée dans le silence de la méditation de l'étude.'[47] More importantly, the curriculum was to be revitalized by a new emphasis being given to subjects generally neglected. On the one hand, medical students were to be given a good grounding in the ancillary sciences of chemistry, natural history and botany, as far as they related to medicine. On the other, the instruction traditionally available in hygiene and practical medicine was to be greatly extended, 'car l'Hygiène, telle que l'on l'a professée jusqu'ici dans les Ecoles, ne contient que des vérités triviales; et l'enseignement de la Médecine pratique désirée depuis long-temps est encore inconnu parmi nous.'[48] Vicq d'Azyr envisaged a separate professor who would teach physics and hygiene, two professors of practical medicine who would give a two-year course in acute and chronic diseases, and two professors of practical surgery, one of whom would give a course in midwifery. In addition, he demanded the erection of courses in legal and forensic medicine, and a course in the history of medicine where the professor would give an exposé of the different medical 'schools' of the past and explain to his pupils their failings. 'Il fera connaître les grandes causes qui ont amené constamment des erreurs.'[49] At the same time the professor of the history of medicine was to teach his charges how they could perfect their knowledge of the art of medicine by reading and observation.

The courses in practical medicine and surgery were to be henceforth hospital-based. This was the primary desideratum in all the proposals concerning curricular reform. Medical students had to be introduced to real patients before they were let loose on the outside world, and the reformers were unanimous that the hospital was the ideal institution to serve their purpose. The hospital was to become the centre of medical teaching.[50] Vicq wanted each medical college to be annexed (the direction of the association is significant) to a 'grand hôpital', which would contain an amphitheatre, dissecting rooms, a cabinet of natural history, a library, a *jardin des plantes*, a pharmacy, and a menagerie (for animal experiments). The practical courses were to be based around clinical wards, whose patients were to be drawn from both sexes and different age-groups, and reflect a wide variety of ailments. The course was to consist of two parts: the clinical course proper where the professor would comment on patients during the round of the clinical wards, and a separate lecture series given in the amphitheatre where other diseases could be described and discussed beyond those seen in the hospital. To ensure the broadest possible acquaintance with specific diseases, it was crucial that the professor was also a hospital doctor, so that he and his students could have access to all the wards. [51] Vicq had nothing particular to say about the manner of clinical teaching, but it can be supposed that he approved of the 'hands-on' method of instruction, promoted by other reformers. According to Tissot it was essential that students did not just observe the sick but were required to look after patients themselves, even to the extent of performing the autopsy if their charge died. The professor should delegate two students to a bed, and each day on his rounds demand an account of the patient from those responsible. Students walking the wards with the professor would pay much more attention when their peers were in charge.[52]

Besides the official clinical courses taught in the school hospital, Vicq hoped that similar courses would be put on in other hospitals, both civil and military.[53] He was equally hopeful that students would be allowed to follow hospital doctors and their assistants on their rounds throughout the hospital network. In this way the hospital would become an integrated institution for practical learning and healing the sick. Vicq believed that the two tasks were complementary. 'Ici le bien des malades est tellement d'accord avec celui de l'instruction, qu'il est impossible de rien prescrire de véritablement avantageux pour l'un, qui ne soit immédiatement applicable à l'autre.'[54]

The extent to which the medical school and the hospital were to become synonymous was made even clearer in the discussion of the teaching to be provided by the provincial *écoles pratiques*, which were also to be located in an appropriate hospital. Departmental doctors did not need to be learned in the manner of the college-trained physicians. In consequence they were to follow only an abridged course in the natural sciences and medical and surgical theory, and the central point of their teaching was to be the hospital-centred course in clinical surgery and physic. Indeed, pupils in the *écoles pratiques* were not just to attend the hospital courses but were expected to serve there as interns to help the permanent staff, for '[d]ans les Sciences-Pratiques on n'apprend bien [que] ce à quoi on participe'.[55] Presumably, Vicq hoped that the college-trained doctors would also gain hospital experience before they began to practise privately, but this is never stated specifically, and there is no general discussion of the number of interns per hospital and their method of appointment. He contented himself merely with saying that a form of hospital service traditonally open only to trainee surgeons should now be extended to all tyro medical practitioners.[56]

Although Vicq placed such emphasis on revitalizing the faculty curriculum, he laid down no conditions as to how long the would-be medical practitioner had to attend a medical college or *école pratique*, or in what order he should pursue his studies. Indeed, it was not even compulsory to have attended a medical school for Vicq accepted that students could train at home.[57] To become a legal medical practitioner all that was required was that a candidate should demonstrate his sufficiency in a series of examinations. To become a faculty graduate contemporaries had to submit to a number of oral examinations in private on their medical knowledge, which were conducted in the form of a question-and-answer session. On several occasions, they also had to sustain in public (over several hours) the arguments laid out in a thesis or dissertation that they had supposedly composed. Generally these examinations were conducted in Latin.[58] Vicq found both methods of testing students unsatisfactory, claiming that the examinations were often perfunctory (too many physicians were graduated 'à la hâte'), and that theses could too easily be composed by other people.[59] Instead, he wanted a series of written examinations instituted which would last over a period of days where the student would answer a number of questions chosen by lot in the silence of the examination room. The first would be a three-day examination on the preliminary medical sciences, the second a five-day examination on medical theory, and the third a five-day examination on clinical medicine and surgery. This would be followed by a day's practical examination on surgical operations, which would be carried out on a cadaver, and a three-day practical examination on clinical medicine, where the candidate would be taken on to the wards and asked to write reports on specified patients. Vivas were not to be totally abandoned, for the candidate was also to be subjected to oral interrogation after each written examination (presumably to clarify points made in the written paper). It was made quite clear, however, that an ability to express oneself fluently (essential in performing to effect when sustaining a thesis) was not a talent needed of the medical practitioner. Medical practitioners were not lawyers. Nor did they have to know Latin, for both the oral and written examinations were to be in French. Anyone who satisfied the examiners, whatever his form of training, would be awarded a doctorate and allowed to practise throughout France.[60] How candidates for the departmental doctorate were to be assessed was not made clear, but presumably Vicq would have wanted them subjected to a similar type of examination, if of a less gruelling kind.

Vicq's aim that the *Plan* should be the basis for the *comité de salubrité's* reform recommendations to the National Assembly was duly realized, for the committee's final report drawn up by the physician Guillotin (1738–1814) and printed on 6 August 1791 adhered closely to the programme outlined above. In the short term, however, Vicq and the other reformers were to be disappointed, for the National Assembly and its successors had other priorities besides reforming the medical system, and the programme was put to one side. [61] Indeed, the one change that was made to medical practice in the early years of the Revolution was to create the worst of all possible worlds from the reformers' point of view. From March 1791 all entry qualifications to the liberal professions and artisan crafts were abolished, with the result that thereafter anyone could practise medicine: the legal distinction between the quack and the medically trained no longer existed. Moreover, when the faculties and surgical colleges were officially closed in September 1793, it became virtually impossible to receive institutionalized medical training anyway.[62] Nevertheless, the campaign for the reconstruction of medical practice continued, and reform proposals, especially reiterating the value of hospital-training, continued to be published.[63] Eventually, furthermore, although Vicq himself never lived to see the triumph of his ideas, the reformers' programme was adopted by the politicians and became the basis for the French medical system of the nineteenth century.

The revolution occurred in two stages. First, on 7 and l4 Frimaire Year III (late 1794), the Convention, on the urging of a former member of the *Société Royale*, the physician–chemist Antoine François Fourcroy (1755–1809), established three new *écoles de santé* whose curriculum was to place the emphasis on clinical, hospital-based instruction.[64] The primary aim of the reform was to produce as quickly as possible trained military doctors, since casualties among this group had been particularly high in the European war that had begun in 1792. Initially, then, there was no attempt to limit medical practice to those who had attended the *écoles* or even let the new medical schools issue a certificate of competence.[65] Nine years later, on the other hand, under the more conservative regime of Napoleon, a medical profession was legally reconstituted along the lines the reformers proposed, Fourcroy again introducing the reform to the Convention's Napoleonic successor.[66] Medicine and surgery were united into one profession and only certificated doctors could henceforth practise in both town and country; doctors were divided into those who could practise nationally and those limited to their local *département*, their status dependent on whether they had attended one of the three *écoles de médecine* and gained a degree there,[67] or trained locally; finally, pharmacy remained a separate profession with its own *écoles*, if equally divided into two branches. The chief divergence from Vicq's plan was that there was no attempt to establish stipended doctors of the poor, and the examination-system remained based on a series of orals and a Latin thesis. Essentially, though, it was the plan of 1790. The heirs of the small coterie of physicians who had begun to agitate for a reform of the professsion in the 1780s had finally seen their programme put into effect by the state.[68]

Medical Reform and the Enlightenment

The argument so far has treated the medical reformers of late eighteenth-century France as if they were a nationally isolated group. In truth, this was far from being the case, for there were proponents of medical reform, in particular supporters of the introduction of hospital-based clinical training, all over Europe in this period.[69] Moreover, in the two decades before the French Revolution, reformers outside France were much more successful in making their voices heard in the establishment. In the Austrian empire in particular the state embraced a sweeping restructuring of medical education, which dated from the mid-century reforms of the Viennese faculty by the physician and education minister Gerhard Van Swieten (1700–72), and culminated in the establishment of the course of clinical medicine given by A. Störk (1731–1803) at the Trinity Hospital in 1774.[70] Had Joseph II lived there is no doubt that the medical profession would have been completely reformed. The emperor's plan for the relocation of the Louvain medical faculty at Brussels included the establishment of one training centre for all official medical practitioners in the Austrian Netherlands, the division of the profession henceforth into two – doctors of medicine/ surgery and vulgar surgeons – and the creation of a two-tiered curriculum and examination system.[71]

The French reformers, therefore, were in many ways attaching themselves to a pan-European bandwagon, a fact that was duly acknowledged in the continual references to the activities of the Viennese school. Significantly, the first French physician reformer to publish a detailed account of the value of clinical medicine was the Strasbourg Protestant, G. Christophe Würzt (1756–1823), who lived in a town that was culturally linked to the German bank of the Rhine, not France at all. Similarly, the second book-length work on reform to be published in French was by the Protestant Swiss, Tissot, who had been temporarily in charge of establishing clinical teaching in another part of the Habsburg dominions, Pavia in Lombardy.[72] Indeed, the fact that medical reform was associated in French minds with Germanic culture (there was virtually no homage paid to the Edinburgh clinical school) may well explain the fact that it was the end of the 1780s before the movement began to find public converts in France. German cultural developments of any kind were little known and less appreciated in eighteenth-century France.[73]

Nevertheless, if open French interest in reform was relatively tardy, there can be no doubt in the long term that the French contribution to the published debate was particularly extensive. Nor can there be any doubt that the reformers had their greatest success in France. Whereas a completely new French medical system was in place from the very beginning of the nineteenth century, in other countries reform was slow and piecemeal. This was especially the case in England where the Apothecaries Act of 1815 merely confirmed the existence of a variety of routes to becoming licensed, and where the nineteenth-century medical profession never succeeded in making unlicensed medical practice illegal.[74] As a result, France in the first half of the nineteenth century was a country to which medical reformers elsewhere looked to as an example, and Paris in particular became a medical school to which students from all over Europe and the United States were drawn.[75]

Obviously, the dramatic success of the reform movement in France is closely associated with the Revolution. In the climacteric of the Revolution all extant institutions were subject to scrutiny and a novel emphasis was placed on recreating society *de novo*, epitomized by the decision that the overthrow of the monarchy in August 1792 should constitute the beginning of time itself. The reform of medicine was just one of a series of institutional and administrative upheavals to which France and her growing band of satellite states would be subject in the 1790s and 1800s, as the Revolution spread through Europe in the knapsacks of French soldiers.[76] Countries where the armies of France were kept at bay and where reform quickly became synonymous with revolution would similarly show little enthusiasm to implement change in the medical field or carry it further. But the Revolution only explains the circumstances which made root-and-branch medical reform possible. It does not explain why reform was placed on the political agenda in the first place, in France as elsewhere. As we have seen, what differentiated medical reformers from their contemporaries was their ability to propose a novel way of solving the definite tensions within the existing medical system, one that required not redrawing existing boundaries or drawing them more tightly but completely altering the system. What enabled reformers to do this all over Europe and what underpinned the essential features of the reform programme was primarily the fact that the reformers had come into contact with the Enlightenment. Just as the Enlightenment underpinned the wider changes wrought by the Revolution, so the Enlightenment was the ideology of medical reform.

Any attempt to offer a brief definition of the Enlightenment is fraught with danger, as it becomes increasingly obvious that the movement was extremely complex and heterogeneous, defying national let alone pan-European statements about its identity.[77] It is, however, possible to generalize about its underlying features, as a way of demonstrating the degree to which the medical reform programme was nurtured on its roots. The Enlightenment was an attempt to create a secular science of man, to establish independently of Revelation, custom or prejudice, the fundamentals of human nature and human needs, and to sketch the contours of the ideal society and system of government in which morally autonomous individuals could realize their humanity without harming their fellows in the process. The Enlightenment's tool of enquiry was reason (both inductive and deductive), its building-blocks experiential observation, and its methodological inspiration the activities of contemporary natural and experimental philosophers. The *philosophes*, moreover, were not armchair philosophers but social critics who objected to any contemporary institution which, they felt, detracted from man's natural end. Throughout the Continent, the *philosophes*, if they agreed on nothing else, agreed on two points. First, although the Christian religion was not necessarily evil, the Christian Churches, where there was a confessional monopoly, were dogmatic, intolerant and corrupting in that they downplayed the possibility of human moral and material amelioration. Secondly, the hierarchical, corporate nature of contemporary society, which subsumed members of the élite within a privileged caste or protected corps was a hindrance to individual happiness. The champions of the Enlightenment, therefore, made war on institutionalized religion and corporatism as the twin-pillars of individual subjection and the twin-constraints on human progress. As a result, the *philosophes* were bitter critics of their contemporary world, and as such always a minority within the élite, however much in the second half of the century, they began to dominate public opinion and win the sympathies of princes and politicians.

The French medical reformers of the late eighteenth century for whom we have more than sketchy biographical data were all in some way linked with the Enlightenment. Vicq d'Azyr, Pierre-Jean-Georges Cabanis (1757–1808), and Philippe Pinel (1745–1826), for instance, had close links with leading Enlightenment figures, such as Condorcet and Destutt de Tracy, through their membership of Madame Helvetius's salon at Autueil outside Paris. Thereby (and this was particularly true of Cabanis) they belonged both before and during the Revolution to the *Idéologue* movement, a group of philosophers and scientists wedded to the experientialist epistemology of Condillac and devoted to the amelioration of mankind through practical instiztutional reform.[78] In contrast, the medical propagandists of the first half of the century had either had no link with the burgeoning Enlightenment in France at all (as was true of the Jansenist Hecquet), or had kept their allegiance secret, apparently willing to argue in favour of change or the *status quo* within the traditional corporatist framework. No one reading La Mettrie's savage attacks on the Paris physicians in the 1730s and 1740s could have expected him to turn into the iconoclastic author of *L'Histoire naturelle de l'âme* and *L'Homme machine* of 1745 and 1747.[79] Supporters of the Enlightenment within the medical community before the final quarter of the eighteenth century may perhaps have envisaged a reconstruction of the medical system, but they did not publicize their radical opinions in a period when the wider movement had yet to generate much enthusiasm in professional and governmental circles.[80]

It is not difficult to see how the Enlightenment informed the reformers' critique of the existing medical system. First, it underlay the attack on the corporate medical system. The *philosophes* (in France as elsewhere) promoted the establishment of an open, meritocratic society where individuals were free to prosper according to their talents. But especially in the chief cities of eighteenth-century France the right to medical practice was a privilege conferred by wealth, birth and patronage. In consequence, to a medical practitioner under the Enlightenment's spell, or an embittered 'outsider' ready and able to use Enlightenment ideology to burst the system open, the traditional organization of the official medical community no longer had any legitimacy; it was an offence to individual freedom. Vicq's commitment to a medical system based on the new values of personal talent and competition was implied in the *éloges* that he prepared for defunct members of the *Société Royale de Médecine* in the period 1776–89. The right to belong to the Society, it was stressed, was determined not by family background or the membership of a prestigious corps, but on the successful medical practice of the individual concerned. Members were the brightest stars of the medical firmament.[81] In the heady atmosphere of the Revolution, Vicq's anti-corporatist feelings were made crystal clear. Corporations were not only detrimental to the individual but society as a whole, for they had the effect of isolating citizens from one another and undermining public spirit. Set up as a method of mutual self-regulation, they had become inquisitorial tribunals.[82]

Secondly, the Enlightenment helps explain the novel interest in extending the official medical system to the urban and rural poor, what *Annalistes* have dubbed 'medicalization'. By placing a novel emphasis on achieving fulfilment and happiness in this world, rather than the one to come, the *philosophes* justified the individual making his or her health a central concern. As Diderot insisted in a 1748 letter to the Paris surgeon, Saveur-François Morand (1697–1773), without good health a man could not be truly happy.[83] If then, the aim of the enlightened was to maximize the happiness of all, it was immoral that trained medical personnel should only be available to the few. Of all forms of knowledge, medical science was the most useful for the general good. The people had to be rescued from the charlatans. The fact that Vicq and others promoted a two-tiered medical system, on the other hand, did not mean that their commitment to the maintenance of the people's health was less than sincere. This was a reflection of a wider Enlightenment belief that the rural poor in particular were healthier than the urban rich. The closer to nature, argued Diderot in 1774, the fewer diseases: 'Les animaux ont peu de maladies. Les maladies des habitants de la campagne sont moins nombreuses et plus simples que les nôtres; plus nous sommes éloignées de la vie champêtre des premiers âges du monde, plus la vie moyenne s'est abrégéc.'[84] This did not mean that the countryside was to be given inferior medical care, but it did encourage the belief, enunciated clearly by Tissot in his 1776 memorandum on rural surgeons, that country doctors need only know how to deal with commonplace acute diseases and chronic maladies especially found in the village, such as scrofula.[85]

Thirdly, the influence of the Enlightenment explains the reformers' interest in uniting the professions of medicine and surgery and restructuring medical education. The division of the two branches of the profession made sense in an early-modern society which equated medical competence with theoretical learning. In the eyes of those who defended the medical *status quo,* medical practice was to be limited to those who understood the cause of disease, for the good physician treated the cause not the symptoms. This necessarily meant that medical practice should be monopolized by graduate physicians, trained in the faculties in theoretical medicine. The surgeons, in contrast, might be dexterous operatives but they had limited theoretical knowledge, for they were trained primarily by a system of apprenticeship. They certainly could not be allowed to diagnose and prescribe, even in cases requiring surgical intervention, but were to be made to work under the physicians' supervision. It was not a question of the surgeons' ability to cure diseases (although it was always suggested that this was scant), but rather their ability to explain scientifically what they were doing. To practise medicine without scientific knowledge was immoral.[86]

The wisdom of limiting the right to practise to the learned physician was immediately brought into question, when the credentials of a good practitioner were examined from an Enlightenment perspective. Most medical professors in Europe before 1750 were systematizers, who devised logically coherent but speculative accounts of the body's internal structure in health and disease, based on a handful of non-negotiable first principles. What differentiated the eighteenth from the sixteenth and seventeenth centuries was that the professors had exchanged one set of dogmatic principles – Aristotelian formalism – for another – Cartesian mechanism.[87] To the *enfants terribles* of the French Enlightenment in particular, heavily influenced by the experientialist epistemology of Locke and Condillac, system-building of all kinds was suspect. Science in their eyes had to be worker-science, whose value was judged by its efficacy, and all knowledge had to be evidentially grounded. Consequently, *philosophes* who meditated on the status of contemporary medical science were highly critical of its claims. Many *philosophes* were downright cynical about the ability of learned physicians to cure at all. Voltaire, for one, was continually dismissive of contemporary medicine, especially the fad for sending patients to spas, like Forges on the Normandy/Picardy border. 'There is more vitriol in a bottle of Forges water than in a bottle of ink, and frankly I don't believe that ink is very good for the health.'[88] Even those not so dismissive of contemporary medicine, such as the Chevalier de Jaucourt (who had himself studied medicine at Leiden), were far from sanguine. Jaucourt in the *Encyclopédie* (1765) asserted that medical science had not really advanced since Hippocrates and that medical practice in France in particular was in a state of decay. The fault was judged to lay with both doctor and patient: '... la fausse méthode des académies, des écoles médicinales, l'exemple, la facilité d'une routine qui borne à trois remedes [unstated]; la mode, le goût des plaisirs, la manque de confiance de la part des malades; l'envie qu'ils ont de guérir promptement; les manières & le beau langage qu'on préfère à l'étude & au savoir; la vanité, le luxe d'imitation: le désir de faire une fortune rapide...' Progress in medicine could only come by accumulating knowledge through medical practice and gaining a proper knowledge of the physics of the human body, again through experience.[89]

Most *philosophes*, on the other hand, had a much more positive view of contemporary surgical practice. While physicians were accused of giving their patients at best a cursory examination in a peremptory manner, wrongly confident that their theoretical knowledge was sufficient for a successful diagnosis,[90] surgeons were portrayed as hands-on practitioners who actually cured their patients.[91] Surgical knowledge, unlike medical science, was deemed to be useful and experientially founded, and thus consistent with Enlightenment epistemology. The fact that the skill and ingenuity of the Paris surgeons had clearly increased by leaps and bounds in the first half of the eighteenth century only confirmed this belief.[92] Not surprisingly, therefore, the *Encyclopédie* was used as a vehicle to praise the progress of surgery as much as to decry the decadence of medicine. Whereas the medical articles were entrusted to authors, like Jaucourt, who viewed the contemporary medical scene with misgiving, the surgical contributions were significantly provided by self-confident Paris surgeons, notably Antoine Louis (1723–92).[93]

In the light of the *philosophes*' tendency to turn the contemporary medical value-system on its head, the eagerness of enlightened medical reformers to unite the professions of medicine and surgery becomes immediately explicable. The good doctor was no longer the learned physician but the 'hands-on' medical practitioner, who could best demonstrate his adherence to the new cult of practical experience and utility by successfully performing complex surgical operations. Diagnosis and delegation were no longer sufficient public witness of competence: the good doctor was not just a man of science but a virtuoso. In good Enlightenment fashion, the unity of the two professions was not just something the medical reformers promoted, but something they actually 'lived' through their own practical dedication to the surgical arts. Although none of the physicians may actually have practised surgery, the group included a number of notable anatomists and professors of surgery and obstetrics, especially Vicq d'Azyr and Antoine Petit.[94]

The novel emphasis on a practical medical education based round the hospital obviously also reflected the new experiential ethic. If a good doctor was someone with patient-experience, not someone stuffed full of theory, then it was essential that medical students had access to sick people before they were licensed to practise. The introduction into the medical curriculum of hospital-based courses in practical medicine and surgery made perfect sense. Large hospitals were full of poor people suffering from different diseases. In the course of a year or two's study, they offered the student the chance to observe real patients with real diseases in considerable numbers. An alternative, as the reformers recognized, would have been to apprentice students to practising physicians, but this was generally rejected out of hand. Physicians might refuse to cooperate; there would be too many students to go round; above all private patients would not accept the presence of a third party. According to Vicq, 'la plupart des malades ne consentiroient point à recevoir auprès d'eux des hommes qu'il ne connoîtroient point, et qui n'auroient pas leur confiance'. Such sensitivity was attributed by Chambon de Montaux in terms redolent of Montesquieu to the inevitable lack of public spirit in a monarchy. The alternative plan could only be applied in a republic where patients were not self-obsessed.[95]

Moreover, although these went unstated, there were clear pedagogical advantages in making the hospital the school of medical practice. Students had not just to see patients before they began to practise themselves, but they had to learn to observe properly and carefully. Otherwise, as Vicq emphasized in his *Discours sur l'anatomie,* they learnt nothing. 'Voir et décrire sont deux choses que chacun se croit en état de faire, et dont cependant peu de personnes sont capables. La première suppose une grande attention et des lumières acquises dans le genre auquel appartient l'objet que l'on observe.'[96] Clinical hospital-based courses provided the opportunity for uniform, guided practical tuition, where students would learn what to see and what to make of their observations by personally looking after patients as well as listening to the professor at the bedside. Students would be the beneficiaries of a properly worked-out system of active learning, which the medical reformers, as disciples of the Enlightenment, accepted was the best way to assimilate knowledge.[97]

Furthermore, through hospital training the reformers could be assured that the students were not just learning a good or bad bedside manner, but that they were gaining an objective knowledge of the course and proper treatment of different diseases. The relationship between the doctor and the hospital patient was entirely different from that between the doctor and private patient. The hospital patient was a pauper who was strictly under the doctor's control; the private patient in contrast was his or her own master or mistress,who obeyed or disobeyed the doctor's prescription at whim, and constantly changed practitioners. Above all, even if the private client was singularly obedient and faithful unto death, the family would be unlikely to deliver the patient's body for dissection.[98] The student, then, would have little chance to examine the internal effects of disease through post-mortems. In the new hospital-based medical schools, on the other hand, the poor would pay for their free keep by giving their bodies to science.[99]

But the hospitals were to be more than schools of practical instruction. The enlightened physicians accepted that medicine was a retrograde science in a state of decay, and they were committed to its revival. This, it was agreed, could only happen if medical philosophers turned their back on airy theorizing and established the science on empirical foundations. The new medicine was to be based on observed facts, and the institutional locus for gathering data was to be the hospital. The same reasons that made the hospital an ideal educational institution made it an ideal research centre: the inmates were numerous, captive and passive. Whereas private patients would usually accept only traditional remedies, hospital inmates could be used as guinea-pigs.[100] Drugs, new and old, for instance, could now be subjected to proper clinical trials, and therapeutics could become a 'modern' progressive science. It was through the hospital and the opportunities it afforded for experimentation that surgery had become a useful science, and it would be through the hospital that physic would reestablish its reputation.[101]

The reformers' aim, therefore, was to use the hospital to complete the work already begun in a haphazard fashion by the correspondents of the *Société Royale de Médecine.*[102] In 1794 the foundations of this medical revolution were formally laid, when Fourcroy decreed that the professors of the new medical schools were to be researchers as well as teachers. 'Ce n'est pas seulement à l'enseignement de ce que l'on sait que se bornent leurs fonctions; elles ont encore pour objet les recherches les plus étendues sur toutes les branches de l'art de guérir; pour but l'avancement de toutes les sciences qui peuvent éclairer la physique animale.'[103] What this new medical science would look like, however, was a matter of some disagreement within the reforming camp. Thus, for a Dulaurens medicine as an empirical science would be essentially reduced to the sciences of nososlogy and therapeutics, the science of knowing when to let nature heal herself and when and with what to intervene. He saw little point to detailed anatomical knowledge, claiming that the developments in the science over the last two centuries had little helped medical practice. The more anatomical knowledge a practitioner had, the more timid the practice. The greatest French physician-anatomist of the eighteenth century, he maintained, Jacques-Bénigne Winslow (1669–1760), had shaken when he prescribed.[104] Others, like Vicq and Pinel, disagreed, and believed that the new medical science would provide as of old an understanding of the internal cause of disease, not just an account of its manifestation and method of treatment. But it would be a science founded on genuine empirical knowledge whose key was comparative and pathological anatomy.[105] In the long run, of course, it would be the second position that would triumph and find realization in the work of Bichat, Laennec and other members of the the early nineteenth-century Paris medical school.[106]

The two positions seem to have reflected where the reformers had originally trained. In the final decades of the eighteenth century the medical faculties of France no longer taught an iatromechanical theory of medicine but were divided in their response to an alternative medical ideology that was at that date sweeping Northern Europe: vitalism. This was a medical theory which predated the Enlightenment and was first developed at the turn of the eighteenth century by Georg Ernst Stahl (1660–1734) at Halle. Essentially, vitalism challenged the iatromechanical theories in vogue in the first part of the century by insisting that living organisms were not machines but only machine-like: their physiology was ultimately controlled by the soul or some vital principle, whose vitiation or exhaustion could cause death or disease. The doctrine was introduced to Montpellier in the 1730s by François Boissier de Sauvages (1706–67) and from 1760, reworked in a more materialist guise by Paul-Joseph Barthez (1734–1806), it was the dominant medical theory there. Elsewhere in France, especially at Paris, faculty professors were less enthusiastic, although they did recognize in the final decades of the Ancien-Régime that attempts to explain health and disease mechanically or chemically had hitherto proved chimerical.[107] The two groups had different views about the value of anatomical investigation. Montpellier professors, like Barthez, were sceptical of any attempt to construct a science of physiology and pathology based on detailed anatomical research, and emphasized in their courses the need rather to build a new experimental science of therapeutics. Paris professors, on the other hand, unconvinced that life was simply a vitalist mystery, continued to emphasize the need to investigate internal lesions, albeit more empirically, and attempt to construct at least an account of the state of the bodily parts in health and disease.[108] Reformers like Dulaurens were Montpellier trained; those with a passion for anatomy, like Vicq d'Azyr, attended the Paris faculty.[109]

It might seem, then, that if the Enlightenment encouraged the medical reformers to turn their back on building theoretical castles in the air and to develop a new science of medicine based on controlled observation, the actual content of this new science was determined by ideological currents internal to the history of medicine. However, such a conclusion neglects the fact that vitalism and the Enlightenment were interconnected. Vitalism as it developed in France in the mid eighteenth century was a medical philosophy with radical religious and political implications. Not only was it implicitly materialist,[110] but the emphasis that Louis de Lacaze (1703–65) and others placed in their pathology on the role of institutions in upsetting the delicate balance of the animal economy through over- or under-stimulation gave it a subversive social edge. Vitalism developed Hippocratic environmentalism in a dangerous direction.[111] Vitalists, moreover, were not simply theoreticians; the Montpellier-trained Paris physician, Théophile de Bordeu (1722–76), based his powerful critique of the iatro-mechanical conception of glandular secretion on just the kind of careful empirical enquiry that the *philosophes* applauded.[112] Not surprisingly, then, the *philosophes* found vitalist ideas a useful weapon in their critique of the *status quo.* Diderot in particular was their friend,[113] and vitalists, especially the Montpellier professor Gabriel-François Venel (1723–75), contributed most of the medical articles to the *Encyclopédie:* hence their dismissive attitude of medical achievements to date.[114] In some ways, indeed, vitalism can be seen as *the* Enlightenment medical philosophy, if most *philosophes* would probably have eschewed the erection of a vitalist system *à la* Barthez in favour of the more cautious agnosticism cultivated by the Paris faculty in the last decades of the Ancien Régime.[115] In other words, there was certainly no absolute tension between the Enlightenment and the medical theories taught in French medical faculties on the eve of the Revolution. The medical reformers might feel that the curriculum was overly theoretical and speculative, but they were not as alienated from their teachers as they would have been if the *philosophes* had dismissed vitalism as just another vainglorious abstraction. Their teachers were able to have an influence on their formulation of the new medical science, because in the eyes of the Enlightenment those teachers were not unenlightened.

The Triumph of the Physicians

The specific medical reform programme promoted by French physicians in the 1780s and 1790s can clearly only be understood as part of a wider movement generated by Enlightenment epistemology and humanitarianism. Only in France, however, was the reform programme broadly put into effect, because only in France were the reformers able fully to gain state support for its implementation. Before 1789 both in France and other countries, governments came under the influence of the Enlightenment and often displayed sympathy with the reformers' aims, but only during the Revolution were the forces of the *status quo* sufficiently undermined to ensure wholesale reform of the medical system.[116] The Revolution gave full reign to critics of Ancien-Régime institutions who used Enlightenment ideas to demand a wide variety of cultural, social and political reforms. The revolutionary assemblies that came to dominate France in the 1790s were filled with politicians who were themselves committed to the enlightened ideal of an open, meritocratic society.[117] Anxious to build society anew they welcomed criticism of existing institutions with open arms, and once the Revolution was broadly secure after 1794 began the task of positive social reconstruction, as far as state finances in a time of war would allow.[118]

It remains to consider who, within the traditional medical system, were the intended beneficiaries of the medical reform programme. This is a question that must be addressed, for although there is no reason to doubt the commitment of the reformers to the Enlightenment, there can equally be little doubt that their programme was designed to bolster the influence of a particular constituency. There is always more than one way of transforming an ideology into a practical programme, and the path that reformers actually choose reflects material interest. Revolutionaries are not altruists. It must not be forgotten that the reform programme was an attempt to resolve the tensions within the medical system outlined in the opening section. As a result of its implementation, there were certain to be winners and losers. Paradoxically, the answer to this question would seem to be that the purposed beneficiaries were to be the 4,000 odd faculty physicians.[119] Although the reform movement was led by a coterie of renegade physicians associated with the supra-corporative *Société Royale*, and although the reforms that they proposed completely destroyed the existing medical system dominated by their incorporated peers, nevertheless the movement is best understood as a putsch to secure and extend physician power.

Admittedly, this is a controversial conclusion, for the current orthodoxy, particularly developed by Gelfand, is that the new medical system created by the Revolution placed the surgeons in the saddle.[120] In the course of the eighteenth century, it is argued, the status of surgery was greatly enhanced thanks to the advances in operational technique, the Enlightenment's idealization of useful knowledge, and the state's patronage of the art (primarily for military reasons).[121] At the same time, the Paris surgeons in particular, through the establishment of independent, practically orientated medical courses at the new école de chirurgie and the creation of hospital-based clinical instruction in practical surgery and pathological anatomy, epitomized by Desault's course at the Hôtel-Dieu, laid the foundations for the new curriculum of the *écoles de santé*. The Revolution afforded the surgical élite the opportunity to reform the medical system and medical education in such a way as to privilege surgery and the surgical pattern of education. With the collapse of traditional patterns of professional formation in the chaos of the 1790s, tyro physicians, like Bichat,[122] chose to study under leading surgeons, such as Desault, and in the period 1794–1803 a new medical system was evolved modelled on the dynamic aspects of the Ancien-Régime surgical profession.[123]

This argument, however, does not fit the facts. To begin with it was the physicians who led the reform movement. There were surgeons who joined the public debate, but they were few.[124] More importantly, the physician reformers showed little sympathy for the great mass of Ancien-Régime surgeons, the general consensus being that the profession was full of ignoramuses.[125] No reference either was made to the curricular innovations of the eighteenth-century Paris surgeons in describing the ideal medical education. It may have been the case that the curricular reforms had been anticipated in the manner Gelfand suggests, but, were this so, the physician–reformers were slow to acknowledge their debt. At best, it must be concluded that the physicians were stealing the surgeons' clothes and deliberately keeping quiet about the theft. Much is made of the fact that the new Paris medical school of 1794 was housed in the recently erected buildings of the college of surgery. This, though, should not be read as a symbolic statement of approval on the revolutionaries' part of the medical teaching formerly given there. When Fourcroy, himself a physician–reformer, announced the chosen location in his address to the Convention, he disparaged the college and its activities by associating it with the Ancien Régime and its discredited values: 'Le despotisme & la vanité qui avoient fait elever ce monument, ne s'étoient point occupés de le meubler'.[126]

It is more sensible, therefore, to see the physicians' reform programme as an attempt to undermine the achievements of the eighteenth-century Paris surgeons rather than give them their seal of approval.[127] Arguably, the physicians were attempting to regain their monopoly of medical education and eradicate the newly constituted surgical élite which challenged the physicians' traditional place in the medical hierarchy. This could never be achieved simply by advocating the closure of the surgeons' colleges and attacking the profession's power-base: the independent surgical corporations in the big cities. A frontal assault of this kind had got nowhere in the eighteenth century, for the surgeons had been able to use the increasingly politically-correct language of utility to justify their independence. The way forward was rather to obtain the closure of the city surgical colleges and corporations as part of a much larger medical reform which would make a nonsense of the Enlightenment view that physicians were by and large theory-ridden, useless practitioners. This meant the closure of the medical faculties and corporations, and the acceptance that the practice of physic and surgery were of equal value, but this was a small price to pay, when it could be assumed that the new schools would be dominated by professor-physicians and the graduates of these schools would be physician-surgeons not surgeon-physicians. This was inevitable. Reformers like Vicq naturally expected that they would form the professoriate, while the cost of attending the new schools would mean that their clientele would be socially respectable and hence composed of those who would formerly have been medical students, not surgeons' apprentices.[128]

Thus, on one level, the reform programme was intended to destroy the threat to the physicians' livelihood that was presented by the competition that they faced from a section of the surgical profession. Arguably, it was a way of keeping the number of élite urban medical practitioners limited, ensuring that the right to practise continued to pass from physician father to physician son, while bolstering the solidarity of the profession by ending the internal quarrels precipitated by corporate rights. This interpretation would also help to explain why there was no agitation in favour of uniting the professions of pharmacy and medicine. Eighteenth-century apothecaries, even in the big cities, seem to have stuck to their last. Had Parisian apothecaries taken up the practice of physic with the same gusto as their London peers, then the reformers might well have moved the creation of one single, united medical profession.[129]

The reformers, however, were not simply reasserting the medical *status quo*. They were also intent on extending physician–power in that the reform programme gave future graduate physicians the automatic right and the necessary training to practise surgery, if they so wished, thereby extending their power in the medical marketplace. The physician–surgeon, it must be stressed, was a category of medical practitioner already extant, for the Montpellier faculty had offered a combined degree from 1728. The number of such graduates increased dramatically after 1750, emphasizing that some medical students at least no longer felt that 'hands-on' medical practice was undignified.[130] The move to take 'high-tech' surgery out of the hands of the surgeons had thus already begun, but the development had been understandably met with open hostility from the surgical corporations.[131] On another level, then, the reform programme was obviously intended to regularize and consolidate the burgeoning take-over.

An extension (albeit indirectly) of the physicians' control of the market-place was also intended by the reformers' plan to establish a subordinate professional tier of departmental doctors, who would look after the poor of town and country. Before the Revolution, as we have seen, the majority of the French population relied for their medical care on the services of unlicensed empirics or local surgeons who acted as general practitioners. Outside the big towns, the faculty doctors had little means of controlling the actitivities of these practitioners, for resident physicians were seldom to be found in communities under 2,000 inhabitants. If any group exercised some control over rural medical practice, it was the surgical corps in the larger towns who had the right to license surgeons to serve in the local villages and bourgs. Indeed, one of their number, the lieutenant of the king's chief surgeon had also the right to inspect rural surgeons.[132] Vicq d'Azyr and the other reformers were unanimous in their condemnation of the inadequacy of rural medical practice. The *Plan* of 1790 aimed to purge the countryside of ignorant surgeons and dastardly empirics and provide the rural poor with 'state-of-the-art' medical care. Significantly, however, the new cantonal doctors were to be trained by physician–professors in the departmental hospital-schools, and their activities were to be supervised by departmental *conseils de santé*, dominated (one can presume) by physicians trained in the medical schools.[133]

Bringing enlightened medicine to the majority of the population, therefore, was to be accomplished by extending the physicians' authority. That this was the underlying motive for the structural reform becomes clear when it is realized that the reformers' humanitarian ambitions could have been encompassed in other ways. Indeed, other methods of bringing enlightened medicine to the countryside had already been tried in the second half of the eighteenth century. One way, perfectly in keeping with the *philosophes'* belief in the power of the written word, had been to publish self-help medical manuals. These were aimed specifically at the socially prominent (*seigneurs* and their wives, *curés*, and so on), who could be trained to act as medical outworkers.[134] A second method, much in evidence in the 1770s and 1780s whenever rural communities were hit by epidemics, had been for the local *intendant* to send faculty physicians into the countryside to supervise temporarily the activities of rural surgeons.[135] Both methods had much to recommend them for they worked within the framework of the institutional reality of village life, but, interestingly, neither was normally discussed by the reformers. What they sought was thorough-going structural reform which would extend the permanent control of the physicians, not humanitarian gestures which would encourage the perpetuation of lay medical care or allow independent rural surgeons a new lease of life.[136]

Even the promotion of hospital-based medical education can be read as part of a campaign to extend the physicians' authority (in this case their subordinates', too), as much as to ensure better trained medical practitioners. Eighteenth-century patients, we have seen, were notoriously independent; physicians commonly prescribed according to the dictates of the client, not their conscience. Only physicians, like Antoine Petit, willing and able to charm their patients into submission, could diagnose and prescribe with professional objectivity.[137] But such patient-power fitted ill with the enlightened physician's high view of his professional calling, as did the idea of the physician playing the courtier.[138] Whether his patient were prince or pauper it was the physician's duty to override subjective prejudice and provide the best possible care. A mechanism had, therefore, to be found whereby a new generation of physicians could break free of patient tyranny. Hospital-based training arguably provided an answer. If physicians had spent their formative years watching objective men of science treating with magisterial aplomb a bevy of grateful, deferential paupers, it could be expected that they would have internalized a concept of patient–practitioner relations that would make them far less ready to collude in the prejudices of their clients in the outside world. Hospital-training was thus *de rigueur* for the formation of the good physician, not just because it gave him essential practice in patient-care, but because it would encourage him to take his own decisions and stick to them.

Hospital-training, then, would turn clients into patients, something that had only intermittently happened in the Ancien Régime, usually when the sick were temporarily socially displaced – when they visited a spa, for instance.[139] But the institution of hospital-training and particularly clinical instruction was also essential if the reformers were to achieve their aim of ridding the medical field of the legion of empirics and 'medicalizing' French society in its entirety. In an important respect, the Enlightenment cult of experience that the reformers embraced, and that had clearly already penetrated the existing faculties to a certain extent as part of the vitalist revolution, was a hindrance rather than a help to the extension of physician-power. What had traditionally put the empirical interloper beyond the legal pale was that his medical knowledge was experientially and not theoretically based. If the good medical practitioner was now to be defined as a man with practical experience of medical care, there was a danger that the charlatan would claim that his own credentials were just as sound as the licensed and trained physician's. And he could quote Diderot in his defence. 'J'ai quelquefois pensé que les charlatans qui habitent les faubourgs des grandes villes n'étaient pas si pernicieux qu'on le supposait. C'est l'empirisme qui a donné naissance à la médecine et elle n'a de vrais progrès à attendre que de l'empirisme.' The Enlightenment was not sympathetic to a medical monopoly.[140] The introduction of compulsory clinical training, however, would successfully obviate this objection. On the one hand, it made a clear distinction between experience *tout court* and scientific experience. On the other, by locating scientific experience in a specific institution, the hospital clinic, it ensured that only medical students could benefit from it. The invention of the clinic was certainly a response to the problem of creating a genuine medical science based on controlled observation, but its invention was also vital if the monopolistic powers of the new medical profession were to have any ideological legitimacy. It was a way of dividing in the increasingly enlightened public mind the medical sheep from the empirical goats.[141]

Ultimately, the medical reformers wanted to restructure the French medical system in a manner consistent with both the imperatives of Enlightenment epistemology and humanitarianism, and the preservation and extension of physician-power. Historians have wrongly interpreted the reform programme as a platform for the advancement of the surgical élite and surgical values because they have seen eighteenth-century Paris surgery as modern and enlightened in contrast with Paris medicine, and consequently assumed that any medical reformer in the Revolutionary era must be in the surgeons' camp. This, though, is not necessarily so, and it is perfectly conceivable in an age still very conscious of hierarchy that physician–reformers, even enlightened physician–reformers, wanted to defend the traditional role of the physician through the reformation of medical training and practice. It is surely significant that members of the surgical élite quickly came to feel that the actual implementation of the reform programme gave them very little. By 1815 top surgeons, like J.-C.-F. Caron (1739–1824), were demanding that the two professions be divided again. Surgery, it was argued, was in a state of decay: in the new medical schools (called faculties from 1808) the discipline occupied only a small amount of teaching time, while few graduates were anxious to become specialists in surgery.[142]

This is not to say that the reformers achieved their underlying aim, or even to deny that the medical reforms of 1794 and 1803 were important moments in the history of the modernization and professionalization of medicine (as the terms are now understood).

In fact from the vantage point of the mid nineteenth century the reformers would surely have admitted their failure. The new medical schools were certainly dominated by professors who were physicians rather than surgeons, but by 1820 the number of medical students at Paris alone was three to four times the total number of faculty students on the eve of the Revolution, while the unified profession proved no more able than its Ancien Régime forebear to monopolize medical practice. The first half of the ninetenth century saw the growth of a mass medical profession that had to compete for its clients with an ever-growing horde of astute empirical entrepreneurs.[143] Vicq d'Azyr would have been amazed and appalled. The historian will be neither. Just as revolutionaries are seldom altruists, so they seldom achieve what they set out to accomplish.

Notes

1. The most recent account of the structure of pre-Revolutionary medical practice is Matthew Ramsey, *Professional and Popular Medicine in France, 1770–1830: The Social World of Medical Practice* (Cambridge: Cambridge University Press, 1988), pt i, ch. l and pt ii.
2. A right laid down in the Edict of Marly of 1707: see Isambert, Decrusy and Jourdan, *Recueil général des anciennes lois françaises* (28 vols; Paris: publisher unknown, 1821–33), xx. 510–17 (arts 26–8). Thereafter only licentiates in medicine could practise in France's towns and bourgs.
3. For example, the account of the activities of the surgeon, Jacques Long, in the Dauphiné village of Venterol (pop. 1790, 1363) in J. Demesy-Marant, 'Un maître chirurgien dans la Haute Provence dromoise à la veille de la Révolution', *Cahiers d'histoire*, xxxiii (1988), 43–70.
4. From 1743 no one could practise surgery in Paris unless they had gained an MA; a similar regulation was introduced later into a number of other cities. The royal declaration concerning Paris is given in [François Quesnay], *Recherches critiques et historiques sur l'origine, sur les divers états et sur le progrès de la chirurgie en France* (Paris: C. Osmont, 1744), 519–24.
5. Traditionally surgeons, if they received any formal instruction, attended courses laid on by the medical faculties. The first independent (i.e. surgeon-run) surgical college was established at Paris in 1725: for an introduction to the development, see P. Huard, 'L'Enseignement médico-chirurgical,' in R. Taton (ed.), *L'Enseignement et diffusion des sciences au dix-huitième siècle* (Paris: Hermann, 1963), 171–213 (especially 191–206).
6. From 1730 surgeons who eschewed the barber's art were entitled to be called *notables bourgeois* and enjoy the privileges of liberal professionals: see *Statuts et réglemens généraux pour les maîtres en chirurgie des provinces du royaume* Le Blond d'Olbien (ed.), (5 Paris: P.

F. Didot le Jeune, 1772), 17 (art. vii).

7. Admittance to the Paris college, for instance, required that candidates were doctors of the Paris faculty. As gaining a Paris degree took many years and was highly expensive (*c.* 7000 *livres* = £280 on the eve of the Revolution), admissions closely matched the number of doctors removed from the roll by death: see A. Lelage, *Histoire de la thèse de doctorat en médecine* (Paris: publisher unknown, 1913), especially 128.
8. This is the accepted number of surgical corps; we can presume that there was a similar number of apothecaries' corps.
9. The 1730 *règlement* laid down three types of *maîtrise*: see Le Blond d'Olbien, *op. cit.* (note 6), 28–42 (arts. xxxii–lxiv).
10. On court doctors and their rights, see Colin Jones, 'The Médecins du Roi at the End of the *Ancien Régime* and in the French Revolution,' in Vivian Nutton (ed.), *Medicine at the Courts of Europe 1500–1837* (London: Routledge, 1990), 209–61.
11. Archives Départmentales du Vaucluse (Avignon), D 62, various unnumbered letters and memoirs on the case in a *liasse* marked 1703–80. Avignon was a papal enclave before 1790 and it was a moot point throughout the eighteenth century whether its medical graduates could practise in France.
12. The pamphlet literature is vast and I have only skimmed the surface: see especially the collection in the Bibliothèque Nationale, *Départment des imprimés*, T18 120, entitled *Recueil de pièces et mémoires pour les maîtres en l'art et science de la chirurgie, et pour la faculté de médecine* lst ser. 12 vols in 8°, 2nd ser. 17 vols in 12° (Philadelphia [!], 1760).
13. P. Hecquet, *Le Brigandage de la chirurgie où la médecine opprimée par le brigandage de la chirurgie* (Utrecht: chez les soeurs de C. G. Le Fèvre, 1738). Hecquet was particularly incensed that surgeons were taking over the cure of venereal disease and getting involved in treating maladies specific to women and children. Hecquet was a notorious iatromechanist and Jansenist: see L. W. B. Brockliss, 'The Medico-Religious Universe of an Early-Eighteenth Century Parisian Doctor: The Case of Philippe Hecquet,' in Roger French and Andrew Wear (eds), *The Medical Revolution of the Seventeenth Century* (Cambridge: Cambridge University Press, 1989), 191–221. The dates of medical practitioners mentioned in the text and notes are given when known.
14. Cf. the seven pamphlets of the 1730s and 1740s published by the physician and philosophe Julien Offray de La Mettrie (1709–51); discussed in Kathleen Wellmann, *La Mettrie. Medicine, Philosophy, and Enlightenment* (Durham, NC: Duke University Press, 1992), ch. 2. Arguably (although this point is not made by the author), La Mettrie, an 'outsider' who practised at Saint-Malo, took the surgeons' side because he lacked the wealth to join the Paris college.
15. For the fullest evaluation to date of his non-medical career, see *François Quesnay et la physiocratie* (Paris: Institut National d'Etudes démographiques, 1958).

16. Quesnay, *op. cit.* (note 4), especially pts iii–v. The lengthy work was the surgeons' riposte to the physicians' attempt to get the royal decree (see note 4 above) of 1743 rescinded. There was a grain of truth to his account of the development of the surgical profession in Paris: see below.
17. F. Quesnay, *Examen impartial des contestations des médecins et chirurgiens, considérées par rapport à l'intérêt public* (n. p. , 1748).
18. *Ibid.*, 17–46 (especially 28). In this and subsequent quotations from French texts, the original orthography has been retained.
19. *Ibid.*, 63–86.
20. From hints given in the 1748 pamphlet, Quesnay himself may well have wanted a radical overhaul of the medical system. But, it must be stressed, these were only hints: see below note 31. Quesnay took a medical degree at Pont-à-Mousson in 1744 and eventually became physician to the king and Mme de Pompadour: he made boundary-breaking a speciality.
21. Archives Nationales, Paris, 0[1] 612, nos. 27–31 and 44, various documents concerning the legal case, especially a memorandum for the Paris surgeons entitled: 'Etat des chirurgiens de la maison du roi... Pour servir de renseignements dans l'instance pendant au conseil de S[a] M[ajesté], entre eux [i.e. the household surgeons) et le collège de chirurgie de Paris'. Some of the royal household surgeons were also members of the Paris corps. The number of Paris surgeons declined dramatically after the corps was divided from the barbers in 1743: see Toby Gelfand, *Professionalizing Modern Medicine: Paris Surgeons and Medical Science and Institutions in the 18th Century* (London: Greenwood, 1980), 77. This book is the best account of the eighteenth-century 'rise' of the surgeons.
22. J. P. Goubert and D. Lorillot (eds), *Les Cahiers de doléances des médecins, chirurgiens et apothicaires: 1789, le corps médical et le changement (*Toulouse: Privat, 1984*)*. Of the *cahiers* published in this collection, only the one compiled by the Versailles surgeons asked for the system to be changed. The conservatism of the medical *cahiers* mirrors the viewpoint of the *cahiers* in general: see G. V. Taylor, 'Revolutionary and Non-Revolutionary Content in the *Cahiers* of 1789,' *French Historical Studies*, vii (1972), 477–92.
23. For example, G. C. Wurtz, *Mémoires sur l'établissement des écoles de médecine pratique à former dans les principaux hôpitaux civils de France à l'instar de celle de Vienne.* (Paris: Didot le jeune and Barrois le jeune, 1784); S. A. D. Tissot, *Essai sur les moyens de perfectionner les études de médecine* (Lausanne: Mourer cadet, 1785); Joseph-Michel Dulaurens, *Essai sur les établissemens nécessaires et les moins dispendieux pour rendre le service des malades dans les hôpitaux vraiment utile à l'humanité* (Paris: Royez, 1787); Nicolas Chambon de Montaux, *Moyens de rendre les hôpitaux plus utiles à la nation* (Paris: publisher unknown, 1787).

24. The starting-point for this positive view of the surgeons is O. Temkin, 'The Role of Surgery in the Rise of Modern Medical Thought', *Bulletin for the History of Medicine*, xxv (1951), 248–59. But see especially Gelfand, *op. cit.* (note 21), M.-J. Imbault-Huet, 'Les Chirurgiens et l'esprit chirurgical en France au XVIIIe siècle', *Clio Medica*, xv (1981), 143–57; and Terence D. Murphy, 'The Transformation of the Traditional Medical Culture under the Old Régime', *Historical Reflections/ Réflexions historiques*, xvi: 2–3 (1989), 307–50. Both Gelfand (ch. 4) and Murphy treat the quarrel between the Paris physicians and surgeons in the second quarter of the eighteenth century as one between ancients and moderns. I feel that this position exaggerates completely the radical content of the surgeons' argument in their defence.
25. The best study of the foundation and activities of the Society is Caroline Hannaway, 'Medicine, Public Welfare and the State in Eighteenth-Century France: The Société Royale de Médecine de Paris (1776–1793)', Ph. D. Dissertation, Johns Hopkins University, 1974.
26. Admittedly, the dean and the oldest member of the Paris college were *ex officio* members of the Society, and 20 of the 30 Paris-based *associés ordinaires* had to be members of the college, but there were some 150 members of the Paris college on the eve of the Revolution, so only a small minority ever belonged to the new institution: see Isambert, *op. cit.* (note 2), xxv. 398 (clauses concerning membership in the royal letters patent of August 1778: 395–400).
27. The only detailed study of the work of the committee is H. Ingrand, *Le Comité de salubrité* (Paris: M. Vigné, 1934). Its *procès-verbaux* survive in Archives Nationales (Paris), AF I* 23.
28. 'Nouveau Plan de constitution pour la médecine en France,' in *Histoire et mémoires de la Société royale de médecine 1787–1788*, vol. ix (Paris, 1790), l–201. There is no biography of Vicq d'Azyr. The most recent account of the *Plan* is Caroline Hannaway, 'Caring for the Constitution: Medical Planning in Revolutionary France', *Transactions & Studies of the College of Physicians of Philadelphia*, ser. 5, xiv: 2 (1992), 147–66.
29. Dora B. Weiner, 'Le Droit de l'homme à la santé - une belle idée devant l'assemblée constituante', *Clio Medica*, v (1970), 209–23 (especially 211–14).
30. Toby Gelfand, 'A Clinical Ideal: Paris 1789', *Bulletin of the History of Medicine*, li (1977), 397–411. The 1790 *Plan* discusses a number of other reform proposals, 157–71. I have not seen Chambon's 1789 reform proposal, for it is not in the collection of his unedited papers in Bibliothèque de la Faculté de Médecine (Paris), MS 5143. For his life, see J. Génévrier. *La Vie et les œuvres de Nicolas Chambon (de Montaux) 1748–1826* (Paris: Steinheil, 1906).
31. Quesnay, *op. cit.* (note 17), 206–8. Quesnay expresses a wish in a footnote that the two professions could be united. His practical

suggestion was that the two Paris corps might interchange personnel. Young physicians could improve their surgical knowledge by joining the company of surgeons, while experienced and learned surgeons could be admitted to the college of physicians. He stresses (208) that the faculty would remain the senior partner.

32. Claude-Nicolas Le Cat, *Lettre... sur les avantages de la réunion du titre de docteur en médecine, avec celui de maître en chirurgie et sur quelque abus dans l'un et l'autre art* (Amsterdam: publisher unknown, 1762). Le Cat, an MA and Paris master-surgeon, became royal demonstrator in anatomy at Rouen in 1738; like Quesnay he eventually took a medical degree: see Gelfand, *op. cit.* (note 21), 92, 95, 105.
33. Letter of 6 August, 1787 to Dulaurens, cited in Dulaurens, *Analyse du livre intitulé: moyens de rendre les hôpitaux utiles de perfectionner la médecine.* (Paris: Royez, 1788), 16, n.l. Dulaurens (1726–89) promotes the unification of the two professions in his *Essai*, 60–4 (see above, note 23). Petit was famous for his private lecture-courses on anatomy and surgery. In a 1757 oration he had admitted the advances made by surgery but argued that the two professions should remain separate; Dulaurens deceitfully uses the text of this speech to support his reformist case. The oration can be found in Bibliothèque de la Faculté de Médecine (Paris), *Theses medicae Parisiensis*, 16 vols. in 4°, xiii. no. 39, 'Discours prononcé aux écoles de médecine pour l'ouverture solennelle du cours de chirurgie, 27 novembre 1757'. At this juncture Petit taught the official faculty course in surgery for the benefit of trainee surgeons; it was conducted in the vernacular.
34. Vicq d'Azyr, 'Plan', 4–7.
35. *Ibid.*, 113–19.
36. Cf. the views of Dulaurens, *op. cit.* (note 23), 60–4, who believed that there was little chance of medicine ever becoming one profession. His view of the virtue of the traditional pharmacopoeia is expressed in ch. 6. Another reason for maintaining the *status quo* is suggested in sect. iv below.
37. 'Plan', 104–7.
38. *Ibid.*, 66, 68–73.
39. *Ibid.*, 74–5.
40. A. S. Emch-Deriaz, 'Towards a Social Concept of Health in the Second Half of the Eighteenth Century: Tissot (1728–1797) and the New Preoccupation with Health and Well-Being', Ph.D. Dissertation, University of Rochester, 1984, 236–40, 257–8. A memorandum that Tissot drew up in 1776 entitled 'De l'instruction des chirurgiens pour la campagne' appeared in his *Essai*, 145–65. Tissot's works, written in French were extremely popular in France, so he counts as a French reformer.
41. One physician on the eve of the Revolution who particularly sympathized with the plight of the poor struck down by epidemics was the Caen graduate and Rouen doctor, Louis Lépecq de la Clôture:

see his *Observations sur les maladies épidémiques, ouvrage rédigé d'après le tableau des épidémiques d'Hippocrate, et dans lequel on indique la meilleure méthode d'observer ce genre de maladies* (Paris: Vincent, 1776). The book is an account of a series of rural epidemics Lépecq encountered in 1770: see especially the picture of distress he paints on 96–7.

42. 'Plan', 135–41.
43. Caroline Hannaway, 'Veterinary Medicine and Rural Health Care in Pre-Revolutionary France', *Bulletin of the History of Medicine*, li (1977), 431–47.
44. One physician with a particular interest in animal epidemics was the Montpellier and Paris graduate, J.-J. Paulet (1740–1826); see his *Recherches historiques & physiques sur les maladies epizootiques avec les moyens d'y remédier, dans tous les cas* (2 vols; Paris: Ruault, 1775), published on royal command.
45. There were 24 French universities in 1789 and all but four possessed faculties of medicine. Only a minority of faculties, however, (Montpellier, Paris, Strasbourg, Besançon and Toulouse) received and taught a significant number of students, and half-a-dozen had no students at all: see L. W. B. Brockliss, *French Higher Education in the Seventeenth and Eighteenth Centuries: A Cultural History* (Oxford: Oxford University Press, 1987), 13–19, and the figs. in Dominique Julia and Jacques Revel, 'Les Etudiants et leurs études dans la France moderne,' in *idem, Les Universités européenes du XVIe au XVIIIe siècle: Histoire sociale des populations étudiantes* vol. II (Paris: Ecole des Hautes Etudes en Sciences Sociales, 1989), 260–4.
46. 'Plan', 2–3.
47. *Ibid.*, 20–l.
48. *Ibid.*, 23.
49. *Ibid.*, 22.
50. Hence the title of many of the reformist pamphlets: see above note 23. There were about 2,000 hospitals in France on the eve of the Revolution, ranging from the Paris Hôtel-Dieu with some 4,000 inmates to extremely small hospices in minor provincial towns. They catered for the homeless and dying poor, as much as the indigent sick.
51. 'Plan', 56–8, 94–8.
52. Tissot, *op. cit.* (note 23), 114–44. Tissot's observations were based on his own practice at the University of Pavia where he had established a clinical course in a local hospital. Another reformer to have already used the hospital as an instrument of medical teaching was Chambon de Montaux who had given private clinical lessons at the Salpêtrière hospital in Paris: see the account of his method in Bibliothèque de la Faculté de Médecine (Paris), MS 5143, 'Considérations sur l'enseignement de la médecine en Espagne,' n. d., fo. 8^{v}.
53. There were several large military hospitals in France: one of these, at Rochefort, was where the reformer Dulaurens was located.

54. 'Plan', 80, 92, 94 (especially 80). Tissot was more honest and recognized there was a tension between the needs of the patient and the needs of the medical student: cf. his comments on not tiring patients by multiple examinations, in *op. cit.* (note 23), 119–20.
55. 'Plan', 59–63 (especially 63). Ideally, it was maintained, all medical practitioners should be trained in the colleges, but this was judged too expensive.
56. *Ibid.*, 63. On this point Vicq refers the reader to the memoranda of the Paris hospital physicians, François Doublet (1751–95) and Chambon de Montaux, presented to the *Société Royale*, neither of which I have seen. Doublet was the author of 'Observations faites dans le département des hôpitaux civils', published in the *Journal de Médecine*, lxxxiii (1785). Dulaurens, *op. cit.* (note 23), 151–8, wanted no one to be allowed to practise privately until they had spent three years as an *élève* (i.e. intern or assistant) in a hospital, perfecting their practical knowledge of surgery and medicine.
57. 'Plan', 41–5, where Vicq discusses the programme of studies laid down by other reformers.
58. The nature of the examination system is discussed in L. W. B. Brockliss, 'Before the Clinic: French Medical Teaching in the Eighteenth Century', sect. v. (forthcoming). Actual requirements varied from faculty to faculty.
59. There is no doubt that this did happen: see the information in the article cited above note 58.
60. 'Plan', 45–55.
61. Joseph-Ignace Guillotin, 'Projet de décret sur l'enseignement et l'exercice de l'art de guérir... (August 1791), in A. de Beauchamp (ed.), *Médecine et pharmacie: Projets de lois* (5 vols; Paris: publisher unknown, 1888–95), i. 159–89. The report did not champion Vicq's proposal that stipended cantonal doctors should be established, but wanted the poor to be looked after by an elected committee of four doctors, one pharmacist, and one citizen. The infamous Guillotin, a Paris physician, was one of the few medical practitioners to sit in the National Assembly. He had proposed to the Assembly the establishment of a separate medical committe.
62. There is evidence that some faculties did survive, albeit temporarily, their official closure: see J. Léonard, *Les Médecins de l'ouest au XIXe siècle* (3 vols; Lille: Université de Lille, 1978), i. 217–20.
63. For example, *The Clinical Training of Doctors. An Essay of 1793. Philippe Pinel* (ed.) and trans. Dora B. Weiner (Supplement to the *Bulletin of the History of Medicine*, 3: Baltimore: Johns Hopkins University Press, 1980). Pinel's essay was a contribution to a prize competition set by the *Société Royale*, abolished itself in September 1793.
64. Léonard, *op. cit.* (note 62), i. 222–31. The text of the decree establishing the new schools in late 1794 can be found in *Rapport*

et décret de la Convention nationale sur les Ecoles de Santé de Paris, Montpellier et Strasbourg (Paris, Year III), 25–31: see British Library, R405 (17). The new Paris school quickly gained an international reputation: see especially E. Ackerknecht, *Medicine at the Paris Hospital, 1794–1848* (Baltimore: Johns Hopkins University, 1967).

65. From November 1797 the schools were allowed to issue a certificate. An important development came in 1802 with the establishment in the Paris hospitals of state-supported internships, awarded on the basis of a competitive examination.
66. The reform of 1803, established by the *loi de ventôse an* XI is published in *Recueil des lois et règlements concernant l'instruction publique depuis l'édit de Henri IV en 1598 jusqu'à ce jour. Publié par ordre de son excellence le Grand-Maître de l'université de France* (8 vols; Paris: publisher unknown, 1814–27), ii. 334–43.
67. Students could graduate either as doctors of medicine or doctors of surgery. The curriculum and system of examination for the two degrees was the same, except prospective doctors of surgery had to pass an 'external' rather than 'internal' clinical examination (*ibid.* 335, clause 6).
68. The best account of the new medical system is in Léonard, *op. cit.* (note 62), i. 254–302. Later refinements to the nineteenth-century medical system included the establishment of provincial medical schools to supplement the hospital-based or apprentice-type training of the departmental doctors. This category was finally abolished in 1892.
69. For example, in Austria Johann Peter Frank, *Plan d'école clinique, ou méthode d'enseigner la pratique de la médecine dans un hôpital académique* (Vienna: publisher unknown, 1790).
70. See in particular Othmar Keel, 'Cabanis et la généalogie épistemologique de la médecine clinique', Ph.D. Dissertation, McGill University, Montreal, 1977, Vol. ii, ch. 9, 355–450.
71. See 'Directio pro facultate medica a consilio regio gubernii generalis belgici, 30 Septembris, 1788 praescripto', in J. Molanus, *Les Quatorze Livres sur l'histoire de la ville de Louvain*, P. F. X. de Ram (ed.), pt ii (Brussels: M. Hayez, 1861), appendix, 1082–8. For recent accounts of medical reform in the second half of the eighteenth century in other countries, see notably M. C. Burke, *The Royal College San Carlos. Surgery and Spanish Medical Reform in the Late Eighteenth-Century* (Durham, NC: Duke University Press, 1977), and Thomas Broman, 'The Transformation of Academic Medicine in Germany 1780–1820', Ph. D. Dissertation, Princeton University, 1987. The restructuring of the education of physicians was part of a wider university reform movement. The literature here is vast, but see, as an introduction, many of the essays in James Leith (ed.), *Facets of Education in the Eighteenth Century* (Studies on Voltaire and the Eighteenth Century, CLXVII; Oxford: The Voltaire Foundation,

1977).

72. The works of Würtz and Tissot are cited above note 23. Earlier publications were relatively slight: see the work of the Paris graduates, Claude-François Duchanoy (1742–1827) and J.-B. Jumelin (1745–1807), 'Mémoire sur l'utilité d'une école clinique en médecine', *Observations sur la physique, sur l'histoire naturelle et les arts*, Supplement 13 (1778); and that of Nicolas Jadelot (1738–93), professor of medicine at Nancy, 'Essai sur les moyens de perfectionner l'étude de la médecine,' *Journal de Médecine*, lvi (1781): see Gelfand, *op. cit.* (note 21), 132–4.
73. Mme de Staël in *De l'Allemagne* (1813) was exaggerating when she claimed the French had no knowledge of German letters and philosophy, but she was essentially correct. Of course the arrival of the Austrian Marie-Antoinette as the wife of the future Louis XVI in 1770 must have helped create contacts with Austria. Interestingly, one of the medical reformers, Cabanis, translated Goethe into French in the 1790s.
74. Irvine Loudun, *Medical Care and the General Practitioner 1750–1850* (Oxford: Oxford University Press, 1986), chs 6–8; Susan Lawrence, 'Science and Medicine at the London hospitals: The Development of Teaching and Research, 1780–1815', Ph.D. Dissertation, University of Toronto, 1985, ch. 7. For the development of the medical profession in other countries, see the comparative article by Matthew Ramsey, 'The Politics of Professional Monopoly in Nineteenth-Century Medicine: The French Model and Its Rivals,' in Gerald L. Geison, *Professions and the French State, 1700–1900* (Philadelphia: University of Pennsylvania Press, 1984), 225–305.
75. Cf. the comments of John Thomson in Christopher Lawrence, 'The Edinburgh Medical School and the End of "The Old Thing"', *History of Universities*, vii (1988), 259–86 (at 277). The Anglo-American attitude to Paris (sometimes critical) is explored in John Harley Warner, 'English and American Perceptions of French Medicine in the 19th Century' (forthcoming).
76. The 1803 medical reform was extended to the territories in the Netherlands, the Rhineland and Northern Italy incorporated into the greater French state: medical schools were also to be established at Brussels, Mainz and Turin.
77. The best recent account of the Enlightenment remains Peter Gay, *The Enlightenment: An Interpretation* (2 vols; London: Wildwood House, 1970). It is flawed by its attempt to reduce the Enlightenment to a small, cosmopolitan, clearly defined movement. Above all, too anxious to establish that the epistemological basis of the Enlightenment was Newtonian science (itself no easily definable phenomenon anyway), Gay refuses to include the extremely influential and important German Cameralist movement within its parameters. A laudable attempt to examine the national

manifestations of the movement is Roy Porter and Mikulá Teich (eds), *The Enlightenment in National Context* (Cambridge: Cambridge University Press, 1981).

78. On the *Idéologues*, see especially S. Moravia, *Il Tramonto de l'illuminismo: filosofia e politica nella società francese, 1770–1810* (Bari: Laterza, 1968); François Azouvi (ed.), *L'Institution de la raison. La Révolution culturelle des idéologues* (Paris: Ecole des Hautes Etudes en Sciences Sociales, 1992).
79. La Mettrie died in 1751 so it is impossible to know what contribution he might have made to the reform movement.
80. Cf. notes 31 and 33 above for Quesnay's cautious reformism and Petit's readiness to accept the traditional division between physicians and surgeons.
81. D. Roche, 'Talents, raison et sacrifice: l'image des médecins des Lumières d'après les éloges de la Société royale de médecine', *Annales: économies, sociétés, civilisations*, xxxii (1977), 866–86. Vicq also used the *éloges* to champion the union of medicine and surgery.
82. 'Plan', 8–9.
83. Cited in Peter Gay, 'The Enlightenment as Medicine and Cure,' in W. H. Barber *et al.*, *The Age of the Enlightenment: Studies Presented to Theodor Besterman* (London: Oliver and Boyd, 1967), 375–86 (at 386). Morand wrote some of the articles on surgery for the *Encyclopédie.*
84. Diderot, 'Plan d'une université pour le gouvernement de Russie,' in *idem. Oeuvres complètes* J. Assézat (ed.),Vol. iii (Paris: Garnier *frères*, 1875), 497. This document, 499–505, contains an early description of a revitalized faculty of medicine where the emphasis would be placed on clinical, hospital training, and demonstrates that medical reform was not just of interest to professional physicians; the 'Plan' was prepared for Catherine the Great.
85. Tissot, 'De l'instruction des chirurgiens pour la campagne', published in *op. cit.* (note 23), especially 155–63. Tissot's interest in the 'medicalization' of the countryside stemmed in part from a Calvinist dislike of waste and a mid-eighteenth-century Cameralist fear of depopulation as much as from his humanity: see Emch-Deriaz, *op. cit.* (note 40), pt ii, ch. 2, especially.
86. In defending the monopoly of the learned physician eighteenth-century polemicists like Hecquet reiterated arguments that had been developed in the sixteenth and early seventeenth centuries when the corporate medical system was taking shape. Cf. for example the view of the Montpellier professor, Laurent Joubert, *Première et seconde partie des erreurs populaires et propos vulgaires touchant la médecine & le régime de santé, refutez et expliquez* (Lyon, 1608), especially ch. iv. The belief that medicine was a learned science was defended equally strongly in other countries in the eighteenth century, such as Germany: private communication by Thomas Broman, Department of the History of

Science, University of Wisconsin.

87. On French medical teaching before 1750, see Brockliss, *op. cit.* (note 45), ch. 8.
88. Cited from a letter of 1724 in in T. Besterman, *Voltaire* (London: Longmans, 1969), 103. Cabanis attacked such cynicism in his 'Du degré de certitude de la médecine', written in 1788: see *idem, Œuvres* (5 vols; Paris: Boussanges *frères*, 1828), i. 400–531.
89. D. Diderot (ed.), *Encyclopédie ou dictionnaire raisonné des sciences, des arts et des métiers* (17 vols; [Paris], 1751–65), x, 260–75 (especially 274), article on 'médecine'. Jaucourt wrote large sections of the work, see R. N. Schwab, 'The Chevalier de Jaucourt: Physician and Encyclopedist', *Journal of the History of Medicine*, xiii (1958), 256–9. Jaucourt's medical hero was Boerhaave under whom he had studied.
90. Cf. Diderot's account of the physician called to examine Suzanne in *La Religieuse* R. Mauzi (ed.), (Paris: Gallimard, 1972), 168, and his general remarks on medical practice in his 'Plan', 498.
91. Voltaire was particularly keen to stress the utility of surgery: see his attack on those in the *philosophe* world who were cynical about the abilities of all licensed medical practitioners in *Diatribe du docteur Akakia* (1752–3). His gibes were aimed at Maupertuis but they could just as easily have been directed at Rousseau, who had little faith in any branch of the medical profession: see *The Confessions of Jean-Jacques Rousseau* (ed.) and trans. J. M. Cohen (Harmondsworth: Penguin Books, 1953), *passim.* Voltaire, in contrast to Quesnay (!) saw the reign of Louis XIV as a period of rapid surgical advance: see his *The Age of Louis XIV* trans. M. P. Pollack (London: Dent, 1961), 374–5.
92. Quesnay's assertion of the rise of Paris surgery is perfectly justified, if his explanation is scarcely acceptable: see section i above. Paris in the first half of the eighteenth century was the Mecca of European surgery: see especially *Johannes Gesners Pariser Tagebuch 1727* U. Boschung (ed.), (Bern: Verlag Hans Huber, 1985), 15–186.
93. Louis's contributions appeared in a separate work entitled *Dictionnaire de Chirurgie* (2 vols; Paris, 1777). Louis wrote 70 articles for the *Encyclopédie,* see especially 'Histoire de la chirurgie', the complement to the Jaucourt article on medicine. On the medical authors of the work, see M. Lagnel-Lavastine, 'Les Médecins collaborateurs de l'Encyclopédie', *Revue d'histoire des sciences*, iv (1951), 351–8; and P. Astruc, 'Les Sciences médicales et leurs représentants dans l'Encyclopédie', *ibid.*, 359–68.
94. Caroline Hannaway is completing a study of Vicq d'Azyr as an anatomist, and maintains that comparative anatomy was his consuming passion. Petit through his public and private lectures introduced a whole generation of physicians (including Vicq) to anatomy, surgery and obstetrics: his private teaching is discussed in Brockliss, *op. cit.* (note 58), sect. iv.
95. 'Plan', 102; Chambon de Montaux, *op. cit.* (note 23), see also Claude-

François Duchanoy, *Projet d'organisation médicale* (n. d. but after 1794), in British Library, R 405. For Duchanoy see above note 72.

96. F. Vicq d'Azyr, *Œuvres* J. L. Moreau de la Sarthe (ed.), (6 vols; Paris: L. Duprat-Duverger, 1805), iv. 208.
97. The most famous exponent of active learning was Rousseau: see *Emile* (1762). The *Idéologues* developed a secondary-school curriculum temporarily introduced in the mid-1790s which was meant to train both the eye and the mind: see Moravia, *op. cit.* (note 78), 347–69. For a general account of the new pedagogy, see G. Snyders, *La Pédagogie en France aux XVIIe et XVIII siècles* (Paris: Presses universitaires de France, 1965), especially 345–443.
98. Cf. the comments of Lépecq de la Clôture on the unwillingness of peasants to hand over bodies to him when he attended the epidemic at Gros-Theil in 1770: see *op. cit.* (note 41), 185.
99. Admittedly the hospital would have had to be remodelled to serve its new educational function, for there is plenty of evidence in the eighteenth century that the regular orders who provided the nursing staff disobeyed the physicians' orders and tried to prevent automatic dissections: see especially the comments of Dulaurens, *op. cit.* (note 23), chs l, 5 and 9 (86). General comments Laurence Brockliss and Colin Jones, *Medicine and Society in Early-Modern France*, ch. 10, 'The Hospital in the Enlightenment' (forthcoming).
100. The stubborness of patients, as well as their independence, was noted by many physicians in the last quarter of the eighteenth century, not just reformers: e.g. J. E. Gilibert (1741–1814), *L'Anarchie médicinale ou la médecine considérée comme nuisible à la société* (3 vols; Neuchâtel: publisher unknown, 1772), ii, 105–9. This work by a Lyons physician, who taught medicine in Poland (1775–83), bemoans the state of the medical system at great length and accuses medical students of laziness and decadence, but it does not suggest any structural innovations.
101. Vicq says nothing in the 'Plan' about the role of the hospital in research, but many other reform proposals did: see especially Cabanis, 'Observations sur les hôpitaux' (1790), in *Œuvres complètes*, ii, 316–62 (especially 343–6). The most innovative Paris surgeons had all held hospital positions.
102. It will be recalled that this was primarily a data-gathering body. Hospitals hitherto had not really been used for research purposes, although some physicians were beginning to collect and assess data about the inmates: e.g. Jean Razoux (1723–98), *Tables nosologiques et météorologiques dressées à l'hôtel'dieu de Nîmes depuis le ler janvier 1757 jusqu'au ler janvier 1762* (Basle: J. R. Imhof, 1767).
103. *Rapport et décret de la convention nationale sur les Ecoles de Santé de Paris, Montpellier et Strasbourg* (above, note 64), 17–18: note to Fourcroy's introduction to the law establishing the new medical schools; the research-orientation of the schools was specified in cl. x

of the decree.

104. Dulaurens, *op. cit.* (note 23), 135–9.
105. In 1790 Vicq published the lengthy and positive article 'anatomie pathologique' in *Dictionnaire de médecine de l'Encyclopédie méthodique* (14 vols; Paris: Panckoucke, 1787–1830), ii, 236–612.
106. Especially Michel Foucault, *La Naissance de la clinique* (Paris: Presses universitaires de France, 1963). To Foucault, of course, the Paris school had moved beyond the Enlightenment through its recognition of the individuality of disease-states and the impossibility of explaining organic life in terms of a set of universally applicable physical laws.
107. For vitalism generally, see especially F. Duchesneau, *La Physiologie des lumières: empiricisme, modèles et théories* (The Hague: Nijhoff, 1982). For vitalism in France, see *int. al.* Elizabeth Haig, *Bichat and the Medical History of the Eighteenth Century* (Medical History, Supplement 4; London: Wellcome Foundation, 1984).
108. Details in Brockliss, *op. cit.* (note 45), ch. 8, sects. ii–v, *passim*; and *idem., op. cit.* (note 58), sect. iii.
109. Admittedly the fit is not perfect, for Pinel was trained at Montpellier (after initially studying at Toulouse), and the Paris-trained Cabanis showed little interest in pathological anatomy: see Keel, *op. cit.* (note 70), *passim.* Much is made of the fact that Bichat gained his enthusiasm for pathological anatomy from working with the Paris surgeon, Pierre-Joseph Desault (d. 1795) at the Hôtel-Dieu in the early 1790s. Just as important may have been the favourable attitude to anatomy among the capital's physicians. Had he gone to Montpellier, like his physician father, he would arguably never have matured into the founder of histology. The most important member of the Ancien-Régime Paris faculty who survived to become a leading light of the post-Revolutionary Paris school was the auscultationist, Jean-Nicolas Corvisart (1755–1821), but he made no contribution to the literature of the reform movement.
110. Vitalists in the first half of the eighteenth century agreed with their mechanist opponents that matter was inert; the vital principle lay in the soul; from the mid-century, in contrast, Barthez and others argued that matter was alive, if not necessarily able to think.
111. See the chapter in this volume by Roselyne Rey.
112. Théophile de Bordeu, *Recherches anatomiques sur la position des glandes et leurs actions* (Paris, 1752), in which the triturationist theory of glandular secretion was savaged. Bordeu was a doctor of medicine of both Montpellier and Paris, so could practise legally in the capital.
113. Diderot was the *philosophe* most interested in biology, and produced his own *Eléments de phisiologie* (written in 1776 but not published until 1875). He was a close friend of Bordeu, to whom he attributed a radical transformationist view of life in his *Rêve d'Alembert*, composed in 1769. Bordeu was Lacaze's nephew.
114. Admittedly, some medical articles were written by Diderot's co-editor,

Jaucourt, as we have seen, and Jaucourt was certainly not a vitalist. But Jaucourt's hero was the iatromechanist Boerhaave who epitomized in the Enlightenment's eyes the acceptable face of pre-vitalist medical philosophy: he was seen as cautious and non-dogmatic. See the comments in Wellmann, *op. cit.* (note 14), ch. 3 especially.

115. Significantly Diderot in 1774 had no objection to the theoretical content of the curriculum of the Paris faculty, only the fact that there was no provision for courses in practical medicine: see his 'Plan,' 438.
116. This is not to deny the significant support that the Austrian government gave the movement, as was noted in section iii above, but it was only in post-Revolutionary France that the profession was completely restructured: the role of the Austrian government is explored in depth in Keel, *op. cit.* (note 70), especially chs. 9–11. Keel attributes the particular interest of the Austrian Habsburgs and other German princes in medical reform to the relative underdevelopment of their territories.
117. From the tone of the *cahiers des doléances* presented to the Estates-General in 1789 there is reason to believe that only a small proportion of the educated élite had adopted the *philosophe* programme of radical social and political reform, but there was strong support for change among sections of the nobility, and the deputies to the third estate seem to have quickly come under the influence of a small group of *ultras*; enlightenment ideas underpinned all the major revolutionary documents: see especially Taylor, *op. cit.* (note 22) and G. Chaussinand-Nogaret, *La Noblesse au dix-huitième siècle. De la féodalité aux lumières* (Paris: Hachette, 1976), chs 7–8.
118. Admittedly, the revolutionaries were not always sympathetic to the educational aims of the medical reformers. Revolutionary politicians with an interest in poor relief were often anxious to close the hospitals and have the poor treated either at home or in small parish hospices. This idea was already being canvassed in the 1780s: see Anon [the physiocrat, Dupont de Nemours], *Idées sur les secours à donner aux pauvres malades dans une grande ville* ([Philadelphia]: publisher unknown, 1786). The best survey of the revolutionaries' attitudes to the poor is Alan Forrest, *The French Revolution and the Poor* (Oxford: Oxford University Press, 1981).
119. The number of faculty physicians in 1789 will never be known with certainty; the figure is based on the fact that some 160 doctorates were given a year in the late eighteenth century: explanation and intro. to available data in Jones and Brockliss, *op. cit.* (note 99), ch. 8, sect. D. There may have been from 14,000–28,000 surgeons: *ibid.*, calculation of nos.
120. Gelfand, *op. cit.* (note 21), especially pts. ii and iii.
121. The state's patronage of surgery in the eighteenth century was epitomized by the establishment of the Paris dominated *Académie Royale de Chirurgie* as early as 1731. The physicians had no similar

institution until 1776, and even then it was only called a *Société* not an academy.

122. For Bichat's training, see above note 109.
123. Gelfand, *op. cit.* (note 21), 165, argues that the man really responsible for the 1794 reform was not the physician, Fourcroy, but the surgeon–physician, François Chaussier (1746–1828). Like Quesnay, Chaussier was a boundary-breaker; he was a Dijon surgeon who eventually took an MD at Besançon.
124. Vicq d'Azyr cited one example of a surgeon who had offered a reform programme, Cantin of Nantes: see 'Plan,' 157. Dulaurens claimed support from the king's first surgeon, Andouillé: see his *Analyse du livre intitulé...*, 30 (above, note 33). Also, it will be recalled, the Versailles surgeons favoured unification: see above, note 22.
125. For example Dulaurens, *op. cit.* (note 23), 64, who claimed that young surgeons serving in hospitals could hardly read or write. Vicq, too, implied that there were many surgeons who had had no elementary schooling: see 'Plan', 5.
126. *Rapport et decret de la convention nationale* (above, note 64), 8. The Montpellier school was also housed in a discredited Ancien-Régime institution, the bishop's palace.
127. Gelfand, *op. cit.* (note 21), 192, accepts that it is possible to conclude '[f]rom a superficial perspective of social conflict' that 'the physicians simply "coopted" their professional rivals and erstwhile subordinates'. But he rejects this idea out of hand. He does admit, however, (176) that it is puzzling that the physician–reformers made no reference to the surgical model of professional formation that, in his view, they imbibed.
128. No quantitative study of the social origins of the different branches of the eighteenth-century medical profession has yet been undertaken. But a study of entrants to the highly prestigious Paris college of physicians would suggest that about a third were relatives of college members. See the relevant vols of the college minute book in Bibliothèque de la Faculté de Médecine (Paris), MS l–24, 1391–1789; the last has been published: *Commentaires de la faculté de médecine de Paris, 1777 à 1786* G. Steinheil (ed.), (2 vols, Paris: publisher unknown, 1903). Anecdotal evidence would suggest that most physicians who were not themselves physicians' sons were the sons of bureaucrats, lawyers or *rentiers*, or occasionally well-to-do surgeons (e.g. Pinel and Chambon de Montaux). In the diocese of Auch a third of barber–surgeons were sons of surgeons; others were sons of artisans: see Toby Gelfand, 'A Monarchical Profession in the Old Regime: Surgeons, Ordinary Practitioners, and Medical Professionalization in Eighteenth-Century France,' in Geison *op. cit.* (note 74), 149–80 (at 157).
129. On the emancipation of the London apothecaries, see Harold J. Cook, *The Decline of the Old Medical Régime in Stuart London*

(Ithaca, N.Y.: Cornell University Press, 1986), ch. 6. The number of French apothecaries was possibly on the decline in the eighteenth century, and their corps were continually being forced to go to law to defend their monopoly right to prepare and sell drugs (often against surgeons): see especially Pierre Rambaud, *La Pharmacie en Poitou jusqu'à l'an XI* (Poitiers: Blais and Roy, 1907), ch. xxvi (wide-ranging); this originally appeared in *Bulletin et Mémoires de la Société des Antiquaires de l'Ouest*, 2nd ser., xxx (1906).

130. See Louis Dulieu, *La Chirurgie à Montpellier de ses origines au début du XXe siècle* (Avignon: Presse universelle, 1975), 175.

131. For example the case of one Germillac, holder of the new degree, who was pressed by the corporation of surgeons of Périgueux to become a surgeon's *élève* and take the *maîtrise* if he wished to practise there: see Bibliothèque de la Faculté de Médecine (Montpellier), collection entitled: Archives de la Faculté de Médecine de Montpellier, F 57, unnumbered letter, 28 March, 1772.

132. From 1723 the surgical profession was hierarchically organized under the king's first surgeon, who had the right to appoint lieutenants to each corporation or *bailliage* (administrative district) where no corps existed. The powers of the lieutenants were laid down in the 1730 *règlement* for the profession: see Le Blond d'Olbien, *op. cit.* (note 6), 11–15 (arts i–v).

133. 'Plan', 63–4, 71–2. Vicq gives a list of possible professors of the new departmental schools, all but one correspondents of the *Société Royale* or Montpellier professors. The organization of the *conseils de santé* is unclear.

134. See especially Roselyne Rey, 'La Vulgarisation médicale au XVIIIe siècle: Le cas des dictionnaires portatifs de santé,' *Revue d'histoire des sciences*, 3–4: xliv (1991), 413–33. According to the Dijon physician, Hugues Maret (1726–86), in the introduction to his *Mémoires pour servir au traitement d'une fièvre épidémique* (Dijon: L. N. Frantin, 1775), the then minister of finance believed that the only way 'prévenir les épidémies, étoit d'éclairer ceux que la nécessité des circonstances obligeoit à donner des soins aux Habitans de la Campagne'. Self-help manuals written by physicians had a long history: see Andrew Wear, 'Popularized Ideas of Health and Illness in Seventeenth-Century France', *Seventeenth-Century French Studies*, viii (1986), 229–42. In the mid-eighteenth century one was posthumously published from the pen of Philippe Hecquet: see *La Médecine et la chirurgie des pauvres* (Paris: Veuve Alix, 1740).

135. One such physician sent into the countryside to deal with epidemics was Louis Lépecq de la Clôture, envoy of the Rouen *intendant*, Thiroux de Crosne, on several occasions in 1770: see *op. cit.* (note 41), especially 95 and 238. Vicq d'Azyr's *éloges* of dead members of the *Société Royale de Médecine* refer frequently to physicians attending rural epidemics on the *intendant's* request; Maret of Dijon was faith-

ful unto death: see Vicq d'Azyr, *op. cit.* (note 96), iii. 134–6 (from the *éloge* of Maret). Dulaurens, *op. cit.* (note 23), 157–8, believed that in future the role of epidemic doctors should be filled by junior physicians straight out of the hospital: such service should be the culmination of their training.

136. Rey, *op. cit.* (note 134), 420, points out that the great danger of self-help manuals was that they would teach the readers to criticize and question professional physicians.
137. On Petit's bedside manner, see Lindsay Wilson, *Women and Medicine in the French Enlightenment: The Debate Over Maladies des Femmes* (London: The Johns Hopkins University Press, 1993), 98.
138. According to Gilibert, *op. cit.* (note 100), ii. 108–9, physicians fed up with patient-power preferred to give their services to the poor, with the result that the poor were better served than the rich. One enlightened physician who seems to have concentrated on treating the poor was Cabanis: see Martin S. Staum, *Cabanis. Enlightenment and Medical Philosophy in the French Revolution* (Princeton, N.J.: Princeton University Press, 1980), ch. IV.
139. See L. W. B. Brockliss, 'The Development of the Spa in Seventeenth-Century France,' in R. S. Porter (ed.), *The Medical History of Waters and Spas* (Medical History Supplement 10; London: Wellcome Institute for the History of Medicine, 1990), 23–47 (at 36–9, 43–5). In the last 20 years of Louis XIV's life it would also seem that practitioner-power was established at Versailles through the 'tyranny' (Saint-Simon's word) that the king's chief physician, Fagon, was allowed to exercise over the court: see *idem.*, 'The Literary Image of the *Médecins du roi* in the Literature of the Grand Siècle,' in Nutton, *op. cit.* (note 10), 117–54 (at 133–43).
140. Diderot, 'Plan d'une université,' 499. The more sceptical among the *philosophes* believed that physicians had a vested interest in frustrating medical breakthroughs, so that their income could be maintained: see J. Avalon, 'Une diatribe de Restif de la Bretonne contre les médecins', *Bulletin de la Société française de l'histoire de médecine*, i: 5 (1921), 169–81.
141. Admittedly, Vicq did not demand that hospital-training should be *de rigueur*: see above under the section Medical Reform. There was an evident tension between his liberalism and professionalism. Nevertheless, the reformers uniformly wanted the good doctor in the future associated with the clinically-trained physician.
142. Jean-Charles-Félix Caron, *Démonstration rigoureuse du peu d'utilité de l'Ecole de Médecine...(du grand avantage que l'on a retiré, et que l'on retirera toujours du rétablissement du Collège de Chirurgie* (Paris: Pillet aîné, 1818). Cf. Caron's view of Vicq d'Azyr: 'Homme rare, j'admire tes talens; mais je vois en toi le plus grand ennemi de la chirurgie' (25). For another example, see the arguments against the 1794 and 1803 reforms in M. Léveillé, *Mémoire sur l'état actuel de l'enseignement*

de la médecine et de la chirurgie en France et sur les modifications dont il est susceptible (Paris: publisher unknown, 1816), especially 13–24.

143. The history can be followed in Ramsey, *op. cit.* (note 1), chs. 2–6; Léonard, *op. cit.* (note 62), i, ch. 5 *et seq.* In 1789 there were only 498 faculty students (a minimum figure); by 1825 there were *c.* 2,000 medical students at Paris alone: see R. Chartier, M. M. Compère and D. Julia, *L'Education en France du XVIe au XVIII siècle* (Paris: Sedes, 1976), 274; Ackerknecht, *op. cit.* (note 64), 36.

3

Whose Enlightenment? Medicine, Witchcraft, Melancholia and Pathology

Johanna Geyer-Kordesch

The Enlightenment changed traditional beliefs, habits and customs. Insights into this process are especially significant where popular beliefs confronted enlightened views.

Changes were very evident, for example, in regard to witchcraft beliefs and in perceptions of the body. Both are intimately related to medicine, but also to the larger context of natural philosophy and cultural beliefs regarding invisible nature or the world of the spirit. Definitions of health or illness are thus not entirely medical problems. Medical publications of the eighteenth century reflect these concerns, and, indeed, directly engage them in medical case history literature. This is especially true where medical publications were popular enough to engage the general reader. Thus collections of medical case histories were published in the German-speaking lands; their appeal lay in their close affinity to life-stories and the didactic use of life-stories in the new moral weeklies.[1] In fact this form of journals using true-life stories probably originated as popular reading matter just then.

Be that as it may, the medical case history collections of the Enlightenment, whose market value proved itself after 1721, was *not* of a kind to be hidden on a specialist's corner shelf.[2] Quite the contrary, the patient narratives and their themes, ranging over witchcraft, infanticide, melancholia, poisoning, chronic and acute diseases, as well as physicians' advice in relieving suffering, were an excellent read. Hence they seem a good starting point for examining shifts in mentalities.

True stories or letters to agony aunts are usually prescriptive: they strongly imply what is right or wrong. That quality is also obvious in the medical case history. Not surprisingly, cautionary tragedies and helpful advice entice the general reader, but they are not at the core of the subject-in-hand. The medical case history of the eighteenth century has a complex structure composed of many parts and various voices; these merge to enrich it.

The story derives from a patient telling a relative or local doctor about illness, who writes it down, often with a wonderful sense of drama and a pertinent hold on social detail and beliefs held dear.[3] This was sent to a consultant, after, probably, reading it over to the client, for a written medical opinion. The recipient, usually a medical faculty professor, writes a response, in which he draws together salient points and reaches both a diagnostic conclusion and recommendations for medication and therapy.

Within this settled, but elastic, structure, something quite interesting happens: the same tale is told twice, once by the originators and then again by the medical godfather. Like all good godfathers at baptisms, the baby comes out christened an orthodox believer. Thus the original story is told and recast, as a life narrative the first time, and the second time, the medical view polishes away cultural beliefs that seem to be irreconcilable with it. Witchcraft is laundered in a special way; and melancholia, representative of another facet of spiritual and demonic powers, is reinterpreted by medical diagnostics.

In the following, the uneasy relationship between these elements is explored. Falling ill and seeking relief are subjects not in themselves tidy. Harm and healing were popularly believed to be intertwined with unseen powers in nature. By the mid eighteenth century nature was not yet stripped down to cause-and-effect observations, although the mechanical view of the animal economy was used to excise metaphysical interpretations.[4] Hence medical advice remains haunted, and the themes of metaphysical, spiritual, or popular superstitions weave a fabric in which the enlightened themselves move.

Ideological shifts establish medical and legal claims to Enlightenment. One discernible shift is reductive: medical diagnostics removes the material body from the powers of feelings, imagination and the faculties of the soul and objectifies it. If the body is ill, this must be a tangible illness. The second shift distinguished popular thinking from medical expertise. Thus healing, and falling ill, formerly well imbedded in practices common to many, became a medical enterprise whose parameters were set by medical men.

Embodiment and the 'natural' world

Images and symbols, stories and allegories describe events not otherwise understood, that are none the less deep life experiences. For example, forms and shapes in nature were traditionally seen as manifesting both tangible and invisible reality. The invisible fashioned its own body. The story of the basilisk illustrates this belief.[5] Its bodily shape was of sublime ugliness and it often lived at the bottom of wells, an element (water) congenial to the powers of the unseen and the demonic. The basilisk was very real to the popular mind, and it still has its own pre-enlightenment memorial in a commemorative plaque in the Schoenlaterngasse in Vienna. The legend illustrates the story that its evil was magically tamed by using a mirror. The basilisk died when it saw itself.

In this world of animated shapes and fluid incarnations, the basilisk (a worm-like dragon) sometimes represents the agency of poisoning, that is, an unseen, liquid (alchemical) power affecting the body.[6] The basilisk is the 'body' for unidentified influences whose latter tangible effects are disease or death. Monster shapes and strange 'people' were not aliens to those who lived before superstition became an Enlightenment label.[7]

So-called folklore is usually vilified or separated out from histories concerned with scientific medical progress. But in effect it shouldn't be. Images and symbols, stories and allegories synthesize and explore life experiences, especially of illness, as much as a medical diagnosis does. Analytically and historically the medicine of the Enlightenment reacts and feeds on a common imagery and projected encounters with nature, visible and invisible.

One sure instance of this was French and German cultured and learned men and women's pleasure in collecting fairy tales. Charles Perrault published many fairy tales (they have become known as the Mother Goose stories) for a court audience in 1697. The Arabian Nights were introduced from 1704 to 1717 in a French edition using oriental material. A collection called the *Cabinet des Fees*, in 41 volumes, was published in Geneva and Paris from 1785–9; and the Brothers Grimm published their *Kinder-und Hausmaerchen* in 1812.[8] Angela Carter, deeply familiar with fairy tales, wrote about this eighteenth century fascination: 'And it was a sophisticated hand that polished and rationalized the old stories, adding the moral tags that temper their darkness and magic with good-natured cynicism.'[9] Obviously darkness and magic were pervasive; the moral tags and the 'cynicism', or distancing from embodiments of the unseen, were indicative of a divisive thrust. Rationalism was not going to tolerate other loves. 'Pure' reason was dissociative of emotions.[10]

Popular beliefs were, after all, not so very irrational. If no clear science of cause and effect mechanisms is forthcoming, it is a questing mind that visualizes what may transform the familiar. In the lengthy medical case narratives, hideous and long-drawn out illness and its physical deformities, whether acute or chronic, are recounted in spectacular detail.[11] Familiar people become unrecognizable, and if poison is suspected, the manner of dying, so often described, visualizes in the reader's mind the vomiting, pain, and defecation that goes with it. The autopsy sections don't suppress the body's discoloration, the inflamed stomach and intestines and what it all looks like. The features of deformity, monstrosity and ugliness are plain to see. The popular stereotype of the witch as old and ugly is not really far removed from this narrative material. Many fairy tales turn on ancient equations of beauty and ugliness either evocative of evil and good, or as delusions that are transcended and cured (happy endings!) by another unseen element, the power of love and endurance.

'Popular' reading and its subjects were used for the evocation of the unseen both in narrative and visual representation. In many palaces built in the eighteenth century, a central architectural feature, the grand staircase, made any assent an allegorical one: the carriage entrance guarded by caryatids, representative of forces active underneath the earth, the climb up the steps showing a ceiling of skies, peopled by the gods, the ancient figures of Apollo and Dianá prominent amongst others.[12] The four corners of the ceiling displayed allegories of the (then known) four continents. This symbolical world surrounded mere mortals who ascend from the underworld to the heavens with each step, be they aristocrats or domestic servants. The arts acknowledged the sciences, but the imagination was not empirical.

These examples serve to show the pervading interpretative closeness to seeing invisible powers and powerful incarnations that were Nature's imaginative natural history. Depictions, stories and narrations of the time can't be less than the elements that surround them. Medical case histories published throughout the eighteenth century are suffused with the beliefs also traceable in folklore (fairy tales) and symbolic and allegorical approaches to the 'natural' world.

Medical Case Narratives

Medical consultation letters and *consilia* abound in printed collections. Their observations of illness are close to the language, perceptions and experience of the patient when they explain what they suffered. The second part of the case histories, the doctor's summary as a medical response (advice) retells the story to fit diagnostic identifications. This is the 'enlightened' medical blueprint for interpreting illness.

Closely allied to these narratives are the forensic cases.[13] These contain letters and judicial records (inquisition by the courts) in place of the initial letter. The second part of these case histories is the *consilium* or *responsum* of (again) the learned member of the medical faculty who writes authoritative assessments on matters brought before him. As in the consultation letter and the response to it, the latter written opinion usually brings an 'enlightened' viewpoint.

Medical narratives thus provide an opportunity to explore change in belief structures and superimpositions of enlightened ideology. The thematic focus most useful for an analysis of Enlightenment seem to be cases of witchcraft and psychological disorders.

The medical case histories regarding witchcraft and melancholia cited below are taken from Friedrich Hoffmann's *Medicina Consultatoria* (1725–39), a many-volumed work of cases originating from his own case load as an official consultant of the medical faculty of the University of Halle in Brandenburg-Prussia.[14] These are *bona fide* cases, all from contemporary practice; none were borrowed by Hoffmann from any previous literature.

The first case of 1718 concerns a young male aristocrat of 22 years.[15] The letter to Hoffmann describing his illness draws together in a fluid narrative the young man's mental and behavioural symptoms. These are linked in a series of vignettes of his profound disturbance. The story begins with the young man's inability to learn to walk until he was seven years old. He is characterized as weak and over-sensitive from early on and 'could not be brought up properly'.[16] During early adolescence he smoked and drank heavy spirits. The illness narrative remarks his doing this in isolation, not in the company of peers. The next episode highlights a fatal and climactic incident, his relationship with a 'disreputable woman' at the age of 13. He pledged marriage to her with an oath written in blood. The mother thinks he has been bewitched. His mother and his Lutheran confessor confront him. Thereupon he disavows his actions, battering the woman physically until she returns to him the oath written in his blood. The narrative recounts other critical episodes, such as his loud praying and ostentatious sighing within sight and sound of his parents' guests at social functions. He develops paroxysms that lead to catatonia and cold sweat, but which also cast off, as the writer notes, his pervading fear. These incidents occur 10 to 12 times per day, after which he is observed to be catatonically speechless. To quote the narrative: 'He cannot be moved, even by the greatest force, from where he is, because he imagines he would insult God if he were to move one foot in front of the other. When he eats, he stops in the middle of swallowing because he thinks he will choke to death on the morsel in his mouth and then spits it out vehemently.'[17] Other eating disorders are mentioned, but the catatonic religious fear and subsequent burst of spitting is obviously the central dramatic climax to this psychological illness narrative. The suspicion of witchcraft is understated, but adds to the texture of strangeness and behavioural abnormality so well portrayed. The whole story conveys the grotesque reality of behavioural illness; a narration that fits well with what fairytales present as ogres or incorporations of consuming monsters. The unfathomable, and indeed, exotic proportions of disturbance are the key elements of the narrative. Because of this the story is also familiar, recounting disease as if it were a tale of admonishment, akin to the moral tales told in *Straw Peter* with their horror stories of what happens to bad children.

The disjunction in narrative purpose enters with Hoffmann's judgement *(consilium)* on the case. He recasts perception of illness into diagnostic parameters. This forces the re-interpretation of 'darkness' and hateful 'magic' (oaths in blood) to a sane orderliness devoid of shadows. Hoffmann is imposing medical control. He writes: 'This *morbus* is called *pro affectu melancholico,* originating in feebleness, especially of the brain and nerves, when the whole *systema nervorum* is weak by nature, perhaps also *ex dispositione haereditaria,* compounded by a rotten diet of tobacco and spirits, that was afterwards aggravated through an over-scrupulous conscience ('Gewissens-Angst') and lengthy depression ('Bertruebnis'); all this contributed to disorderly *motibus spasticis,* resulting in an action of the blood. ... '[18] Hoffmann continues his minute linking of mental symptoms with a mapping of pathophysiological symptoms. He ends his medical recasting of the dramatic behavioural life-story by his emphasizing: 'Because this disease has fully natural causes, there can be no indication of supernatural [causes] or witchcraft.'[19] His prognosis is for a difficult cure, because the illness had become habitual. His treatment provides for a rigorous daily regimen of proper food, no smoking or drinking, riding and exercise and the taking of Hoffmann's medicines. If this doesn't bring results, the patient is to try a spa cure (the *Egrische Brunnen*).

Clearly the aim of Hoffmann's *consilium* is to suppress 'speculation' involving invisible powers in nature and to reduce even overt behavioural disorders to by-products of circulatory or nervous disease. He disparages explanations not covered by current medical pathophysiology. A strong division is made between illness in medical terms and illness described any other way, however much this is a believable story for the wider audience. Such a tense trade-off between different forms of narrative stagings of illness is basic to the cases in the *Medicina Consultatoria.*

Hoffmann is not above using plots within a plot to eradicate witchcraft beliefs, dating back to the *Hammer of Witches* (1484).[20] This seminal book on witchcraft prosecutions lists, amongst other items, the 'induction of evil love in a man for a woman and a woman for a man'[21] as one of the major ways in which witches injure humanity. Obviously the Church-based prosecution of witchcraft cannot be equated with other beliefs, those of 'white' and 'black' magic from more traditional sources. But by 1700 much had been run together. The version eliminating 'evil' love has the programme of sexual purity and disparagement of women behind it that aided witchcraft prosecutions.

In a case cited for 1695, *Exhibens judicium de falso philtri imputatione,* a woman is accused of 'poisoning' a member of the high aristocracy. A philtrum made of menstrual blood is described as having been given to the man. The man died, apparently in a fever.[22]

Hoffmann prints only his *consilium* judgement. This is a superb narrative refutation of occult causes. The strategy is akin to that of the barrister summing up. Can reasonable and medical grounds support the use and known effects of a philtrum? Not at all, Hoffmann states, because up to now no dedicated or prudent medical man would allow that philtra or so-called love-potions, 'usually prepared *ex sanguine menstruo*', could have the effect of inducing passionate love for a certain person, even though it is well known that these substances can produce *mentis turbationem, inordinatum spirituum motuum et furorem* (in other words, a disturbed nervous condition).[23] The suspicion of having applied a philtrum must be accompanied by immediate symptoms, states Hoffmann, such as feeling nauseous, wanting to vomit, restlessness, meaningless laughter, delirium, incoherent speech, lack of modesty in the expression of the eyes, insomnia and loss of strength. Hoffmann here plays the card of empirical evidence. If the pattern of recognized medical symptoms is not there, neither was the poison.

So, he states, the alleged victim had a fever for two years and not an observable sudden alteration due to a philtrum. The medical grounds for the accusation have thus disappeared; and to make sure causal links between love-potions and witchcraft are disposed of, Hoffmann introduces a witty common-sense anecdote of how men normally fall in love. Where there are manifest causes one doesn't need the occult: history relates the story of the Macedonian King Phillipp who loved a beautiful woman and wished his Queen to believe he was bewitched. The Queen summoned the woman and dryly observed on seeing her: *'valeare calumniae! Tu in te philtra habes.'* (What strong calumny! You contain the love-potion in yourself.) Hoffmann adds laconically: not everything need be ascribed to evil when there are simpler explanations.

Hoffmann's purpose in the case literature is to demonstrate medical expertise. He resumes *his* story with a minute consideration of the autopsy report: *pulmones scirrhosi, cor flaccidum* with a *polypo, viscera corrupta,* intestines and stomach very flaccid and full of damp and black substances. A normal fever and *polypus cordis* cannot derive from a philtrum. These findings come from a bad state of the body *(cachexia)* and from *phthisis.* Hoffmann continues with an explicit post-mortem re-examination of the man's former illnesses and only duly returns to the witchcraft allegation to refute a report by a certain Agricola Libertus *('sub nomine ficto').* A. L. is irresponsible when he concludes even '*ad suspicionem*' [that a philtrum had been given] when there are *causas manifestas et actualis,* and he omits them, to imply occult powers'.[24] A. L. is accused of citing indiscriminately and without the scientific stringency of causal links between pathiognomic patterns and specific diseases.

That is the crux of the matter and the reason for Hoffmann's detailed diagnostics; his lengthy exercises in narrating the minute progress of an illness, its complications and its physiological 'signs' substitute scientific explicitness in cases where stories turned the mind toward the occult. Hoffmann's tales show exactly how enlightenment medicine deflected witchcraft (no exact causal link, only incidental syncronicity) and established secularized disbelief.

This did not, however, eliminate contemporary needs for narrative exploration of illness, even though it anchored the claims of medical Enlightenment. Myths are not, of themselves, medical explanations, but, like essential story telling traditions, viz. the cultural hold of Grimm's Fairy Tales even today, a means of defining horrendous and unfamiliar events, be they in nature or in the soul.

A Case of Melancholia

Hoffmann's strategy used medical narrative to ban witchcraft from medical considerations. It did not quite ban the 'darkness' of another state of illness closely associated with witchcraft. Johann Weyer, the sixteenth-century medical doctor who was an early opponent of witchcraft trials, tried to deflate the witchcraft argument by linking melancholia to a disturbance of the imagination rather than supporting the belief of it being intrinsic to the phenomenon of witches' powers.[25] In his view the medical disease, melancholia, alone distorted the senses and altered the mind.

In Hoffmann's *Medicina Consultatoria* a forensic case illustrates how medical arguments played a role in Enlightenment medical reasoning. In a case of 12 July, 1717, Hoffmann writes the Medical Faculty opinion on a juridical case of child-murder.[26] In Halle a man murdered the child of a woman serving in the same household. The medical question put to him was whether the murderer was suffering from a psychological disturbance caused by melancholia or whether he was juridically accountable.

The place of the initial patient letter is here taken by the transcript of direct questions put to the accused. The man had no history of physical illness, alcoholism, nervous disability ('Herzklopffen'), but instead was of an extremely retiring nature, mindful of daily prayers and church attendance. Further questions, however, begin to reveal unsettling traits. The accused relates 'that he received too little pay and feared he could not support himself, and meditated for several weeks that if he murdered the child, he could depart this world'.[27] When asked about lack of pity for the poor child he answered: 'It had been dark in the room ... if he had seen the child, he could not have done it ... so he struck blindly with great fury without feeling anything, and cut himself, but did not feel anything.'[28]

The questions then reveal supernatural experiences. They explore the accused's dreams and sightings of apparitions. The man had a recurring dream of wading in deep water and he sleep-walked. One evening in another town he was fearfully startled by the apparition of an enormous woman approaching him. He feared such ghosts. On the night of the crime he testified that, although the door was locked, his pillow and bed-clothes had been removed from under him and he found them the next morning lying on the floor.

The medical explanation, given by Hoffmann, skilfully weaves these events into a watertight diagnosis of melancholia. Hoffmann's medical sleight of hand makes the ogre of these terrifying projections disappear into the framework of a rational label, that of medical pathology. This is done step by step, proceeding from given medical definitions of melancholia right down to the mind's profound dependence (in essence Hoffmann's theoretical view of 'mechanical' physiology) on the body. Hoffmann gives three related definitions of melancholia: 1) the common medical understanding; 2) the Hippocratic definition; 3) the manic phase as it relates to depression.[29] All three of them cover the behaviour brought out in the protocols. The common definition is: 'a melancholic is a person who insists on the truth of imagined dissonant and crazy things but is otherwise clever'.[30] Hippocrates defines it as 'a person who without necessity or cause feels fear, depression, terror, anxiety, and has desperate thoughts and *taedium vitae,* and this lasts for some time'.[31] Melancholia can change into mania when the person loses all sense of perception, thought and understanding. True mania is present when the person is driven to enact violence through an inner necessity unrelated to a cause.

Hoffmann links these diagnostic definitions to physiological findings, typical for post-Harveian circulatory explanations. The movement of the blood and its 'thickness' is seen as causal in creating particular tendencies toward restless sleep, anxious and heavy dreams, terror and fear. The accused, according to Hoffmann, suffers from 'thickened blood' and (in a curious circular argument) this caused his dreams of wading through water; his restless sleep-walking are also symptomatic of his bodily disfunctions. Hoffmann even states that the accused's vision of ghosts are attributable to his bodily condition. The murder itself resulted from the flip of depressive melancholia to its manical side. Hoffmann concludes, in his final judgement, that the accused did not act out of malicious intent and that his melancholia is still in an incipient stage. He recommends treatment through diet and medicines 'so that the potential of medical help may be realized while there is still time to cure'.[32]

What seems a pathological horror story is seen as medically enlightening by Hoffmann. By way of reasoned deduction, psychiatric illness is related to contemporary ideas of circulatory disorders. Hoffmann is able thus to somatize psychological illness. The medical text achieved enlightenment through a materialistic reduction to bodily dysfunction.

Enlightened it seems to be, even though, in this case, not everyone would agree, least of all his colleague George Ernst Stahl (1659–1734).[33] Hoffmann rationalizes what even the trial evidence does not record as intrinsically imaginary or fictional. The medical view of the imbalance of mind that spent itself, like an electrical storm, in the reprehensible act of child-murder, does not, in the end, entirely eliminate the question of invisible powers or the dark constellations of the soul.

Enlightenment

The patient narratives summarized here by no means stem from peasant or village folk; they are told by and about the middle classes and the aristocracy. Common to them, however, is the acknowledgement of the emotions, positive (love) and negative (melancholia) which underlie a case history: an ensuing illness, harm done to the mind and body, a resultant murder. The linkage in popular narrative thinking interweaves invisible powers with life and fate. In this sense they are true narratives, tales of the unexpected.

These observations on the style of narratives, points, I think, to an important aspect of what also occurs in the relationship of patient narrative and medical explanation (the consultation letter). Even though the patient narrative, in the Hoffmann cases for example, is decidedly middle class, it contains direct incorporation's of beliefs and cultural norms, plus, through its dramatic structure, the lure of the story.

The aim of learned doctors is to rationalize and medicalize through learned commentary. In the Hoffmann cases we see how he retells the story of the ogres of disease, the skeins of witchcraft, the visions of the melancholic in terms of specific diseases and somatic disorders.

If I now return to the question: Whose Enlightenment? The following points can be made: 1) medical enlightenment is geared towards common sense. Certainly the therapeutics arising from the medical commentary expound the simple and the abstemious. 2) In the illness narratives two different agendas interact. Talking about illness, as far as patient narratives are concerned, include beliefs in the supernatural. The patient narratives relate these perceptions to the drama of illness. The medical narrative, however, disclaims such interpretations. In Friedrich Hoffmann's case histories ideas about the supernatural and mental disorders are somaticized.

The Parts and the Whole

In Hoffmann's case histories he develops the rationale of the medical Enlightenment by using overt symptom observation and an internal physiological explanation of the body's functions as overriding medical concerns. Hoffmann tries to demonstrate the causal connection between symptoms and specific pathological diagnosis. The theory of physiology and pathology was used as an instrument for solving analytical medical questions as *systems,* that is, finding the common denominators linking health and illness. In regard to the living body the learned physician was confronted with the specific dilemma of having to speculate about dynamic processes, as, for example, those internal workings that result in secretions and excretions. Or, indeed, to try and ascertain what the movement of the blood and other fluids in the body and the 'fibres' (a term encompassing muscles and other tonic or active tissues, such as organs) really was. In order to tell this scientific story, learned medicine had to create theoretical systems descriptive of physiology and of pathological 'reality'.[34]

The word often used as a descriptive tool in the eighteenth century for this problem is *pathiognomic*.[35] As in the word physiognomic, more familiar from nineteenth-century readings of facial characteristics that were thought to indicate basic traits of personality, pathiognomic readings refer to the 'picture' or 'face' of disease. Such a reading of the shape or 'gestalt' of a disease describes more than random symptoms or signs; it locates a characteristic pattern of illness.

To return to a case mentioned earlier, the child-murder committed by the man diagnosed as suffering from melancholia, melancholia was medically seen to originate in the obstruction of the blood-flow through the *vasa cerebri*. The *commercio anima et animae cum corpore* could no longer function in its normal tonic balance (fluids and fibres), and this 'stagnation' and lack of proper circulation led to 'heat' in the head, and this, in turn, caused fear, depression, feelings of terror and intense worry (*Furcht, Betruebnis, Angst und Sorge*).[36] Although we might dismiss the crudeness of such materialist ideas today, the basic principle Hoffmann tried to set up for medical explanation holds some truth. He was seeking to establish mental and physical links in such a way that particular disorders in the material functions of the body could be identified as causing a disease state, in this case the nervous disorder of melancholia.[37] It is a functionalist model and it illustrates well what is meant by 'mechanical' medicine, the new theoretical speculation about internal physiology extolled by most mainstream physicians of the medical Enlightenment.

The theoretical systematization in physiology and pathology in medicine represented the political agenda of the profession. It cut across story-telling with its appeal to 'guardian' healers, its ogres and witches, and produced the Enlightenment we recognize, where the mysteries of life are tagged and labelled with morals and explained by science. Rationality was the agent for making the constructs of popular belief seem like so many chimeras.

Whose Enlightenment? is answered by saying it was the professionals who imposed explanations by fixing parameters. Of course, it didn't last. Anti-Enlightenment writers like E. T. A. Hoffmann (no relation to Friedrich) dipped their pen into an acid scepticism regarding rationalism when they took up the question of illusory appearances. In *Der Goldene Topf* (The Pot of Gold) E. T. A. Hoffmann uses the ambivalence between illusion and reality to unsettle flat common sense.[38] As Walter Benjamin writes in his famous book on baroque tragedy: 'Ghosts, like deeply meaningful allegories, are apparitions from the realm of grief; through those who grieve, the melancholic who ponders over symbols and the future, the subjects conjured make their appearances.'[39] These are the associations that Friedrich Hoffmann missed: the power of the mind to elucidate complex emotions. Feelings conjure sensual images and stories hold them.

Thus the world of learned medicine created a 'whole' based on the 'animal economy', rather than the soul. The popular culture of the body and what it could embody by way of spirit, mind or soul, was supplanted. But traditions in the popular mind (such as folklore) retained gods, spirits and saints, a story-telling insight into the soul's dialectic with 'active' substances. This enabled the imagination to forge symbolic awareness of a world of nature not reducible to exact science: apparitions, visualizations and emotions as symbols of the whole do relate to subjective 'ghosts', that is, illness perceived as a personal experience of the body *and* mind.

Whose Enlightenment? has to be a two-way street, a twice-told tale. In the medical life-narrative of the eighteenth century the story creates its own narrative space. It is moulded into another shape, the mechanical model, but like Alice in the looking-glass, it can be read backwards to reveal other depths.

Notes

1. W. Martens, *Die Botschaft der Tugend, die Aufklaerung im Spiegel der deutschen Moralischen Wochenschriften* (Stuttgart: J. B. Metzler, 1968). See also, for a different approach: T. Laqueur, 'Bodies, Details, and the Humanitarian Narrative', in L. Hunt (ed.), *The New Cultural History* (Berkeley, 1989), 176–204.
2. Published collections of medical case histories, and periodicals that also printed cases, began to flourish in Germany in the eighteenth century. The starting point is probably the 1708 publication of cases documenting the therapeutic efficacy of the *essentia dulcis,* see C. F. Richter, *Merckwürdige Exempel sonderbahrer durch die Essentiam Dulcem (von Anno 1701 bisz 1708) geschehenen Curen* (Halle: Waisenhaus Verlag, 1708). For those collections cited for this essay see below. Medical case-history literature of the life-narrative kind continues to be published throughout the century; only when the hospital case record was introduced is diagnostic reduction, of 'irrelevant' information, practised. Collections of case histories of the narrative type were obviously widely read, otherwise the book market would not have been keen to publish such volumes year after year.
3. See *passim:* F. Hoffmann, *Medicina Consultatoria,* Theile 1–12 (Halle: Renger, 1721–39).
4. J. Geyer-Kordesch, Medizinische Fallbeschreibungen und ihre Bedeutung in der Wissensreform des 17. und 18. Jahrhunderts,

Medizin in Geschichte und Gesellschaft, Heft 9, 1991, 7–19; *idem*, 'Chemie and Alchemie: J. J. Becher, G. E. Stahl, J. S. Carl und J. C. Dippel', in G. Fruehsorge and G. Strasser (eds), *Johann Joachim Becher 1635–1682 (Wolfenbuettel, Wolfbuettler Arbeiten zur Barockforschung*, in press 1993).

5. E. Fischer-Homberger, *Medizin vor Gericht, Gerichtsmedizin von der Renaissance bis zur Aufklaerung* (Bern: Hans Huber, 1983), 308–82.
6. Fisher-Homberger, *op. cit.* (note 5), particularly her chapter on 'Doctors and Demons', 134–52. Other writings by Fischer-Homberger, listed in her book are illuminating on the link between early psychiatry and medicine.
7. See especially the exhibition catalogues: Oesterreichisches Museum fuer Volkskunde, *Die Groteske in der Volkskunst* (Vienna: 1975); *Niederoesterreichische Landesausstellung, Groteskes Barock* (Stift Altenburg: 1975).
8. S. Thomson, 'The Folk-Tale since Basile', in N. M Penzer, *The Pentamerone of Giambattista Basile*, 2 vols (Oxford: John Lane, The Bodley Head Ltd, 1932) 286–304.
9. A. Carter, 'About the Stories', in *Sleeping Beauty and Other Favourite Fairy Tales* (London: Gollancz, 1991), 125–8; for this quote, 126.
10. J. Geyer-Kordesch, 'Passions and the ghost in the machine: or what not to ask about science in seventeenth- and eighteenth-century Germany', in R. French and Andrew Wear (eds), *The Medical Revolution of the Seventeenth Century* (Cambridge: Cambridge University Press, 1989), 154–63.
11. See, for example, Hoffmann, *op. cit.* (note 3), 1721; cases of poisoning: Decade I, cases: I, VI, VII. But most cases give graphic bodily observations.
12. For baroque and rococo, see A. Blunt, A. Lang, C. Tagdell, K. Downes, *Baroque and Rococo, Architecture and Decoration* (first published 1978; Ware, Hertfordshire: Wordsworth Editions, 1988); J. Seznec, *The Survival of the Pagan Gods, the Mythological Tradition and its Place in Renaissance Humanism and Art* (Princeton: Princeton University Press, 1972).
13. Hoffmann, *op. cit.* (note 3); forensic cases are interspersed with consultation cases. See also: M. Alberti, *Systema jurisprudentiae medicae* (Halle: Vol. I: 1725; Vol. II, Fulda, 1729; Vol. III, Schneeberg,1733; Leipzig, Vol. IV, 1737; Leipzeg, Vol. V, 1740; Leipzig, Vol. IV, 1747).
14. It should be noted that the Hoffmann cases are different from the traditional collections because they are *not* republished from previous medical literature. They, in effect, largely represent Hoffmann's private practice observations and consultations.
15. Hoffmann, *op. cit.* (note 3), Decade 4, Case I, 151–5.
16. *Ibid.*, 151. The translations from the German are my own.
17. *Ibid.*, 152.

18. *Ibid.*, 153.
19. *Ibid.*
20. J. Weyer, *De praestigiis daemonum. Witches, Devils, and Doctors in the Renaissance* (Medieval and Renaissance Texts and Studies, Vol. 73, Centre for Medieval and Early Renaissance Studies, Binghamton, N.Y.: 1991). Therein see John Weber, 'Foreword', LI.
21. *Ibid.*
22. Hoffmann, *op. cit.* (note 3), Theil I, Deade III, Case VIII, 142–5.
23. *Ibid.*, 142.
24. *Ibid.*, 145.
25. Weyer, *op. cit.* (note 20), LXIII.
26. Hoffmann, *op. cit.* (note 3), Decade I, Case IV, 16–23.
26. *Ibid.*
27. *Ibid.*
28. *Ibid.*
29. *Ibid.*, 19.
30. *Ibid.*
31. *Ibid.*
32. *Ibid.*, 23
33. J. Geyer-Kordesch, 'Georg Ernst Stahl's Radical Pietist Medicine and its Influence on the German Enlightenment', in A. Cunningham and R. French (eds), *The Medical Enlightenment of the Eighteenth Century* (Cambridge: Cambridge University Press,1990), 67–87.
34. The eighteenth century created a systematised theory of medicine; in reference to Germany, major texts include: G. E. Stahl, *Theoria medica vera* (Halle: Waisenhaus Verlag, 1708), F. Hoffmann, *Medicinae rationalis systematicae* (Halle: Renger,1718–20, 2 vols) and the works of Albrecht von Haller.
35. For a contemporary definition, see J. Storch, *Praxis Stahliana* (Leipzig: Eyssel, 1732), 153ff.
36. F. Hoffmann, *op. cit.* (note 3), Decade I, Case IV, 20.
37. *Ibid.*, also A. O. Goelicke and J. P. Burggrau, *De existentia spirituum nervosarum* (n. p., 1725).
38. E. T. A. Hoffmann, *Gesammelte Schriften* (Berlin, Georg Reimer, 1871–3) Bd. VII.
39. W. Benjamin, *Ursprung des Deutschen Trauerspiels* (Frankfurt am Main: Suhrkamp Verlag, 1963): This quote cited in R. Alewyn (ed.), *Deutsche Barockforschung, Dokumentation einer Epoche* (Berlin: Kiepenheuer und Witsch, 1965), 398. The translation is my own.

4

Sarah Stone: Enlightenment Midwife

Isobel Grundy

'Enlightenment midwife' sounds like an oxymoron. Midwives of the eighteenth century and earlier are often presented as forces of darkness: ignorant, superstitious, resistant to change and progress, even when not actually heavy drinkers or practisers of witchcraft.[1] Male take-over of birth procedures was constructed by the takers-over as improvement or reform. This construction is no longer universally accepted as self-evident; as Adrian Wilson remarks, it depends on one's point of view whether the replacement of midwife by male midwife is seen as heroic revolution or tragic decline. Wilson, however, is symptomatic. Presenting himself as impartial balancer of these two viewpoints, he nevertheless takes it for granted that a man would succeed where a woman would fail.[2]

The Enlightenment, though like other movements it was too complex and disparate to be easily definable, implies the testing and often the discarding of tradition. It suggests a shift from faith to reason, from authority to experiment, from tales or annals to analysis, generalization, and abstraction. This shift has been read by both orthodox and feminist scholars as inimical to the female.[3] Nature is a female body exposed to the gaze, intervention and control of the male scientist. That which is replaced by scientific, objective knowledge is categorized as 'old wives' tales'; modes of knowledge possessed by women are downgraded as insufficiently logical or specialized.

Rare indeed is the male enlightenment scientist who recognizes women's claim to knowledge even of female phenomena. One such exception is the anatomist James Drake: declining to stoop to refuting rumours that menstrual blood has harmful or poisonous properties, he remarks that the rumours serve 'to shew what things have been superstitiously taken up upon Credit, without sufficient Examination by Men of great Authority, who have been prevail'd upon to believe, what the Women at all times would laugh at.' Drake, unusually, had a sister who possessed both medical knowledge and feminist sentiments (and who may, indeed, have edited his great work on anatomy after his premature death).[4]

None the less Sarah Stone, who trained in midwifery late in the seventeenth century, and practised until at least 1737, was both a champion of her sex and a disciple and advocate of the Enlightenment. Nature is her watchword: a very Enlightenment nature, non-numinous, knowable, requiring intellectual effort and cooperative guidance from human beings. Ignorance is the dragon which Stone heroically combats and often vanquishes. Outspoken about the ignorance of local, traditional midwives, she is yet more critical of the male upstarts who, claiming to represent science, really stand for a new and pernicious form of Authority ranged against Experience. Proud of having, unusually for a woman, 'read Anatomy' and 'seen several Women open'd', not averse to carrying out her own investigatory dissections of infant corpses, she none the less rates her practical apprenticeship to her mother as her most valuable qualification; without that, she says, she would have remained ignorant.[5]

The battle for control of the birth-chamber, argues Wilson, was not a simple old-new, female-male contest, but instead a conflict belonging exclusively to men-midwives, among whom it pitted against each other 'forceps practitioners and Deventerians'. For Wilson, these two groups *share* their superiority to female practitioners: 'Earlier male access to difficult births meant the delivery of a living child, rather than a dead child.'[6] This reading assumes the non-existence of skilled women, and the impracticability of Stone's project for properly qualified women to train others, so that male help (with or without forceps) might remain a rare last resort.

Her *Complete Practice of Midwifery*, finished in 1736, printed with her name after her move from the provinces to London in 1737, has received little attention in the current debate over reform versus decline.[7] She is a figure inhabiting many margins: a female devotee of reason and science, a Christian believer who invokes God at moments of crisis yet has no patience with more fatalistic piety, a professional who pursues career moves upwards yet chooses to write about her first and poorest practice. Her preface defines herself in contrast to the new male midwives; her case studies define herself in contrast to local, female ones. She balances esteem for 'men of erudition, grave and sedate', with indignant contempt for 'young Gentlemen pretenders' with no knowledge of the healthy female body but only of dissection (xvi, xi–xii).

She was practising in Bridgwater, Somerset, by about 1701, after six years as deputy to her mother, a renowned midwife (xix, xxiii).[8] She moved to Taunton about 1703, soon after her mother's death, and practised for more than 17 years there and across a wide swathe of Somerset, latterly bringing 'at least three hundred Children a year into the World'. The damaging pressure of overwork drove her, she said, to move to Bristol (138–9). Ambition as well as self-protection may have been involved: as the single midwife of any training or standing in a rural-industrial area without male practitioners, she would have met with little informed appreciation or remuneration. Recognition and a higher income, as well as the sharing of burdens and responsibilities with many colleagues – or rivals – of both sexes, awaited her in opulent and fashionable Bristol. When, after 16 more years, she moved with her husband to London, she had a daughter with ten years' experience as a qualified midwife, and had already drafted her book on the subject. She was impelled to write, she says, by Bristol experience of over-rated male practitioners and over-used forceps.[9] Her text, however, gives very little space to the years after 1720. It frames its bulk of Taunton and rural cases with an opening four cases from Bridgwater and a closing three from Bristol, the last one dating from only four years before she wrote of it.

Her lengthy sub-title expounds her themes: her belief that difficulties occurring naturally are outweighed by those created by human rashness, ignorance, or lack of experience. Her dedication to Queen Caroline (who was to die that year, repeating Elizabeth Cellier's bad luck in dedicating to James II in 1688) indicates her Court Whig sympathies; Wilson links this political stance with progressive views but also with Hendrick van Deventer, and with coolness towards forceps but also with males. Stone's preface gives her new address: Piccadilly, 'over-against the Right Hon. the Earl of *Burlington*'s' (xx). Printing a letter to her husband from the 'justly celebrated' Dr Allen establishes a link with a higher rung of the medical profession, and corroborates Sarah's account of her career with a brief, flattering resumé (xxi–xxiv).

Ignorance, as Stone perceives and attacks it, is an anti-Enlightenment trait. She certainly does not favour technical ignorance (neither of dissection, for instance, nor of forceps use), but such ignorance is not a moral failing in the way that ignorance of anatomy is. Anatomy is nature, and ignorance of nature is more damaging than ignorance of art, for nature subsumes art: knowledge of art *alone* is just another form of ignorance.

Knowledge of Nature, not inborn but learned by arduous experience, gives us the terms of female heroism. Stone's text is unlike most midwifery treatises in the importance to it of the author's self-construction. Generically multiple, it is both autobiography or apology and collection of tales, as well as advertisement, polemic, scientific report and teaching text. It demands literary analysis, not only because of the literary skill it displays, but because of the degree to which it is shaped by techniques borrowed from heroic romance and scriptural narrative. Stone fashions herself as a hero, whose labours, like those of Psyche rather than those of Hercules, involve a non-climactic series of patient, resolute cooperations. Stone as romance hero proves invincible against her personified adversaries, Ignorance and Rashness, as she repeatedly encounters them in other people, and even in their internalized forms. Like the hero tested by specious disguises, she rejects the temptation of internal rashness when it falsely masquerades as courage, and she steadily diminishes the area of her own ignorance over the course of her work (both her practice and her writing). Even the last case in the book recounts her mastery of a new skill, a new piece of knowledge.

Though the preface asserts the equal or greater rashness and ignorance of trendy young male midwives (among whom Stone had worked, at Bristol, almost as long as she had in a region free from them), the book effects no such exposé of them as of the outdated women of Somerset. Perhaps Stone was unwilling to make gender the leading determinant in her construction of herself as practitioner. Or perhaps she simply failed to complete a Bristol section of her observations. While each tale, as they stand, deploys a firm closure of death or survival, the collection as a whole breaks off abruptly. The last ends on 'a difficult work; and it is not to be done without knowledge and resolution; but, praised be the Almighty God, I accomplished it': a resounding closure to this one case, yet still a lame one for the series as a whole (163).

Stone's contextualizing of birth practices is also unusual, even though her attention to social detail is intermittent. Her clients (some of her own, some taken over in emergency, in a manner which Wilson connects with male midwives only) include gentlewomen (six mentioned), women with specified occupations, and others defined by their husband's occupation. Stone specifies the employment of only three women (weaver, washerwoman and schoolmistress). Of these the first two are back within two or three weeks of giving birth at the work which Stone blames for their failure to produce a living child. She probably mentions their trades for this reason, rather than because they were unusual in having trades.

The 27 husbands' occupations mentioned (besides, presumably, six gentlemen and a perhaps unemployed 'poor man') comprise a remarkably homogeneous society sustained by animal husbandry and its offshoots the wool and leather trades. Combers (seven) balance farmers (six). Two smiths, a shepherd, a butcher, and a soap-boiler (dependent on agriculture) balance two weavers, a tucker, a serge-maker and a tailor (dependent on wool) and a tanner, a cobbler and a shoe-maker (dependent on leather). Least closely tied to the land is an innkeeper. In this tightly-knit society, where a well-developed grapevine links genteel with ungenteel houses (97–9), the midwife seems to be at home everywhere. She is not a scientifically detached observer of this society, but adds some social protest: against the prevalence of 'illiterate and unskilful' midwives (who need to be trained, not done away with), and against the rigours of weaving and combing (which cause 'many Wrong Births and Bad Labours ... among the poorer sort' of Somerset women: xiii).

Stone's range spanned 15 or 20 miles from north to south, and from east to west: it covered the wetlands of Sedgemoor (commons and moors in eighteenth-century terminology), rich lowland pasture, and villages tucked under the Quantock and Blackdown hills. Unlike male local writers, she has little interest in natural description (she notes dirty roads or mean houses, not productivity or improvements), and none in genealogical or ecclesiastical matters.[10] Her gentlewomen remain as anonymous as her washerwoman. She never mentions whether a baby being born is an heir, nor whether, if born in distress, it is baptised at once. She seems not to think, like William Smellie, of obstetric killing in terms of 'destroy[ing] the hopes of the parents'.[11] Her babies, born in rooms full of attendant women, are not yet socialized into patriarchal society. Stone presents this in no rosy light, but presents it as fact.

More systematically and variously than any other contemporary writer, she puts flesh and bones on statistics of childbirth perils. These nearly 50 births (four of the 42 observations detail more than one case) are not, of course, a representative selection from the several thousand she must have attended in Somerset. By definition they are problem cases (trouble-free birth is mentioned only once, and then only because it runs concurrently with someone else's problems), and they are also Sarah Stone's triumphs. They recount three maternal deaths in childbed or soon afterwards; 25 infants do not survive. Of 44 maternal survivors, a majority experience a more or less close brush with death: 'with the symptoms of Death in her face, and all spectators pronouncing Death against her' (11–12); 'to all human reason expiring' (15). Once Stone demurs at taking on a patient who is such a bad risk, but agrees to out of compassion (18). Many women are described as low-spirited or despairing during labour: one says she won't be touched, but 'chose to die, rather than go through any more Pain in that manner' (27); another, enduring nine days of violent pains, 'often begg'd the Women to kill her' (102). Six or eight miscarriages before bearing a living child are not uncommon (148–9). Of 14 labours to which Stone is summoned because they are going badly, the average length has been very near three days and nights. Even omitting one nine-day labour (in which the baby died early and putrified), the average is still above three days and two nights.

As protagonist of her own stories, Stone relates to her clients with compassion as well as with succour. She relates, however, as a professional; she does not mention her own childbearing experiences, though they must have overlapped with this part of her career. She relates to the rural midwives with forthright and rigorous professional judgement. Her assessments are not a whit gentler than those of the strongest advocate of male appropriation, but for the most part they avoid rhetorically explicit condemnation. It is the midwives' lack of resources, lack of an agenda for action, to which Stone addresses herself.

Midwives' blunders are recorded in most of her observations, together with those of the relations, neighbours, female servants or 'Handy Women (as they call them)' (28), who are almost indistinguishable from midwives proper. (Where Smellie compares the practice of London and Paris, Stone records the practices of Hatch and Creech and Curry Mallet, putting forward no other authority for her own better practice besides its conformity with nature and its experiential success.) The first observation presents a midwife 'in a sound sleep' while her patient, after three days in labour without ever going to bed, is 'reduced to the utmost degree of Weakness .... her Spirits quite exhausted'. Stone dislodges the baby from the *os pubis* and delivers it in three hours, 'to the grand surprize of her Midwife, when awake, who seem'd glad the Child was born alive, she believing it dead the day before' (1–3).

The dry humour of 'when awake', the tone of restrained understatement or *satire manqué*, is characteristic of Stone; the midwife is typical too. Country practice was to keep women in labour out of bed, though more alternatives were available than many historians note.[12] Stone mentions the use of a birthing-stool, or a close-stool filled with warm water ('The first Child fell into the pan of water; notwithstanding which, it was alive when I came there': 65–6), or kneeling (a usual but 'wretched' way: 71), or 'leaning forward on the back of a chair' (85), or standing up (which proves doubly fatal in a case – not one of Stone's – involving an unusually short cord and a 'feeble ancient' midwife: 55). Though Stone thinks it best to give birth in bed, she values a free choice for her client more highly than a 'correct' one.

Sometimes what midwives lack is manual skill. Two of them spend a day and a night trying vainly to turn a child, before Stone does so 'with a great deal of ease in less than ten minutes' (85–6). Their inability was not unusual: Drake writes that if 'a *Hand*, a *Foot*, a *Knee*, or an *Elbow*' presents, '*Delivery* is impractable, and unless the *Midwife* has the Address and Skill to turn it, as they boast that they do sometimes, either Mother or Child, or both, must be lost' (312). But this skill, implies Stone, can be taught by her book: the midwives had been trying vainly to force the infant's presenting arm back into the mother's body, causing her terrible pain. Stone finds 'liberty enough, with gentle proceeding and strength, to pass by the Arm, and come at the Feet', as she has always succeeded in doing in such cases.

More frequently the obstacle is simple ignorance of anatomy. Most midwives are unable to ascertain, as Stone can, when the baby is stuck on the *os pubis:* one 'could give me no account, whether the Child was [lying] right or wrong' (81). 'The practice of Midwives, in general', with a child wedged on the pubic bone, is to press hard on the back part of the body (9), or to 'press back the *Os Sacrum* with all one's strength, the breadth of one's hand', or else to urge the mother to push harder and harder although, as Stone tartly observes, 'it was impossible it could come through the bones' (144). Another common practice in a difficult labour is to work on stretching the anus, 'opening the outer gate ... to help the inner' (24).

Ignorance extends beyond bone-structure to the processes of parturition itself. Often such things as colic or constipation or even smallpox (62–4, 89, 94) are mistaken for labour pains: 'Forc'd Deliveries in these Cases, have destroyed many Lives' (75). One midwife is unable, after premature birth, to bring the afterbirth away (14); most are powerless to stop haemorrhaging. Tight lacing is advised in pregnancy, even when the woman 'was usually sick, and fainted three or four times a day'; two week-long labours producing dead babies are diagnosed as 'owing to her not lacing straight enough'. (In this case it is the husband, appealed to for his authority, who risks breaking with tradition: 127–8.)

Lack of knowledge results in lack of control; this in turn encourages reliance on superstition or on medication (which seem to rank about equally in Stone's bad books). Sometimes in extremities a midwife will do nothing because she 'waited for Pains' or 'God's time was not come' or (in the case of a second twin) 'when the other apple was ripe, it would also fall' (27, 45, 66). Such passivity seems more likely to stem from not knowing *what* to do than from the old medical belief that it is the child in the womb which makes its own way out. Stone finds it usual, though 'intolerable', to administer 'hot forcing things' or 'strong waters' (48, 82). She makes no distinction between new commercialism and traditional nostrums, between proprietary brands like Dr Stevens's (132), which produce fevers, and the much-favoured 'Husband's Water with the juice of Leeks', which is 'a horrid Medicine, and as often mischievous as prescrib'd' (96, 132, 103–4).

Local superstitions, recorded by Stone in the manner of an anthropologist, clearly reflect the desire to find meanings and patterns; they stand in for the missing anatomical and physical knowledge. Repetition (or consistency of experience) is expected. A woman whose first pregnancy ended after eight months (in stillbirth) is certain that her second will last no longer – and so are 'her Midwife and Women' (113). A shoemaker's wife (his second) is given up for lost because his first wife 'was in the very same case as this, and she died undelivered' (11). A more specific fear of the unknown or aberrant is particularly potent: long hair on a child in the womb signals a bad time for the mother (46); a woman reads the breaking of her waters a month early as 'a token of her death, because her Children always followed her Waters' (124). Stone causes alarm and disapproval (not in either case to the patient but to gossips and advisers), once because the delivery is too quick and once because it is harder than that woman's former ones (140).

She herself entertains some unfounded beliefs: that a pregnant woman witnessing an abnormal birth will reproduce the same abnormality herself (21–3), and that to long for anything in pregnancy and not get it will endanger both mother and child (74). These beliefs (unlike the ones about long hair or a second wife repeating the experience of a first) could be compatible with belief in a physical rather than a magical universe. A foetus might respond to its mother's emotional experience in a nature which adhered strictly to its own laws, assuming such laws decreed close and physical interconnection of body and mind.

Midwives lack teaching not only in anatomy but in any code of professional conduct. Several try to conceal their mistakes. One of St James's parish, Taunton, caught as it were *in flagrante*, after a two days' labour, the child dead in the womb with one 'Arm hal'd out as far as the Shoulder', slips off home once Stone has been sent for, leaving other women instructed to deny that any midwife had been present. When summoned to return, she refuses, since Stone 'had been often after her bad works, and could not help condemning her for keeping Women long in hand, as she usually did, not suffering me to be sent for till the Child was dead, and the Woman in great danger' (41–2). A child presenting face-foremost has an eye put out and her 'upper Lip tore quite hollow from the Jaw-bone'; the midwife seeks refuge in the transparent falsehood that 'the Mother fell down two days before she was in Travail, and, as she thought, hurt the Child' (52). Another tries to conceal from Stone a baby not only dead but mangled ('the left Arm was tore off, in a most indecent manner'), by sewing it up in a piece of flannel and covering it with flowers for burial (83).[13] But Stone does not use such horror stories as argument for putting female midwives out of business. This one, at the remote distance of 11 miles from Taunton, accepts admonishment and advice, 'acknowledg'd what I said was very just', and promises not to 'proceed so rashly for the future' (84). Even here enlightenment, it seems, is a viable project.

Only one of Stone's stories, the last, shows men so incompetent and uncandid: two of them, when a woman-midwife has failed to return a prolapsed womb into position, try to do this themselves but cannot, and take refuge in blaming the woman. Stone makes no comment on their record, but says the woman midwife 'should have presently sent for farther advice' (159–62). The line which she seeks to draw between the skilled and unskilled does not separate one gender consistently from the other. Nor does it separate written from unwritten authority: the futile practice of exerting pressure on the *os sacrum*, Stone says, is recommended in many books (156).

With her humdrum yet sensational raw material, Sarah Stone weaves a series of tales which possess the complex, compelling shapes of narrative art, and which succeed in realizing the experience of birth-attendance in a manner extremely rare in the literature. All but one begin with some variant of 'I was sent for': the first-person singular is given pre-eminence, the sender deprived of agency.[14] The reader is led with Stone *through* each case, in several stages of process: journey (sometimes), first impression ('I found her very low and weak'), listening (often) to the testimony and emotional outpouring of others, then through first-hand investigation and findings ('I then thought it highly necessary to inform myself of the reasons of her violent Flooding; and Touching her found ....' Threat and danger is reduced by learning and understanding into a problem to be solved. This particular narrative is succinct, concentrated, uninterrupted (92–3); more frequently the exposition leads into a developed sequence of struggle, alternating gains and reversals. Often the action is varied by dialogue between Stone and others present, by expression of her feelings, or by analysis of the case in relation to others or to general principles, with professional and moral lessons drawn. Closure often combines the resolution of specific action ('The Child had been dead some time, but the Mother recover'd': 86) with comment. This ranges from a mere placing reference ('which is common in those Labours': 54) to statement of authorial purpose: 'This Observation I have set down to caution those professing the Art of Midwifery, to be well assur'd of a True Labour, before they begin their Work' (91–2).

Defeat and triumph jostle together in the tales. Often a child's death, recorded as a grievous blow, is softened by its mother's survival, apparently against the odds. Most striking of these is the case of the schoolmistress's baby, which 'suck'd my finger in the Womb, which concern'd me; fearing it impossible for the poor Infant to be born alive'. Here the midwife has to override her merely human compassion. 'But recovering my thoughts, I resolved to do my duty for the poor Woman's sake, and leave the event to the Omniscient God.' The effort required is of two parallel kinds: 'resolved with all my [physical] strength, and a full [mental] resolution, to accomplish what I was about.' Despite limited finger grip and repeated cramps in the hand and arm, Stone manages to drag out the child's feet:

> then I wrapt them in a linnen cloth, and gave them to two strong Women, and desir'd them to draw in a strait line, whilst I took care of the Woman's body, to prevent any injury, and secure the Child that it might be brought off whole; which, thro' mercy I compleated. ... The Child had not the least appearance of life, and 'twas impossible it should .... I don't remember above four such terrible Labours, in all my practice. The Woman did well. I have set this Observation down as plain as possible, to encourage Midwives, that they may with justice and safety go thro' the most difficult part of their work, as well as that which is easy. (77–80)

The observation closes on the physical pain which this delivery causes the midwife-heroine for 'near a week'.

Her concern to bring out this lifeless body 'whole' is one seldom addressed by either eighteenth- or twentieth-century discussions of forceps use. Drake, without mentioning male practitioners, writes that in the 'deplorable Case' where a child cannot be delivered, 'the Life of the Mother is generally preferr'd to that of the Child, and the Child, by means of Instruments, has been brought away by Piecemeal' (312–13). Stone, who claims to support the use of forceps in cases of real need, reveals here a reason for regret, at least, over their use even in stillbirth.

The very rare *wholly* bleak endings to her tales make their effect through surprise and shock. When 'the Life of the Mother, and two Children were lost for want of judgment, and good management', that follows Stone's delivery of undiagnosed twin sons, alive, from a woman near death after three days' labour. All three, in surviving the birth, pass the borders of Stone's power; and all die. The model here is near-epic telling of a gallant, doomed attempt, without the warning or punitive note common in other writers' case histories of disaster. When, for instance, the French midwife Louise Bourgeois writes 'Of a Woman, that because she would not be ruled in her Lying in, died', she concludes with a general assertion of her powers: 'See here how ill a thing it is to be opinionated; for I could easily have delivered her, if she would have been ruled by me.'[15] Stone does not make such claims, which would sit badly with her posture as representative of the broader values of reason. She seldom condemns midwives, and never mothers, as sweepingly as this. In her tales ignorance typically meets with enlightenment, not punishment, 'encouragement', not deterrence. A defeat for Judgement is a defeat for Stone as champion of Judgement; a disaster to mother or child is a disaster to Stone, as centre of subjectivity in her own narrative.

A typical sequence is for Stone to arrive at a case, listen, *touch*, and deliver. The word 'touch', as technical term for skilled manual internal examination, is hardly a matter of choice; yet it sounds also like a deliberate echo of gospel accounts of Christ's life-saving miracles.[16] (Listening and delivering are also, of course, divine activities.) The allusion is confirmed in Observation Five, where the women tell Stone 'That had I been with the first wife, she had not died' (12), in an echo of words spoken by both Martha and Mary, sisters of Lazarus (John, xi, 21, 32). This points the parallel. Stone makes, of course, no claim to Christ's power to undo death: there is no question of a raising like that of Lazarus for the shoemaker's long-dead first wife, no possibility of granting the mute appeal of the schoolmistress's doomed baby. The human healer treads consciously in the steps of a divine master; but she neither emulates Christ nor fathoms the apparently harsh decrees of God.

The regularity with which Stone is proved *right* suggests a parallel with a particular breed of modern hero, the fictional detective. Like her namesake by birth, Sherlock Holmes, the midwife-heroine makes no serious errors of judgement, and invariably emerges vindicated (though often puzzled or emotionally shaken) where others are baffled. Like Holmes, she credits her art or science, not herself. But unlike his (or Christ's) her system of knowledge is limited, never to be counted on as perfect except as it is renewed, verified, and extended by each successive case.

The narrator's self-presentation, therefore, is crucially unstable, constantly needing renewal by one tale after another. A claim to authority which is not (like a man's) institutional or conferred by degree, but is based on experience, is not achieved but in process. The successful midwife, delivering her clients, also depends on them for her knowledge and power. At her outset she is 'thought too young' (3). Through her attendance on others is mediated her discipleship, not to any teacher, but to Nature. For them she hopes, through her book, to continue her beneficial influence 'when in my grave' (138–9). She expresses this hope in Observation 39, which sums up her time at Taunton and justifies her leaving it on health grounds. Bedridden herself in this tale, she receives steadily escalating calls for help all night, and finally at 5 a.m. has herself supported by two people to and from the childbed. This expenditure of her own body in pursuit of her calling is a vital element in her construction of her midwife identity as one combining care and vulnerability with power.

In her last few observations, Stone presents herself as still learning, her art still living, self-shaping, not perfected. She marks the difference of her new milieu from Somerset with medical, not social, detail. Her pre-Bristol cases have mentioned only three physicians, each summoned in dire emergency, none of them strikingly effective. One is helpless in face of smallpox (96); one is able to halt bleeding but not to prevent its recurrence (105–6). The last orders fomentations and prescribes 'a great many proper medicines' for a case of postpartum pain and urine retention; but he seeks diagnostic advice from Stone and another midwife, and leaves it to Stone to institute regular use of a catheter. It seems magnanimous of her to attribute the woman's recovery, after two weeks at death's door, to his care rather than her own (134–6). Perhaps her text conceals some personal loyalty to this 'Gentleman of E[r]udition and Judgment'.

In Bristol, midwife-doctor relations are touchier, and the last few observations are more interrupted than others with digression, comparison and self-justification. The first physician encountered there differs in opinion with Stone as to whether or not to deliver a woman who is six months pregnant and repeatedly haemorrhaging: Stone is vindicated since the mother sides with her, and becomes a grateful and regular client (145–8). In the second Bristol case which she relates, Stone repeatedly urges that a man-midwife should be sent for, who, she apparently assumes, would use an 'Instrument' to unbrain the child and save the mother; although her confidence ebbs and flows, on balance she expects saving the mother to entail killing the child. She shows her distaste for instruments as unexpectedly vindicated when she manages to turn the child by hand and thus save both parties (149–54). On the other hand, she leaves herself open to criticism for having tried hard to hand over the case to a man only too likely, by her own account, to prove a killer. Yet this story captures the fear and loss of confidence under whose influence women were likely to call for forceps and men were likely to use them. By enacting fear and uncertainty, Stone's tales put the affect – the terror and the pity – back into midwifery. In doing so they realize for us some reasons for the spread of forceps which are essential to understanding the history of childbirth, but which are largely erased from contemporary treatises and theoretical writing, and from the historical record.

Sarah Stone is a daughter both of the Enlightenment and of a tradition of female solidarity; she seeks to bring the two streams together, by amelioration, not revolution. Professionalism for her entails moral qualities like patience and courage, which often spell the difference between survival and death. It also entails a commitment to teaching and improvement. Her book constructs its author: a woman who works with women, who works with brain and brawn, with study, emotion and prayer. It is a useful corrective to any belief in traditional midwives as generally wise or in traditional childbirth as 'natural' or joyous. It is a corrective, too, to any idea that such beliefs are the corollary of a sympathetic view of midwives. Stone resembles dozens of women writers of the Enlightenment in attacking 'custom'. But where they generally refer to areas like marriage law or gendered education, where men are obviously the shapers and women the victims of custom, the midwife needs to debunk and reform a set of customs practised by women.

Stone wants women midwives not downgraded but uplifted to education and professional standards: liberated out of custom into knowledge and understanding. This is a project typical of the Enlightenment in what one might call its female manifestation: in tune with systematizations of data and the birth of statistics, but even more in tune with charity schools, inoculation for smallpox, the popularization of science, and the campaigns against slavery and cruelty to animals. It represents childbirth, and even a range of known complications of childbirth, as a matter of human passions and morals, in which the personalities of mother and helpers are of vital significance, which is highly dangerous but non-medicalized, continuous with active life. It recounts an ongoing, uncompleted mission of education and improvement for traditional female care-givers, instead of the polemic against the new ways which its preface seems to promise.

It may be that extraneous reasons like ill health or canny politics prevented Stone from narrating further cases from her Bristol practice. She might have feared to antagonize male practitioners, or she might have thought her own portrait shone more brightly flanked by ignorant women than by men who were sweeping all before them. But literary or generic reasons alone suffice to justify her ending where she does. The tales depict the midwife-hero as scrapping many victories or half-victories from her unequal antagonist, death; as cultivating, in a social context which had been backward even in 1720, a grassroots enlightenment that might have brought her 'Sisters Professors in the Art of Midwifery' into the modern scientific world, enabling them to docket hard as well as easy cases, 'finish'd with credit' (xix, 111).

By 1737, when Stone reached London and her already-drafted book reached print, this agenda was already *passé;* midwifery was dominated by a different plot, that of male appropriation. Smellie, publishing 13 years later, has much in common with Stone. He too can turn a child by hand and deliver it by the feet; he too thinks that real problems number single figures to a thousand births; he agrees with Stone on the best position for giving birth (though he has less value than she has for maternal choice); he too wishes to keep 'instruments and violent methods' to a minimum, and advises 'young practitioners' against them; he too disapproves 'strong fermented liquors' as causing fevers; he too holds that knowledge of anatomy, and experience of labours, are crucial (194–6, 199, 241, 258, 397, 4[4]6, 447). His single major disagreement with her is his certainty that competence is gendered. A female midwife, he advises, 'ought to avoid reflections upon male practitioners, and when she finds herself difficulted [sic] candidly have recourse to their assistance'. A male, on the other hand, 'instead of openly condemning her method of practice, (even though it should be erroneous) ought to make allowance for the weakness of the sex' (448). Excellent advice, no doubt, so long as the male has skill and the female has none; but useless to the skilful woman or the unskilful man, both of whom alike are stricken from the record.

Stone's preface reflects awareness of this trend, and gives some hint of the book she might have written about it. But the book she did write has the unusual plot of Woman as Enlightenment Hero. Many things would have been different if, as she wished, a woman-centred scientific training had become established in the field of childbirth. We shall improve our present understanding of the Enlightenment, as it did historically occur, when we recognize the complexities which have been concealed by insistence on gendering it male.

Notes

1. Cf. D. N. Harley, 'Ignorant Midwives: a Persistent Stereotype', *Bulletin of the Society for Social History of Medicine*, xxvii (1981), 6–9, and 'Historians as Demonologists: The Myth of the Midwife-witch', *Social History of Medicine*, 3 (1990), 1–26.
2. Sir George Clark, *A History of the Royal College of Physicians of London* (Oxford: Clarendon, 1964) ii, 501; Wilson, 'The Politics of Medical Improvement in Early Hanoverian London', in Andrew Cunningham and Roger French (eds), *The Medical Enlightenment of the Eighteenth Century* (Cambridge: Cambridge University Press, 1990), 35. Laurel Thatcher Ulrich assumes a golden age of midwifery: *A Midwife's Tale: The Life of Martha Ballard, Based on Her Diary, 1785–1812* (New York: Knopf, 1990). Thomas McKeown and R. G. Brown argue that the results of the forceps 'on the mortality of mother and child were extremely bad': 'Medical Evidence Related to English Population Changes in the Eighteenth Century', *Population Studies*, 9 (1955), 122.
3. Cf. Ruth Salvaggio, *Enlightened Absence, Neoclassical Configurations of the Feminine* (Chicago: University of Illinois Press, 1988).
4. James Drake, *Anthropologia Nova; or, a New System of Anatomy* (London: Samuel Smith and Benjamin Walford, 1707), 321–2: preface completed by Judith Drake, for whom see Virginia Blain, Patricia Clements and Isobel Grundy, *The Feminist Companion to Literature in English: Women Writers from the Middle Ages to the Present* (London: Batsford, 1990).
5. *A Complete Practice of Midwifery. Consisting of Upwards of Forty Cases or Observations in that valuable Art, selected from many Others, in the Course of a very Extensive Practice. And Interspersed With many necessary Cautions and useful Instructions, proper to be observed in the most Dangerous and Critical Exigencies, as well when the Delivery is difficult in its own Nature, as when it becomes so by the Rashness or Ignorance of Unexperienc'd Pretenders. Recommended to All Female Practitioners in an*

Art so important to the Lives and Well-Being of the Sex (London: T. Cooper, 1737), xv.

6. Wilson, *op. cit.* (note 2), 35–6. This recalls the views of Thomas Laqueur and Robert E. Erickson about the shift from one-sex to two-sex models of the body: that both doctrines were the property of male physicians, and that medically articulate women like Louise Bourgeois and Jane Sharp simply went along with this male orthodoxy (Laqueur, *Making Sex: Body and Gender from the Greeks to Freud* (Cambridge and London: Harvard University Press, 1990), 68; Erickson, review of Laqueur in *Eighteenth-Century Fiction*, 4:3 (April 1992), 271).
7. Less than the Chamberlen family, William Smellie, John Burton, William Hunter, Bourgeois, Sharp, Elizabeth Cellier or Elizabeth Nihell: e.g. James Hobson Aveling, *English Midwives: Their History and Prospects* (London: Churchill, 1872; repr. London: Elliott, 1967); Jean Donnison, *Midwives and Medical Men: A History of Inter-professional Rivalries and Women's Rights* (New York: Schocken Books, 1977; 2nd edn London: Historical Publications, 1988); Robert Erickson in Paul-Gabriel Boucé (ed.), *Sexuality in Eighteenth-Century Britain* (Manchester: Manchester University Press, 1982); Edward Shorter, *A History of Women's Bodies* (New York: Basic Books, 1982); Jean Towler and Jean Bramall, *Midwives in History and Society* (London: Croom Helm, 1986); Barbara Brand Schnorrenburg, 'Is Childbirth any Place for a Woman? The Decline of Midwifery in Eighteenth-Century England', *Studies in Eighteenth Century Culture*, x (1981), 393–408; Donna Landry and Gerald MacLean in *Eighteenth-Century Studies*, 23:4 (Summer 1990). Stone does not appear in Valerie Fildes (ed.), *Women as Mothers in Pre-Industrial England, Essays in Memory of Dorothy McLaren* (London and New York: Routledge, 1990), though her testimony would have been relevant more than once. Barbara Ehrenreich and Deirdre English in *Witches, Midwives and Nurses: A History of Women Healers* (New York: Feminist Press, 1973), give only a paragraph to seventeenth- and eighteenth-century midwives.
8. She is listed, but no further information given, in P. J. and R. V. Wallis, *Eighteenth Century Medics* (Newcastle-upon-Tyne: Project for Historical Bibliography, 1988). Nothing is said there of her mother ('the famous Mrs. *Holmes*' of Bridgwater, 'the best Midwife' ever known to Dr John Allen of Bristol), or of her husband, whose 'Profession' and 'Qualifications' Allen does not specify (*Complete Practice*, xxii–xxiii) – or of other women, like Judith Drake and Jane Barker, whose texts claim that they practised informal medicine.
9. Wilson locates the male take-over, 1720–50, in London (34).
10. As evinced in, for instance, *A Compleat History of Somersetshire* (Sherborne, 1742 [1743]). The Bodleian catalogue says this is extracted from *Magna Britannica et Hibernia, antiqua et nova* (in parts, 1715; 6 vols, 1720–31), by Thomas Cox; the Eighteenth

Century Short Title Catalogue ascribes it to John Stuckey.

11. Smellie, *A Treatise on the Theory and Practice of Midwifery* (London: D. Wilson, 1752), 194.
12. For instance Shorter, *op. cit.* (note 7), 57.
13. Shorter quotes Percivall Willughby on midwives concealing mistakes (81).
14. The only real exception, when someone else initiates the action, is Obs. XXXVI: 'A Farmer's Wife that lived two Miles in the Country [the tight-lacing woman], came to speak with me' (126).
15. Stone may well have taken her term for her case histories from Bourgeois, *Observations diverses* (1609). She would have known this from its incorporation in Thomas Chamberlen's long-term best-seller, *The Complete Midwives Practice* (1656), a likely source for the title of her book itself. I have quoted from Chamberlen's 4th edn (1680), as probably the one used by Stone's mother and therefore first known to herself. Its case histories, set into discursive exposition, are too few to amount to a composite narrative like hers.
16. For instance Matthew, viii, 3, ix, 29; Mark, i, 41, viii, 22; Luke, v, 13; cf. Smellie, 180.

5

Developing Medical Expertise: Medical Practitioners and the Suspected Murders of New-Born Children

Mark Jackson

Introduction

Throughout the eighteenth century, medical practitioners of all persuasions became interested, and influentially involved, in investigations into the suspected murders of new-born children. Physicians, surgeons, apothecaries and both male and female midwives examined women suspected of having given birth to bastards, inspected and dissected the bodies of dead new-born children, and gave evidence at inquests, at magistrates' hearings and at the assize courts. In addition, medical practitioners were prominent in promoting a new, ostensibly more humane, account of the behaviour of women accused of this crime.

The extent of medical interest in cases of suspected new-born child murder ran contrary to the general neglect of legal medicine in this period, a neglect marked by the absence of legislative provisions for the admission of medical evidence at inquests or in the trial courts, by the lack of English texts on medical jurisprudence until the end of the century, and by the low status of the coroner and his inquest.[1] Elsewhere I have argued that the major reason for medical interest in these cases was the construction of a statute of 1624, which directed that any woman found to have concealed the death of a bastard child was to be found guilty of murder unless she could prove that the child had been born dead.[2] Both initial use and later disuse of the statute focused the attention of the courts on signs of still and live birth. I do not wish to discuss the medico-legal implications of the statute and its application here. Instead I wish to examine the manner in which medical practitioners became practically involved in the examination of suspects and suspected victims, and the extent to which they contributed to a novel construction of the behaviour and guilt of accused women.[3]

Examining Suspects

Once suspicions that a woman had given birth to, and possibly murdered, a bastard child had spread through a village, township or parish, the woman's neighbours made every effort to discover 'what she had done with the said Child or where she had hid or concealed it'.[4] The neighbours' approach was ruthless. They interrogated the suspect, searched the woman's rooms or house for evidence of delivery and for the body itself, and arranged for a physical examination of the suspect for signs of recent delivery. Occasionally, in the north of England, this bodily examination was carried out by a 'Jury of Matrons' carefully selected from the neighbourhood as experts in the matter by virtue of their own experience as child bearers:[5]

> they were warned and requested by Mr. Robert Proud of Hovingham aforesaid the Constable as well as eleven other respectable Matrons of different Townships or villages all having had Children and Child bearing women to wait upon Frances Harrison ... Singlewoman with an Intent and on Purpose to inspect and examine her state and condition whether she had lately been delivered of a Child or not.[6]

In most cases of suspected murder, however, the physical examination of a suspect was performed by midwives, or by male medical practitioners (that is, surgeons, apothecaries, physicians and man-midwives), rather than by members of the public. During the course of the eighteenth century, the pattern of involvement of these practitioners in the examination of suspects changed. Before the middle of the century, it was customary for both the local community and courts to call in a female midwife in order to confirm that a suspect had been recently delivered of a child, and to give an opinion about the body of a dead child. Male medical witnesses rarely appeared in the Northern Circuit courts before 1750 and, when they did give evidence, confined their comments to opinions about the corpse.[7]

The midwives called in to examine suspects and to testify in court were usually well-practised in midwifery. In 1771, for example, Elizabeth Catchasides testified that 'she hath practised as a Midwife for the Space of Eighteen Years now last past and hath herself bore several Children'.[8] This level of experience may have been considered a material factor in a midwife's ability to determine whether or not a suspect had been delivered of a child: in 1757, for example, Isabel Hudson referred to the fact that she was 'lookt upon as a Judge, haveing many Years practic'd the Art of Midwifery.'[9]

Since nearly 60 per cent of the midwives testifying before magistrates and coroners signed their depositions, compared with only one quarter of the suspects and remaining female witnesses, it is also likely that most midwives were better educated than the majority of the other women, and some of the men, involved in these cases.[10] Significantly, however, even those midwives who were unable to sign their names, and who may well have been lower in the social scale than their clients, were nevertheless established in the neighbourhood.[11] The official reliance on midwives in this way suggests that contemporary views (and historical accounts) of midwives as witches and bawds failed to recognize the status of midwives in some local communities.[12]

Although the midwives involved in cases of suspected new-born child murder appear to have been more respectable and more influential than some accounts of midwifery in this period would suggest, and although they spearheaded many local investigations, it is clear that in the course of the eighteenth century their contribution in these cases was limited by the expanding role of male medical practitioners. In the second half of the eighteenth century, neighbours called in far more surgeons and apothecaries than midwives to examine and interrogate suspects and inspect dead bodies. In addition, in the courts, male practitioners gave opinions about all aspects of these cases, including those that required intimate internal examination of the suspects. Although midwives continued to be involved, particularly in the early local stages of an investigation, they were increasingly subordinate to male medical practitioners. Their contributions were sometimes limited to witnessing the examination performed by a surgeon, and on occasions they referred the case to a male practitioner:

> Mary Hopwood Midwife is of the Opinion that Hannah Turner had Boarn a Child but was not willing to have the Jury Depend on her Judgement alone, and Desired that an Apothecary should be sent for.[13]

This transformation in the use of medical witnesses reflected both broad changes within the practice of midwifery and changing attitudes to the body as a source of evidence. Until the eighteenth century, child-birth was the almost exclusive preserve of women. During the eighteenth century, however, in spite of considerable opposition both from male medical practitioners and from midwives, an increasing number of men began to practise midwifery, largely at the expense of the reputation and practice of women. The gradual rejection of the value of female experience and tradition in child-birth which this process entailed is reflected in the growing use of male medical witnesses in suspected cases of new-born child murder.[14]

The declining use of midwives as experts can also be attributed to developments in medical jurisprudence and to changing attitudes to the body as evidence. When the statutory presumption of 1624 fell into disfavour in the middle of the eighteenth century and a greater number of trials were conducted at common law, the courts placed greater emphasis on medical evidence that the child had been born alive. This evidence required some form of post-mortem dissection. Since women were traditionally excluded from the use of surgical instruments to probe bodies in this way, it was male medical practitioners who were requested to examine the body and give evidence in murder investigations. Consequently, as male practitioners became more prominent in investigations, it became convenient for both a woman's neighbours and the courts to ask medical men, rather than midwives, not only to open the corpse but also to search the body of a suspect for signs of recent delivery.

What signs then constituted evidence of recent delivery? For a suspect's relatives and neighbours, the discovery of blood and the general disorder of delivery were the signs most likely to give rise to suspicion. But the signs most frequently discussed by medical writers and witnesses, and which when taken together were considered as proof of delivery, were: relaxation or distension of the vagina; swelling of the genitalia; the flow of the lochia or 'Cleansings'; the open state of the *os uteri;* a flaccidity or laxity of the abdomen; swollen, hard breasts which produced milk on pressure or suction; and extended *areolae.*[15] In practice, neither the results of internal examination nor the presence of 'the Discharges usual with lying in women'[16] were viewed by medical witnesses as conclusive because 'Feminine Disorders or Delivery of Children' could both produce the same appearances.[17] Proof of recent delivery therefore depended almost exclusively upon demonstrating the presence of milk in a suspect's breasts:

> Upon Examination found the Os Tinse or Passage into the Uteris, the Discharge in a State to suspect some substance has passed, No Child appearing was ready to pass the most favourable Construction on the Affair and said she perhaps had had a Miscarridge but gave directions to look to her Breasts for Milk which might Ground Suspicion more strongly.[18]

The presence of milk was demonstrated by pressure or suction on the breasts:

> the examinent says he ordered a Woman then present to Draw or

> suck her Breasts and findeing Milk it was put into a Tea Cup and the Milk so taken out of Ann Bennison Breast was sufficient to Certify that she had had a Child.[19]

Milk in a supect's breasts was regarded by witnesses as the most 'certain Proof' of recent delivery.[20] Although *Aristotle's Compleat Master-Piece* reiterated a traditional belief that virgins and the non-pregnant could have a type of milk in their breasts, witnesses were convinced that only pregnancy could produce the milk found in the women examined by them: in 1755, Mary Thompson, midwife, testified before a magistrate that 'she found Milk in her [Ann Stockdale's] Breasts which she never knew any to have that had not been with Child'.[21] Corroborated on occasions by the presence of milk on a woman's shift 'opposite to the Nipples',[22] milk in the breasts encouraged neighbours to continue their search for a body and to urge the suspect to confess to recent delivery. Indeed, this form of evidence was regarded as so conclusive that many suspects ceased to deny the fact and readily confessed to the birth once milk had been drawn from their breasts: 'this Deponent telling the said Martha that as She had Milk in her Breast She must have brought forth a Child very lately, upon which the said Martha Gleadhill did Confess that..... She was delivered of a Male Child'.[23]

The damning nature of milk in the breasts led some women to find ways of drying up the flow artificially. In 1768, Elizabeth Woodman was reported to have asked a fellow servant 'if there was not a Method to carry of[f] Milk from one that had bore a Child of the Breast'.[24] At least one surgeon, having failed to find milk in a woman's breasts, did believe that there were methods to achieve this end. In 1752, Francis Taylor, a surgeon, gave evidence before a magistrate that 'it is very possible in his Opinion for the Milk in a Woman's brest to be Dried away by Art in a Day or two time'.[25] This possibility was questioned by midwifery writers. Although Pierre Dionis and William Smellie both described the use of various applications to drive back milk in women who were 'not willing to give suck' and who wanted to put their children out to nurse, both writers doubted the efficacy of such measures:

> We must not be so credulous as to believe that a Linen-Rag dipt in any Liquor, and applied to the Breasts, will drive back the Milk, and change the ordinary Course of Nature.[26]

In practice, most women later accused of murder had failed to stem the natural flow of milk or to provide convincing alternative explanations for its presence,[27] and the discovery of milk convinced neighbours and local officials that a woman strongly suspected to have been pregnant had finally been delivered of her bastard child.

The demonstration of milk in a woman's breasts also helped to determine further issues for the courts. In contrast to some seventeenth-century writers who asserted that women could have milk in their breasts early in pregnancy,[28] in the eighteenth century the presence of milk was taken to indicate that the mother had gone to her full time. It was therefore used to rebut a woman's claim that she had been miscarried of a premature, and therefore still-born, child. In 1790, for example, Hannah Pullen testified to a justice of the peace that she had been delivered of a substance 'like a lump of Flesh' only eighteen weeks after she had had 'connections with a person who had carnal knowledge of her Body'. The surgeon who had examined her disagreed:

> he was sent for to examine Hannah Pullen who it was said had Miscarried that on examining her from milk being in her breasts and thus full and distended and from having the Discharges usual with lying in women he has been led by experience to believe that she was at or near her full time nor does her situation agree with the account she gives of the period of pregnancy.[29]

The value of medical testimony concerning recent delivery was recognized throughout the course of an investigation into a case of suspected new-born child murder. It was not only routinely admitted at coroners' inquests and in the trial courts but was also employed to facilitate the local interrogation and examination of suspects by relatives and neighbours. In some cases, for example, the simple intervention of a midwife or male medical practitioner clearly encouraged a suspect to confess that she had borne a child. Accordingly, some women accused of murdering their new-born children openly expressed their fear of the testimony of midwives and surgeons. Thus, in 1757, Margaret Young, a midwife in Northumberland, 'was called upon to see the said Sarah Newitt, who (upon sight of this Informant) spoke, what! are you (meaning this Informant) come here to swear away my Life – No said this Informant if it had been in my power to have preserv'd your Life and good Name I'd done it'.[30]

Examining the Body

The discovery of a new-born child's body in a privy or dunghill, in a field or river, or hidden under a mattress, caused a neighbourhood to suspect that a local woman had murdered her child. In many cases, the location of the body had been elicited from a suspect by interrogation, but on occasions the body was discovered accidentally by men on their way to work or by children playing in a garth. In these latter instances, the mother had usually already been provisionally identified by her neighbours, but if her identity was not immediately known, a coroner or justice of the peace could order a general search of 'all Suspected persons' for the signs of recent delivery.[31] On a number of occasions, neither local knowledge nor a search of local single women uncovered the mother's identity and an inquest verdict of murder 'by person or persons unknown' could be pursued no further.

The body of a dead child provided both a focus for local inquiries and an important source of evidence for the courts. Inquisitive neighbours made every effort to see the body for themselves and were quick to draw their own conclusions about the cause of the child's death. Of necessity, the body was also examined by the coroner and his jury at the inquest.[32] In addition, medical practitioners were requested by neighbours or local officials to examine the body for signs of live or still birth and for evidence that the child had been murdered. In spite of constraints on the development of legal medicine in this period, evidence derived from viewing the bodies of dead children in this way formed an increasingly prominent part of the evidence presented locally at inquests and later in the trial courts.

In practice, the nature and quality of investigations performed by medical practitioners on the bodies of dead children varied considerably, partly as a result of variations in experience between medical witnesses. Although most coroners in the north of England had investigated a considerable number of suspicious infant deaths,[33] few medical practitioners had extensive experience of these cases. Of the 82 surgeons, apothecaries and physicians named in the Northern Circuit court records between 1720 and 1799, only eight practitioners had certainly examined bodies and presented evidence at an inquest more than once.[34] Even in those cases, however, greater experience did not guarantee a more detailed post-mortem examination.

Variations in post-mortem technique, from superficial inspection of the body to extensive dissection of its internal cavities, can also be attributed to the fact that, in spite of an increased awareness of the medico-legal issues in these cases, there were no comprehensive guides to the post-mortem investigations that should be performed. However, even after Samuel Farr's modified translation of Johann Faselius' *Elementa Medicinae Forensis* was published in 1788, few medical practitioners adopted the systematic and comprehensive approach proposed by Farr.[35] Medical evidence presented at inquests and discussed in the trial courts in the eighteenth century was generally restricted to three topics: evidence of prematurity and still birth; the results of the lung test for live birth; and evidence of violence.

Throughout the eighteenth century, medical practitioners examined the bodies of dead children for evidence that they had been still born. Supported by case precedent, and by the authoritative opinion of Matthew Hale, evidence that a child had been born with no hair or nails, or that it had been unduly small, was accepted as evidence of prematurity and probable still birth.[36] Since such evidence exempted a suspect from trial under the statute of 1624 and left her to be tried under the more problematic common law rules of evidence, signs of prematurity and still birth also usually ensured the supect's acquittal in this period.[37]

In the middle decades of the eighteenth century, when the courts increasingly required evidence at common law that the child had been born alive and subsequently murdered before convicting a suspect, it became increasingly common for medical practitioners to examine a child's body for signs of live birth. Although a number of tests of live birth were discussed in the courts and in medical literature during the century, it was the process of removing a child's lungs to see if they floated in water (that is, the hydrostatic lung test) that attracted the most attention. However, even the lung test failed to establish live birth to the court's satisfaction in most cases. The varied practical application of the test, an awareness that certain circumstances limited the test's validity as a signifier of live birth, the problems inherent in establishing guilt at common law, and a general reluctance on the part of male medical practitioners to consider the test as conclusive, particularly when a woman's life might depend upon it, all limited the extent to which medical examination of a dead child could clarify whether or not a child had been born alive and murdered.[38]

In the light of limitations on medical evidence relating to live birth, medical practitioners attempted to determine the cause of death by further examining the bodies of dead children for marks of violence. Evidence of violence was particularly important in trials at common law, since, as Hale had insisted, if the case lay outside the statute of 1624, it was to be 'left to the jury to inquire, whether she murdered it or not, by those circumstances, that occur in the case, as if it be wounded or hurt, &c.'[39]

In practice, the presence or absence of marks of violence could clearly influence a coroner's or trial jury's verdict. In 1749, for example, an inquest jury found that 'the Child Scull was broke and other suspistious marks of Violence of the inside of its Right Ear,

And so the jurors on their Oath say that the Male Child was Feloniously Murdered by some person or persons as yet unknown'.[40] Similarly, evidence of violence could contribute to convictions at the assize courts by overcoming both evidence of prematurity and the difficulties of convicting married women at common law. Although married, Mary Morgan was found guilty of murder at the Old Bailey in 1724 because she was unable to give a satisfactory account of two stab wounds in her child's belly.[41] Conversely, the lack of evident violence was frequently noted by witnesses and contributed to acquittal on occasions: 'There appeared no Marks of Violence upon the Child the Jury acquitted her.'[42]

Perhaps as a result of verdicts acknowledging the significance of marks of violence, the presence or absence of such marks constituted a major focus for neighbours who found a body. Witnesses frequently commented on the state of the corpse and interpreted manifest evidence of violence, such as a severed limb or head, neck wounds and bruises, and fractures, as proof that the child had been murdered. At an inquest in 1744, Elizabeth Cooper testified that she had seen the dead child of Elizabeth Conney and that 'such marks of violence appeard upon the body of the said Male Child as put it out of doubt of its being murdered'.[43] More significantly, midwives and male medical practitioners viewed marks of violence in the same light. In 1762, Sarah Weatherhead, midwife, testified at an inquest 'that she sees no Marks of Violence whatsoever upon it save a little Bruses about its Neck which she this Witness imagined something bad.' And in 1780, William Pawlett, surgeon, deposed that 'from some Marks which he observed around the Neck of the said Child, there is too much reason to believe the said Child had been wilfully Strangled.'[44] As with the discovery of milk in the breast, suspects feared the perceived association between marks on a child's body and murder. Accordingly, some accused women insisted, even before the body had been found, that they had not inflicted any violence on the child.[45]

Although medical evidence of violence on a child's body could result in conviction, there were several problems concerning this type of evidence that became more apparent in the last half of the eighteenth century. The first problem concerned the difficulties of relating the time of the injury to the time of death. In law, neither the infliction of violence after death nor the destruction of a child in the birth were criminal. Evidence of violence could, therefore, be negated by the inability of a medical witness to establish to the court's satisfaction that the child had been born alive and that the injury had been received after birth. In 1771, a surgeon at the Old Bailey gave his opinion that a deep neck wound, almost severing a child's head from its body, had been a mortal wound. However, he could not say with certainty that the child had been alive after birth. When he was cross-examined by the prisoner's counsel, he further admitted that if the child had been born alive and then wounded, 'there must have been ten or twenty times more blood than I perceived'. The small amount of blood present raised the possibility that the wounds had in fact been inflicted on a still born child and could not, therefore, have caused the child's death. The woman was acquitted.[46]

The second problem facing the courts was the possibility that a child's injuries, in particular those to the head and neck, had been sustained accidentally during labour, especially if the labour had been difficult or if the woman had been so surprised by delivery that the child had fallen from her on to the floor or into the privy. The possibility of accidental injury was acknowledged by medical witnesses,[47] and although bruises, swellings and skull fractures aroused suspicions of murder in the neighbourhood, or at least suspicions that the woman had been negligent in failing to call 'proper assistance',[48] they were increasingly attributed by medical and legal writers to birth trauma or to sudden delivery: 'Proceeding to remove the scalp, the bones of the skull were covered with clotted blood, this being removed, both parietal bones were found fractured across; these are phenomena, however, sometimes produced by the violence of a woman in labour.'[49]

The final problem relating to violence concerned the state of the child's umbilical cord or navel string, which first attracted comment in the Northern Circuit courts in the 1760s, precisely when medical evidence of live birth and murder was becoming increasingly important. A torn or cut, but untied, navel string was regarded by some medical witnesses not only as a cause of death but also as a mark of violence: 'Saith that he can discover no marks of violence upon the Body excepting that the Navel String has been separated by some sharp Instrument and was not afterwards tied up, the want of which wou'd in his opinion produce the death of the Child by Bleeding.'[50] It was also significant that the cord had been cut and not simply torn: 'If it is rent or torn off, or bit off, I believe it will cease to bleed spontaneously, as in other Animals.'[51] It was also important, according to Samuel Farr, to recognize that the failure to tie the umbilical cord could only be the cause of death if 'a mortal haemorrhage' had ensued.[52] Lack of evidence for such a haemorrhage, and the possibility that the cord might break spontaneously as the child fell from the woman in labour, reduced the weight of this evidence. As in the case of most other marks of violence (and indeed much of the medical evidence in these cases), an untied umbilical cord was insufficient evidence of violence or intent on the part of the mother to prove murder even though it was often interpreted as evidence of neglect by her neighbours.[53]

Developing Medical Expertise and the Reappraisal of Suspects

During the sixteenth and seventeenth centuries, it was customary for both writers and the courts to refer to single women who had given birth to, and concealed, bastard children as lewd and unnatural murderers.[54] Such opinions were evident in poor law and bastardy legislation, in the construction of the 1624 statute, and in a miscellany of religious and medical literature. Similar assessments of the characters of accused women persisted through the eighteenth century. In the early part of the century, Daniel Defoe and Joseph Addison referred to suspects as 'merciless mothers', 'wicked murderers', and 'monsters of inhumanity'.[55] The opinions expressed by witnesses in the courts and by the writers of broadsheets and local newspapers also remained condemnatory throughout the century, referring to the 'unnatural perpetrators' who were 'guilty of this horrid crime'.[56] Finally, such attitudes found clear expression in the evangelical morality prevalent at the turn of the nineteenth century, a morality explicated by the Reverend Christopher Hodgson in his discussion of the murders of bastard children in 1803.[57]

From the middle of the eighteenth century, however, such preconceptions about the character and conduct of accused women were increasingly challenged by writers who sought to account for suspects' behaviour and responsibility in broader social terms. In many eighteenth-century discussions of new-born child murder, accused women were portrayed not as cruel and barbaric murderers, but as the modest and virtuous victims of circumstances beyond their control. One of the earliest expressions of this new approach came in Bernard Mandeville's *The Fable of the Bees,* first published in 1714. For Mandeville, it was a young woman's sense of modesty, honour and chastity (inculcated by education), not her supposed cruelty or barbarity, that prompted her to resort to murder in order to preserve her good name:

> the fear of Shame attacks her so lively, that every Thought distracts her. All the Family she lives in have a great opinion of her virtue, and her last Mistress took her for a Saint. How will her Enemies, that envied her Character, rejoice! how will her Relations detest her! The more modest she is now, and the more violently the dread of coming to Shame hurries her away, the more Wicked and more Cruel her

> Resolutions will be, either against her self or what she bears.[58]

It was this interpretation of suspects as modest women endeavouring to preserve their reputation that was adapted by later writers eager to develop a more humanitarian approach to suspects in the second half of the century. Mandeville's initial formulation was, however, considerably reshaped in later discussions. In the works of later writers, the excessive modesty that led women to contemplate this crime was reconstructed as 'a virtue' (rather than a vice, as Mandeville had portrayed it), and the suspects themselves were reappraised as worthy of the 'greatest Pity'. Thus, in 1767, Erasmus Darwin, then practising in Lichfield, responded to a letter of inquiry about a case in the following manner:

> The Women that have committed this most unnatural Crime, are real Objects of our greatest Pity; their education has produced in them so much Modesty, or Sense of Shame, that this artificial Passion overturns the very Instincts of Nature! – what Struggles must there be in their Minds, what agonies! – and at a Time when, after the Pains of Parturition, Nature has designed them the sweet Consolation of giving Suck to a little helpless Babe, that depends upon them for its hourly Existance!
>
> Hence the Cause of this most horrid Crime is an excess of what is really a Virtue, of the Sense of Shame, or Modesty. Such is the Condition of human Nature![59]

Similar sentiments about the modesty of, and sympathy due to, pregnant single women were expressed elsewhere: in House of Commons' debates about the repeal of the 1624 statute in the 1770s;[60] in contemporary newspapers and journals;[61] in the propaganda supporting the establishment and maintenance of both the foundling and the Magdalen Hospitals in the middle decades of the century;[62] and, perhaps most forcibly, by William Hunter, in his essay 'On the Uncertainty of the Signs of Murder, in the Case of Bastard Children', in which he argued not only that women accused of this crime were 'commonly objects of the greatest compassion' but also that, since they were in a state of 'phrenzy, or temporary insanity' at the birth, most women should not be held accountable for the deaths of their new-born children.[63]

Clearly aimed at provoking sympathy and prompting acquittal, this novel explanatory account of women's behaviour was professedly humanitarian. Darwin, Hunter and others were overtly intent on encouraging a more enlightened and more considerate, a less hasty and less prejudiced, assessment of suspects. Unlike Mandeville, for example, commentators such as Hunter did not believe that the majority of accused women were guilty of murder. Indeed, Hunter was openly concerned that *innocent* women were being sentenced to death as a result of 'equivocal proofs and inconclusive reasoning', and hoped that the 'facts' presented in his essay would save such 'unhappy and innocent women' from execution.[64]

Significantly, in the present context, this reappraisal of the character and culpability of suspects was heavily dependent on the experience and rhetoric of medical practitioners. Discussions about the insanity or incapacity of accused women took place within the context of eighteenth-century physiology and psychology, according to which women's proneness to irrationality and insanity was directly linked to their reproductive capacity.[65] In addition, the 'facts' that William Hunter hoped would save innocent women from the gallows were those gleaned from a lifetime of medical practice: 'facts' both about the minds and bodies of women in general and about the medico-legal aspects of new-born child murder in particular.[66] In this way, the new humanitarian account of accused women that was constructed in the last half of the eighteenth century was legitimated by its grounding in the rational expertise and experience of medical practitioners who had examined suspects, inspected bodies, and given evidence at local pre-trial hearings and in the trial courts.

As Thomas Laqueur has suggested in his discussion of what he terms 'the humanitarian narrative', however, Hunter in particular was also making epistemological claims. By highlighting the tendency for women's passionate and irrational natures to cause mental instability during pregnancy and delivery, Hunter was appropriating knowledge of women's behaviour to the medical discourse and restricting the involvement of lay and legal understanding in the determination of guilt. By providing a natural explanation for an apparently unnatural crime, he was therefore 'declaring epistemological sovereignty over the bodies and minds' of suspects.[67] In doing so, Hunter was not only 'staking out professional turf against the laity in general, against ignorant magistrates, and against the legal profession',[68] but was also reaffirming traditional views of rational male agency and irrational female passivity. Accused women were not only the victims of male seduction (a situation criticized by Hunter himself), but, ironically, they also became the passive victims of a professional struggle to maintain male medical superiority.

Given the extensive involvement of medical practitioners in local investigations and trials, the potential implications of this new approach to the character and conduct of suspects were immense. By emphasizing the uncertainty of the evidence and the extent to which defendants were the virtuous victims of circumstances largely beyond their control (such as the force of male seduction), proponents of the new approach raised doubts both about the cause of death and about the culpability of accused women. Since the conviction rate for new-born child murder had already fallen to well under ten per cent by the early decades of the eighteenth century (that is, several decades before the new account of suspects gained prominence), it is unlikely that the opinions of Darwin, Hunter and other writers contributed significantly to the acquittal of women accused of this crime.[69] However, the new approach was not without influence. By providing an explicitly medical framework within which to understand female behaviour and responsibility, and by endorsing the accounts of events put forward by suspects themselves on examination, proponents of this approach encouraged the courts to view supposedly criminal behaviour from a medical perspective and facilitated the medicalization of new-born child murder inquiries that occurred more decisively in the nineteenth century.[70] Together with new rules of evidence and changing standards of proof, the humanitarian account of the behaviour of women accused of murdering their new-born bastard children also provided the background to parliamentary attempts to repeal what was seen by the late eighteenth century as the anomalous statute of 1624.[71]

Conclusion

In his recent comprehensive study of crime and the courts between 1660 and 1800, J. M. Beattie suggested that medical evidence 'became less rather than more important in eighteenth-century infanticide cases, for in itself it could not generally prove that a mother had murdered her new-born child.'[72] Although it is clear that evidence of recent delivery, signs of a child's maturity, the results of the lung test, and evidence of violence could not resolve the problems posed by an increasing number of trials at common law, Beattie's opinion underestimates the significance of, and the changing regard for, medical testimony during the eighteenth century. Locally, a woman's neighbours routinely called in medical practitioners in order to confirm their suspicions about the cause of a child's death, and in the coroners' courts, medical opinion clearly influenced the form and content of inquest verdicts. Although medical evidence generally failed to withstand the greater scrutiny to which it was subjected in the trial courts, its importance was nevertheless acknowledged. In 1781, one of the judges at the Old Bailey criticized a coroner and his jury for failing to send for a surgeon to examine a child's body.[73] And in many trials in the last half of the century, medical witnesses were examined and cross-examined in great depth by court and counsel. By the end of the eighteenth century, court practice and the works of legal and medical writers had not only ensured that medical evidence had become established as an essential component of investigations into the suspected murders of new-born children, but also that these cases were regarded as the paradigm of medical involvement in the court room.[74]

The increasing involvement of medical practitioners in all aspects of investigations contributed to, and was itself encouraged by, a novel appraisal of the character, conduct, and culpability of single women accused of concealing and murdering their new-born children. However, this process of medicalizing new-born child murder inquiries must also be seen within a broader social context. Efforts to develop a new approach to suspects, and replace what William Hunter referred to as 'prejudice and blind zeal' with 'an unprejudiced enquiry', were part of wider enlightenment attempts to establish the supremacy of male reason over female irrationality and superstition.[75] In the present context, these late eighteenth-century concerns are evident both in the replacement of midwives as witnesses by male medical practitioners, and in the adoption of an explanatory framework of female behaviour that not only emphasized female passivity and instability but also carried professional benefits for male medical practitioners.

Notes

1. The gradual development of legal medicine in England is discussed in C. Crawford, 'The Emergence of English Forensic Medicine: Medical Evidence in Common-Law Courts, 1730–1830', (D.Phil. thesis, Oxford: 1987); T.R. Forbes, *Surgeons at the Bailey,* (Yale U.P.: 1985); J.D.J. Havard, *The Detection of Secret Homicide,* (London: 1960), 1–10. See 'An Act for the Attendance and Remuneration of Medical Witnesses at Coroners' Inquests', 6&7 Will.IV c.89, 1836, for the payment of medical practitioners at inquests. On the low status of the coroner in this period, see Matthew Hale, *History of the Pleas of the Crown,* (2 vols, London: 1736), Vol. II, 222; Edward Umfreville, *Lex Coronatoria: Or, The Office and Duty of Coroners,* (London: 1761), v.
2. Mark Jackson, 'Suspicious Infant Deaths: the Statute of 1624 and Medical Evidence at Coroners' Inquests', Michael Clark and Catherine Crawford (eds), *Legal Medicine in History,* (Cambridge University Press, 1994), 64–86. The statute was 21 Jac.1 c.27.
3. Most of the sources for this paper are taken from the Northern Circuit assize court records, held in the Public Record Office: ASSI 41 (minute books); ASSI 42 (gaol books); ASSI 44 (indictment files);

and ASSI 45 (depositions). Other cases are taken from the Old Bailey Sessions Papers (OBSP).

4. See Mary Williamson, 1729, ASSI 45/18/6/76.
5. On the history of the jury of matrons see James C. Oldham, 'On Pleading the Belly: A History of the Jury of Matrons', *Criminal Justice History,* VI, (1985), 1–64.
6. Frances Harrison, 1795, ASSI 45/38/3/51. For other 'Juries of Matrons', see: Elizabeth Pruddam, 1746, ASSI 45/23/2/81–3; Pheeby Cockshot, 1756, ASSI 45/25/4/28–9; Margaret Colley, 1757, ASSI 45/26/1/22–6; Margaret Baker, 1771, ASSI 45/30/1/22–6.
7. I have found only one example of a male practitioner giving evidence in the north of England before 1750. In 1728, William Hornby examined the body of the child supposedly given birth to by Anne Milburne (1728, ASSI 45/18/5/53). According to the printed sessions papers, however, surgeons sometimes gave evidence at the Old Bailey and at the Surrey and Essex sessions in the 1730s and 1740s.
8. Margaret Baker, 1771, ASSI 45/30/1/22–6.
9. Sarah Newitt, 1757, ASSI 45/26/1/97–102
10. Excluding the medical witnesses, all of whom signed their depositions, 20 per cent of the male witnesses could not sign their names.
11. Although Mary Greenside could not sign her deposition, she had practised midwifery for 'betwixt thirrty and forty years': Ann Bateman, 1761, ASSI 45/26/5/2–3.
12. See, for example, Samuel Farr's comments in his *Elements of Medical Jurisprudence,* (London: 1788), 7–8. Farr argued that the determination of pregnancy should not, even on account of decency, be committed to midwives, but should instead 'be entrusted to the more regular practitioner, who being a person of education, would add the influence of his judgment to his examination, and would not be content with a single enquiry, which may be uncertain, but would frequently repeat it, till he had perfectly ascertained the truth.' Similar attitudes to midwives had previously appeared in Percivall Willughby's *Observations in Midwifery,* (S.R. Publishers Ltd., Yorkshire: 1972), *passim,* and in some contemporary novels. For recent views of the midwife as witch and bawd, see Robert A. Erickson, *Mother Midnight, Birth, Sex and Fate in Eighteenth Century Fiction* (New York: 1986); and T. R. Forbes, *The Midwife and the Witch* (Yale U.P.: 1966), 112–32. For an alternative acccount see: David N. Harley, 'Ignorant Midwives – a Persistent Stereotype', *Bulletin of the Society for the Social History of Medicine,* 28, (1981), 6–9; *ibid.,* 'Historians as Demonologists: The Myth of the Midwife-witch', *Social History of Medicine,* 3, (1990), 1–26. Harley has pointed out the limitations of contemporary evidence, noting, for example, that the criticisms expressed by man-midwives were influenced by their eagerness to increase their own practices at the expense of those of the midwives.
13. Hannah Turner, 1778, ASSI 45/33/2/137.

14. The rise of, and controversy surrounding, man-midwifery in the seventeenth and eighteenth centuries is discussed in Jean Donnison, *Midwives and Medical Men A History of Inter-Professional Rivalries and Women's Rights* (London: 1977), 1–59.
15. Farr, *op. cit.* (note 12), 49–50; Bartholomew Parr, *The London Medicinal Dictionary* (London: 1809), Vol. II, 179.
16. The words of William Tindall, surgeon, in Hannah Pullen, 1790, ASSI 45/37/1/176–8.
17. Francis Taylor, surgeon, could not distinguish between these two possible causes of Ann Young's condition in 1752 (ASSI 45/24/4/73–4).
18. The words of John Lincoln, surgeon, after examining Ann Bennison in 1788, ASSI 45/36/2/10–12.
19. *Ibid.;* a description of the procedure by a constable.
20. The opinion of James Armstrong, surgeon, in the case of Hannah Dodd, 1788, ASSI 45/36/2/38–9.
21. Ann Stockdale, 1755, ASSI 45/25/3/99B-H. See also: *Aristotle's Compleat Master-Piece,* 11th edn, (London: 1725), 27–8; William Harvey, *Lectures on the Whole of Anatomy,* (University of California Press: 1961), 155–6, for a discussion of opinions on milk in the breasts of non-pregnant women and men; Audrey Eccles, *Obstetrics and Gynaecology in Tudor and Stuart England,* (London: 1982), 53.
22. Frances Harrison, 1795, ASSI 45/38/3/51
23. Martha Gleadhill, 1749, ASSI 45/24/1/37–38A
24. Elizabeth Woodman, 1768, ASSI 45/29/1/174–8
25. Ann Young/Ambrose Hoyland, 1752, ASSI 45/24/4/73–4. Although Taylor failed to find milk, two midwives did in fact find milk in Ann's breasts.
26. Pierre Dionis, *A General Treatise of Midwifery* (London: 1719), 287; also William Smellie, *A Treatise on the Theory and Practice of Midwifery* (London: 1752), 418–19.
27. Margaret Baker, for example, tried to convince inquirers that her milk was due to her three year old child sometimes sucking at her breasts (1771, ASSI 45/30/1/22–6).
28. Discussed in Eccles, *op. cit.* (note 21), 53.
29. Hannah Pullen, 1790, ASSI 45/37/1/176–8.
30. Sarah Newitt, 1757, ASSI 45/26/1/97–102.
31. See the case of Martha Gleadhill, 1749, ASSI 45/24/1/37–8A. According to Richard Burn, a general warrant to apprehend all persons supsected, at least in the case of robbery, was void – Richard Burn, *The Justice of the Peace, and Parish Officer,* 3rd edn (London: 1756), 725. However, Martha Gleadhill's case and the description of an investigation in a printed broadsheet, *Albertus the Second: or, the Curious Justice,* both suggest that a general search was sometimes used to identify the mother of a dead child.
32. A coroner's inquest could only be held *super visum corporis,* on view

of a body.

33. For example, between August 1790 and December 1795, John Wrightson, one of the coroners for the North Riding of Yorkshire, held inquests into the deaths of at least five new-born children.
34. William Smith, surgeon and man-midwife, for example, testified at the inquest and appeared in court in at least three cases in Newcastle upon Tyne: Mary Hills, 1775, ASSI 45/32/1/121; Elizabeth Bryson, 1775, ASSI 45/32/1/38; and Mary Stolker, 1778, see the indictment and recognizances in ASSI 44/93i–iii.
35. Faselius' work was originally published in 1767. Farr's version seems to have sold well in this country. According to Christopher Johnson in the preface to his translation of Mahon's work, Farr's book was 'now out of print' – Christopher Johnson, *An Essay on the Signs of Murder in New Born Children,* tr. from the French of Dr P. A. O. Mahon (Lancaster: 1813), ix. Chapter V of Farr's translation, entitled 'Of the Murder of Infants', set out a systematic approach to the investigation of suspected murders, based on examination of both the mother and the child. In the conclusion to the discussion (68–9), Farr complained 'that although so much is required, so little is generally done in these cases' and expressed the hope that his work would 'meet the attention of judges and lawyers in this particular circumstance, which so often comes before them, to the shame and scandal of humanity; and that they will be enabled to correct the errors of coroners, or ignorant surgeons, who may have been misled in the depositions they give in. It is a misfortune, that men of eminence in the physical line fly from bars of judicature, as places of trouble and examination. It may be necessary, therefore, to give the courts such checks upon ignorance, as will serve to discover the truth.'
36. Hale, *op. cit.* (note 1), II, 289.
37. See the discussion in Jackson, *op. cit.* (note 2).
38. *Ibid.; idem,* 'New-Born Child Murder: A Study of Suspicion, Evidence and Proof in Eighteenth-Century England (Ph. Dissertation, Leeds: 1992), 78–116.
39. Hale, *op. cit.* (note 1), II, 289; William Hawkins (*A Treatise of the Pleas of the Crown,* Vol.II, 1721, 438) further suggested that evidence of violence itself implied live birth: 'And therefore in such Cases it must appear by Signs of Hurt upon the Body, or some other way, that the Child was born alive.'
40. Martha Gleadhill, 1749, ASSI 44/64.
41. Mary Morgan, OBSP, March 1724, 7.
42. Sarah Nicholson, OBSP, December 1719, 2.
43. Elizabeth Conney, 1744, ASSI 45/22/4/31–3A.
44. Ann Bailey, John Sharp and Elizabeth Sharp, 1762, ASSI 45/26/6/6–7; Ann Holt, 1780, ASSI 45/34/1/55–6.
45. See Hannah Dodd's testimony, 1788, ASSI 45/36/2/38–9.
46. Elizabeth Packins, OBSP No.IV, April 1771, 200–3.

47. See the midwife's testimony in Hannah Bradford, OBSP No. IV, April 1732, 109. See also Ann Ridoubt (OBSP, August 1728, 4), on the impossibility of a child surviving a difficult labour, and Mary Radford (OBSP, January 1723, 6), for the court's opinion that a jaw fracture was sustained when the child fell into a chamber pot at delivery. Elizabeth Warner (OBSP No.II, January 1760, 68–73), was 'Acquitted, as delivered by surprise.'
48. See the depositions of the midwife and surgeon in Elizabeth Ormston, 1763, ASSI 45/27/1/61B-D.
49. From the deposition of a physician and surgeon, quoted by Johnson, *op. cit.* (note 35), 104, fn. In the eighteenth century, both Deventer and Roederer suggested that skull fractures could occur spontaneously in labour; see Erwin H. Ackerknecht, 'Legal Medicine in Transition (16th–18th Centuries)', *Ciba Symposia,* 11 (1950), 1296.
50. Susanna Staniforth, 1799, ASSI 45/40/1/118. The state of the navel string was in fact commented on once prior to the 1760s, in 1742, but interest only blossomed in the last decades of the century.
51. Desmond King-Hele (ed.), *The Letters of Erasmus Darwin,* (Cambridge U.P.: 1981), 41–2.
52. Farr, *op. cit.* (note 12), 62.
53. In 1781, an inquest jury found that an unknown woman 'did neglect and refuse to tie and secure ... that part of the said funis or navel string' (in ASSI 44/97i).
54. The 1624 statute itself, in line with other bastardy legislation of the period, was directed at the 'lewd Mothers' of bastards. In addition, see William Gouge's reference to the 'lewd and unnaturall women' who abandoned their children in *Of Domesticall Duties* (London: 1622), 507. Later in the century, Percivall Willughby and Reverend Oliver Heywood referred to these women as 'the looser sort' and 'light skirts' respectively; see Willughby, *op. cit.* (note 12), 12; and J. Horsfall Turner (ed.), *The Rev. Oliver Heywood, B.A. 1630–1702; His Autobiography, Diaries, Anecdote and Event Books* (4 vols, 1881–5), Vol. IV, 50.
55. Daniel Defoe, *The Generous Protector* (London: 1731), 9; *The Guardian,* No. 105, 11 July, 1713.
56. See, for example, the report in *The Cumberland Pacquet,* 13 March, 1777, 3, which referred to the case of Esther Carlisle and Isabell Spencer, who were tried for the murder of Esther's child at Carlisle in August 1777; the depositions are in ASSI 45/33/1/14P–S. See also: comments in Elizabeth Pruddam, 1746, ASSI 45/23/2/81–3, ASSI 44/60; and the constable's words in Elizabeth Warner, OBSP No. II, January 1760, 72.
57. C. Hodgson, *A Letter from a Magistrate in the Country, to his Medical Friend at Peterborough* (Peterborough: 1800).
58. Bernard Mandeville, *The Fable of the Bees; or, Private Vices, Publick Benefits* (1714; published with a commentary by F. B. Kaye, 2 vols,

Oxford: 1924), Vol. I, Remark C, 75.

59. King-Hele, *op. cit.* (note 51), 42.
60. See the tone of the comments in *Hansard's Parliamentary History,* (1771–4), XVII, col. 453. For a full discussion of the attempted repeal of the 1624 statute, see Jackson, 'New-Born Child Murder', *op. cit.* (note 38), 206–44.
61. See, for example, *The Gentleman's Magazine,* October 1774, 463.
62. For a discussion of the factors influencing the founding of, and support for, the Foundling and Magdalen Hospitals, see: Donna T. Andrew, *Philanthropy and Police: London Charity in the Eighteenth Century,* (Princeton U.P.: 1989), 57–65, 119–27; W. A. Speck, 'The Harlot's Progress in Eighteenth-Century England', *British Journal for Eighteenth-Century Studies,* 3 (1980), 127–39; and Adrian Wilson, 'Illegitimacy and its Implications in Mid-eighteenth-century London: the Evidence of the Foundling Hospital', *Continuity and Change,* 4 (1989), 103–64.
63. William Hunter 'On the Uncertainty of the Signs of Murder in the Case of Bastard Children', *Medical Observations and Inquiries,* 6 (1784), 266–90.
64. Hunter, *op. cit.* (note 63), 280, 290.
65. See, for example, the opinions of: William Battie, *A Treatise on Madness* (London: 1758), 52–3; and John Haslam, *Observations on Insanity* (London: 1798), 52–3, 108.
66. Hunter, *op. cit.* (note 63), 269, 281–2.
67. Thomas Laqueur, 'Bodies, Details, and the Humanitarian Narrative', in Lynn Hunt (ed.), *The New Cultural History* (University of California Press: 1989), 188.
68. *Ibid.,* 187–8.
69. Of nearly two hundred women accused of new-born child murder in the north of England, only six were convicted, and only two hanged, throughout the whole of the eighteenth century. The conviction rate was similarly low in other parts of the country by the early eighteenth century – see the discussion in Jackson, 'New-Born Child Murder', *op. cit.* (note 38), 133–71.
70. On this point, see Roger Smith, *Trial by Medicine* (Edinburgh U.P.: 1981), 143–60.
71. See Jackson, 'New Born Child Murder', *op. cit.* (note 38), 206–44.
72. J. M. Beattie, *Crime and the Courts in England 1660–1800* (Oxford: 1986), 120–1.
73. Elizabeth Harris, OBSP No. V, May 1781, 269.
74. Significantly, when Edward Umfreville, for example, outlined the form of a summons for the assistance of a surgeon at an inquest, the case he chose was the investigation of the death of a new-born child; Umfreville, *op. cit.* (note 1), 510. And, in 1791, Capel Lofft chose surgical opinion on the lung test as his example of 'proof by experts' - L. C. B.Gilbert, *The Law of Evidence* ('considerably enlarged by

Capel Lofft', 1791), Vol. I, 301.

75. Hunter, *op. cit.* (note 63), 267. For a similar effort to establish male superiority in a related field, see William Cadogan's *An Essay upon Nursing, and the Management of Children* (London: 1748).

6

Reflections on Medical Reform: Cabanis' *Coup d'Œuil*

Ludmilla Jordanova

If scholars who work on Enlightenment medicine are agreed about anything it is that a reformist ethos was of paramount importance.[1] It was not that there was consensus about precisely what should change, but a shared sense none the less existed that medical ideas and practices could and should be transformed, that medical practitioners were poised to take on new, socially important roles, and that the manner in which medicine altered required careful, explicit consideration. In this way medicine participated fully in one of the dominant preoccupations of the Enlightenment – a zeal for reform that was carefully thought through and spearheaded by an educated, disinterested group with a commitment to secularized philanthropy. To twentieth-century eyes, programmes for medical reform can appear simplistic, but, despite their naïve utopian invocations, they provide valuable insights into medicial mentalities of the Enlightenment. In order to imagine change, many medical writers surveyed the history of their occupation, assessed the traditions that dominated their field, and contemplated the nature of their own vocation.

I shall examine one example of reformist writing by a key figure of the late Enlightenment, Pierre Jean Georges Cabanis (1757–1808).[2] His *Coup d'Œuil sur les révolutions et la réforme de la médecine* was written in 1795, but not published until 1804. It represents Cabanis' attempt to work out how medicine should change at a time of extraordinary political upheaval in which he was himself a participant. At one level it indicates a high degree of intellectual ambition and of reformist commitment thoroughly characteristic of the Enlightenment, but at another it is negotiating a minefield in search of new visions when revolution, in every sense, was dangerous. Thus in the *Coup d'Œuil* we can see Cabanis working with the problem of giving an account of medical change without making medicine sound like either a subversive or a privileged enterprise. He wished to advance a particular view of the relationship between the state, a properly organized medical profession, and the people's well-being. Cabanis was thus treading an extremely tricky path. In what follows I discuss selected parts of the *Coup d'Œuil* to show how he promoted the interests of a reformed medicine, the practitioners of which would receive esteem and power by virtue of their social value. I suggest that Cabanis sought a gentle vision of the future of his field; he strove to find novelty, change and progress with a minimum of conflict and aggression. Cabanis held a view of government, a view of medical theory and medical practice, indeed, a view of the human race that made immediate change perfectly accessible. In this sense Cabanis drew an implicit contrast between changes in the past, and those in the present and immediate future – the latter came under the category 'la réforme' as well as revolution, and were the result of deliberate reformist actions.

Cabanis' *Coup d'Œuil* was written and published in a context where the discussion of revolutions in science – and for him medicine was, at least in part, a science – was familiar, and where the analogies with political change could be explored.[3] It was also conceived in a context where the project of writing the history of medicine was fairly common.[4] At least part of the book surveys past changes in medicine, passes judgement on the value of major figures and attempts to draw lessons from history. Although very little has been written on eighteenth-century histories of medicine, it is clear that they played a significant part in constructing a medical heritage that gave due respect to (selected aspects of) tradition while outlining an agenda for change. Not surprisingly many such historical sketches had axes to grind, as Julian Martin has shown in the case of John Freind, the Tory Jacobite Newtonian, whose *History of Physic* appeared in 1725 and 6.[5] In tracing the history of writing the history of medicine, Charles Webster pointed to the varied motives that led scholars of the seventeenth, eighteenth and nineteenth centuries to take on such a project. He has identified the work of Daniel Leclerc, *Histoire de la Médecine,* 1696, as the first history of medicine in the modern sense and stressed the richness of German historical scholarship in the eighteenth century – here works were produced that explored questions of progress and revolution in medicine. He judged Cabanis' history to be derivative, a vehicle for the *idéologues,* that loose grouping of intellectuals around Madame Helvétius in Auteuil, who saw themselves as the heirs of Condillac.[6]

Cabanis was indeed a member of this network; he was on

intimate terms with a good many of its leaders, a significant number of whom held prominent public positions in France, especially in the late 1790s and early 1800s.[7] And Cabanis, too, clearly had an axe, or rather several axes, to grind in writing the *Coup d'Œuil*, although, so far as I can tell, these did not derive from any formal *idéologue* programme for medical reform. This group shared certain ideas, particularly about method, about the importance of educational reform, and about the social utility of science and medicine broadly conceived that informed much of their work. All these themes are prominent in Cabanis' text.

Cabanis' biography vividly illustrates his immediate engagement with late Enlightenment reformism.[8] Here was someone who was part of active intellectual and political networks, who thought a great deal about the contemporary situation, who was intensely concerned with medical education, indeed with the role of medical institutions generally, who held moderate republican views, who practised some medicine, but was neither an outstanding theorist nor an exceptional practitioner. In addition to the *Coup d'Œuil* and the *Rapports du Physique et du Moral de l'Homme* – the work for which he is best known, Cabanis published other writings that indicate the nature and range of his interests: *Journal de la Maladie et de la Mort de Mirabeau*, 1791, as Martin Staum suggests an apologetic, not to say defensive account of his treatment of the statesman; *Du Degré de Certitude de la Médecine*, 1798; and *Observations sur les Hôpitaux*, 1790. The *Journal* is an example of Cabanis 'rewriting' the Revolution. It gives a blow-by-blow account of his meeting with Mirabeau (on the day after the fall of the Bastille), of the great man's activities, and especially of his excessive work, his illness and subsequent death. It is a vindication of himself as medical practitioner, and of Mirabeau as a great statesman and so it reveals, in an exceptionally vivid manner, how the political revolution and Cabanis' career were intertwined.

As a member of the Conseil des Cinq-Cents and then as a Senateur under Napoleon, Cabanis was also involved directly in contemporary political debate and some of his speeches survive. As he became increasingly disenchanted with Napoleon's regime, he carefully withdrew from active political life. Cabanis also wrote a number of occasional pieces on matters as diverse as catarrh, apoplexy and the guillotine. We should notice Cabanis' willingness to reflect critically on the state of contemporary medicine, and especially on its epistemological basis. And, this reflexiveness was all of a piece with his interest in education and social reform as well as with his detailed physiological ideas, and the overall style of medicine that he favoured.[9]

In the 'Avertissement' that begins the *Coup d'Œuil,* which was added just before publication, Cabanis set his own work in the context of debates about public education. The key issue for him was how 'analytic methods' could be applied to the study of medicine, presented here as a science, or to be more precise as a science of observation – a common phrase for the life sciences at this time. His sketch of past revolutions was a preliminary step in a search for the general principles that should guide medical reform. Knowledge of the past is a precondition for changing the present – changes that are always presented by Cabanis as both attainable and desirable. These points were further developed in the following short section 'Objet de cet écrit'.

The leading theme here, as elsewhere in the text, is that of order – that is, the need to impose an intellectual framework upon the multitude of observations that form the core of medicine. Cabanis' path was a delicate one; to encourage empirical richness, while avoiding falling into chaos. Accordingly it is not surprising to find that vocabularies of order, arrangement, control, classification, linkage and chains predominated. His argument was that scientific progress brought with it the need to rethink, to reorder, to reform the language of science and its classificatory structures. The novelty was of a gentle kind, that comes to sound more familiar and comforting by the repeated use of the prefix 're': renouvelés, revoir, régénération, réforme. He did, it is true, speak of 'discoveries that shake the very foundations of science', but the purpose remained that of stressing the consequent need for new ways of organizing, presenting and teaching medical materials.[10] The overall sense that Cabanis conveyed was that novelty and change brought with them a potentially overwhelming superabundance, which demanded firm ordering to simplify the data and to weed out the excess. Cabanis deployed a striking image to express the point:

> Science resembles ... an inquisitive traveller who collecting everything that interests him along the way, sees his luggage constantly expanding, and finds himself often forced to go through it, either to get rid of useless articles, ... or to rearrange in a better order those he cannot get rid of, so that they occupy less space, and that their transport or their use becomes easier and more convenient.[11]

He continued: 'If there is a science overburdened .... with superfluous baggage, it is undoubtedly medicine.' The benign, domesticated way in which Cabanis refers to the changes medicine does, and must necessarily, undergo is certainly striking. He went so far as to indicate that medicine is in danger of being 'smothered by this indigestible mass of materials', but this mortal threat is easily recouped by his claim that finding order comes naturally, it seems to happen by itself.[12] Such claims rested heavily on the importance attributed by Cabanis, in typical *idéologue* fashion, to the reform of language as integral to scientific and medical reform. Yet he did not go into this issue in any depth. Rather he used it, rhetorically, to attack vague, obscure and imprecise language, which should be entirely banned, since it is associated with errors in medical thinking on the one hand, and with charlatanism on the other (obscure languages encourage charlatanism to flourish).

The claim that good science was a well-made language was, of course, commonly made by savants in the period, usually by those who acknowledged their indebtedness to Condillac. Cabanis returned to these issues in the final chapter of the *Coup d'Œuil,* entitled 'Objets Accessoires', where he discussed the disciplines related in some way to medicine – natural history, physics, mathematical sciences, philosophical methods, moral philosophy. There he also briefly considered what he called 'Belles lettres et arts', but in fact the discussion mostly consisted of familiar arguments about the centrality of language to medicine.[13] The points he made there are of some interest. He attacked those medical practitioners who condemn literary studies for medical students.[14] For Cabanis, they have failed to see that medicine and science have their own kind of eloquence – that rests on clarity, precision and purity of style – a point driven home by ridiculing the writing style of Georg Ernst Stahl (1659/60–1734). He contrasted Stahl's unacceptable manner of writing with the fine literary qualities of authentic Hippocratic texts.

Like many of his contemporaries, indeed like many French medical practitioners of the nineteenth century, Cabanis was passionately devoted to the Hippocratic spirit. He admired Hippocratic sophistication in clinical matters, and the attention paid to the impact of the environment on human health and sickness. This part of medicine, that is hygiene, was a major focus of interest for French medical practitioners in the late eighteenth and early nineteenth centuries.[15] Having praised the Hippocratic style, Cabanis turned briefly to painting to stress that the arts can present images that are faithful to nature, and hence should not be dismissed by scientific and medical practitioners. He concludes: 'the cultivation of letters and of the fine arts can be harnessed to the more demanding work of the art of healing'.[16]

Cabanis' position on art and literature is, I think, significant in four respects. First, there are a number of references to painting in the *Coup d'Œuil*, the very title of which rests on the idea of looking. Elsewhere he used the verb 'to paint', or the noun 'painting' as a metaphor for the exact representation of nature. Similarly, he frequently referred to 'tableau' to mean a scene, and hence a setting where learning from seeing is the principal issue. Presumably the clinic was a source of such scenes. This is clearly in keeping with the importance of a visual epistemology in the period.[17] Second, Cabanis drew a contrast between pleasure ('arts d'agrément) and strictness ('travaux sévères') in the quotation above. The idea of science and medicine being clearly ordered, tightly argued, with facts closely linked together, to which Cabanis frequently returns in the *Coup d'Œuil*, was the intellectual counterpart of the 'demanding work of the art of healing'. We can perhaps discern a tension here; on the one hand Cabanis wanted to show how medicine can, even should, be allied with literature and art, while on the other he was drawn to emphasize the rigours of medicine, perhaps because he wanted to claim its status as a full science in addition to being an 'art'. It is striking not only that 'art' could be put, in both English and French, to a wide range of uses, but also that its meaning was changing in fundamental ways at this very time.[18]

Third, Cabanis' insistence that medical students should learn about the literary qualities of their chosen field, indicates the importance of writing in medicine in this period. It is misleading to think of medicine at this time primarily in terms of doing, that is working with patients whether dead or alive, in terms of institutions, and in terms of theories divorced from the texts through which they had their being. A large number of medical practitioners in the period were intensely proud of and self-conscious about their literary activities. Both the dominant philosophical traditions and anxieties about their social-cum-cultural standing as gentlemen encouraged this. Many made both money and reputations through writing. There is a need to know far more about the ways in which medical self-images, both individual and professional, were built around cultural activities such as writing, painting, and collecting.[19] It should not be thought that literature and art were peripheral to medicine – quite the contrary, they constituted its very core, provided its languages, and were its basic tools of thought. The imagination was, accordingly, an important faculty for medical practitioners, who lived, after all, in an historical context where there was an intense consciousness of literary and artistic merit. Fourth, we can add to all these points by noting that Cabanis' network included, not only the philosophers of language, as is often pointed out, but a number of literary critics and historians, including, for example, those active in *La Décade Philosophique,* a journal run by an *idéologue* group, in which Cabanis' own works were reviewed, and which paid a great deal of attention to the contemporary French literary scene.[20]

Cabanis' opening section also broached two major issues – therapeutics and the history of medicine – that I shall discuss in turn. They reveal more of the kinds of reforms Cabanis had in mind and the sort of enterprise he took medicine to be. In relation to therapeutics, Cabanis argued that medical education should be organised in such a way that students gained extensive clinical experience. The claim was that therapeutics is the centre of medicine around which everything else should be organised in a co-ordinated fashion. When he said 'organized', he meant both the presentation of medical facts and ideas in the educative process broadly conceived, and also the ways in which medical sub-divisions are formed and related to one another.

These themes are taken up in the penultimate part of the book, entitled, 'Considérations particulières sur diverse branches de la médecine'; one section of which dealt with 'Pathologique, séméiotique, thérapeutique' – a juxtaposition of topics that is highly significant, since Cabanis treated them as inseparable, a natural cluster forming the practical part of medicine.[21] He offered definitions of each one: pathology is the knowledge of morbid conditions, semiotics is the knowledge of signs, and therapeutics is the art of drawing treatment plans from the first two. Here Cabanis was able to unite neatly a number of his favourite themes – the artificiality of many nosologies, the growing importance of bedside teaching, especially in hospitals – a trend he located not in his own Parisian environment, but as deriving from Vienna and Edinburgh – and nature as the ultimate authoritative teacher. And he could at the same time express his admiration of the Greeks:

> Thus the Greeks taught practical medicine by the very beds of the sick; it is for this reason that they gave it the name 'clinic'. Nature provided the text for the lessons... [22]

In this section, the authority of nature was invoked several times, in contrast to useless books and as the teacher who is so effective that learning, through clinical observation in the hospital, is effortless. Cabanis' stress upon the observation of clinical phenomena as the heart of therapeutics enabled him to move perfectly smoothly into the next section on hygiene – an area of practical medicine rooted in observation, where we can see his concern with education, with social improvement, with the Hippocratic approach, and with the 'moral' aspects of medicine beautifully blended together.[23] He expressed genuine vehemence about the ways in which the valuable lessons hygiene has to teach have been shamefully ignored. Hygiene, which teaches us to preserve health, is central to medicine and to 'la morale', which he defines as 'l'art de la vie'. It is so central to human well-being that it should form part of every system of education because it shows people how to develop healthy habits, regulate their passions, follow a good régime. Cabanis developed these points by taking as examples diet, gymnastics, and the changes that come with different ages and environments. His arguments were the familiar ones put forward by hygienists of the time. They stressed the ways in which people's lifestyle could be both understood and changed by drawing on a naturalistic approach to the human body, and this depended upon making reliable associations between how people actually live and their body states – the two terms were linked via habits, and by the rules of hygiene that enable patients to build up a healthy *manière de vivre.*

We may note that although Cabanis' account, like all medical works on hygiene, gives a certain privilege to medical knowledge and advice, it also contains a model of health where the patient has a large degree of responsibility for her or his own condition. And we can grasp more fully the significance of this when we appreciate that for Cabanis the ultimate goal was the 'general perfectibility of the human race'.[24] The stakes in medical reform broadly conceived in this way were rather high – together therapeutics and preventative medicine could bring enormous changes to the human race, not only because of the utopian goal of human improvement, but because responses to environmental conditions affected even national characteristics. Cabanis pursued here a dual strategy. First, he insisted that human beings were strong, not weak, animals, well able to adapt to a variety of circumstances. Second, he pointed out that overall health depended both on mental and on physical habits, even on the habits, or dispositions, of one's parents. People are potentially powerful, yet also potentially vulnerable.

By presenting it in this way, Cabanis both gave voice to the enormous reformist optimism of his time, where reform was the natural successsor to the new perceptions a revolution makes possible, as the title of his book suggests, and, at the same time, demonstrated that medicine, as an organized, state-supported activity, is the essential agent of human improvement. It did not lessen the authority of nature to recognise that perfectibility does not come automatically, that it requires medicine to help it along. We can now see how, through its therapeutic capacity, medicine is envisaged as the handmaiden of nature, its messenger and mediator. Not only did Cabanis find ways to talk about medical revolution and reform without mentioning the violence, pain and savagery of political revolution, but his remedies enabled him to have state sanction for an official, authoritative, professionalized medicine, while the interests of both the ordinary citizen and the collectivity were being perfectly served.

Cabanis had a vision of the past, the present and the future, in which medicine played a significant social role. It acted progressively to improve the well-being and happiness of the people, it contributed to the perfectibility of the human race; accordingly he looked forward to a situation where medicine received enhanced esteem. But his vision could only be fully realized with government help. Three reasons for this are implied. First, Cabanis assumed that medical *education* was an area where the state should directly intervene, and indeed the context in which he was writing reinforced this conviction. Second, he believed that medicine had to be protected from the threat of quackery; he drew an explicit contrast between 'true doctors' and charlatans, whom he characterized in terms of 'brigandage, unreason and fury' – a language that powerfully evokes the sense of a mob out of control, and that echoes the writings of those opposed to the Terror.[25] Third, the very nature of medicine, according to Cabanis, required, as he put it, more surveillance and more support and encouragement than other fields, presumably because it touches so directly the welfare of citizens.

His intention in the *Coup d'Œuil* seems to have been to rouse his readers' feelings, to create an idealistic mood in which medicine was closely linked to a greater good. It was fitting that his conclusion to the work as a whole tried to harness a patriotism, an idealism, a sense of progress and betterment to which the zeal of medical practitioners would make a major contribution.[26] He actively resisted, however, the potentially negative implications of privilege to which such a rousing call to arms could be vulnerable, by stating the importance of the social bonds between individuals and the capacity of everyone, even the simplest artisan, to contribute to the common good.

Despite his protestations, Cabanis' vision did assign a special place to medicine, not just by virtue of its humanitarian qualities, discussed in highly emotive terms, but because of the necessarily wide intellectual compass of medicine. Its study, he claimed, 'embraced practically all knowledge of physical and moral processes'.[27] The professionalism of medicine rested not merely on state support and on effective clinical practice, but also on its broad scope, on medicine as a way of apprehending all aspects of the human condition at both the individual and social levels. The approach to medical revolution and reform developed in the *Coup d'Œuil* was anchored equally in the arguments that medicine was a science, that it was a clinical art and that it was an unusually demanding, wide-ranging and socially valuable endeavour. Cabanis ended the work by presenting these as republican issues. A new era was dawning, he claimed, characterized both by the consolidation of republicanism and by a glorious and benificent medicine. The publication of this specific vision as late as 1804 is indeed striking.

Cabanis' conviction about the role of therapy at the heart of medicine, as science, as art, as an intellectual and humanitarian enterprise, reveals how tightly woven together were intellectual, social and political issues in his thought. Equally, it indicates some of the delicate negotiations his approach required in order to argue for total medical reform while avoiding charges of being factional or openly subversive. He was not, of course, alone in following this route, a route which was made considerably more plausible by appealing to nature as a teacher, to medicine as the teacher's helper. There is a generous, all-embracing quality to such claims, which drew upon decades if not centuries, of ideas about the authority, the goodness and the healing powers of nature.

His arguments also gathered force from an historical orientation and examples – the second issue canvassed at the beginning of the *Coup d'Œuil* that I wish to discuss. It was indeed significant that he decided to use historical arguments, and his particular view of what history entails is revealing. Cabanis' assertions about medical reform in his own time, like his use of humanitarian, political and social themes and of the authority of nature, do not *logically* entail a historical approach. Why then did he begin the book with 'the history of medical revolutions'? At an explicit level, Cabanis' own testimony suggests two closely related reasons. First, the past is a source of direct lessons for the present and the future. For example, he directed the reader's attention to the dislocation, as he saw it, between the progressive developments in medicine as a science during the sixteenth and seventeenth centuries, and the stagnation of medical education in the same period. A totally obvious lesson about the need to keep these two aspects of medicine in harmonious interaction with one another can be taught.

More interesting is the second reason Cabanis provided for studying the history of medicine, namely that it illustrates the context (*circonstances* is his word) in which medical changes take place. He eloquently expressed the idea that medical revolutions are inevitably bound up with alterations in the nature of human societies. It is therefore implicit that medicine is not something static, but that it is, by its very nature, progressive, variable, fluctuating. It follows that it is within the remit of reformers to make medicine better and to make it serve human ends. Two further reasons for the appeal of history present themselves. It helps maintain a suitable distance from delicate and potentially explosive issues, and it can act to sanction novelty and innovation, not merely by showing the possibility or rather the necessity of change, but by offering positive role models from the past – some phases of which can be idealized for productive contemporary ends. We know that this was a widespread characteristic of Cabanis' era, which was a period of (neo-)classicism in far more than the visual arts.[29] Furthermore, enthusiasm for the ancients, especially Hippocrates, was particularly prevalent among French medical practitioners. The past was used by eighteenth- and nineteenth-century medical commentators in diverse ways to explore and advance their own concerns – it was a major cultural resource for them.

Cabanis was perhaps a more acute historian than has been acknowledged. He set out an elaborate programme for the history of medicine, in the full knowledge that his own work could not achieve so much:

> it would be necessary to enter into all the details of (medical) history; to join to that the history of other related sciences, even in some sense to follow the history of all civil society. It is perhaps only in the simultaneous examination of these different issues; in examining the reciprocal influence between the state of society and political events, their shared influence on the general development of the human mind, and the influence of the various sciences on medicine in particular, that one can acquire a precise and complete idea of the state of medicine at all times.... (this kind of history) will shed a new and lively light on several aspects of general human history, with which, at a first glance, medicine seems to have little connection.[30]

It is impossible not to be struck by the capaciousness of his view of medical history. It permitted him to use the intensifying qualities of the revolutionary process he experienced and observed in order to explore the nature of medical change, and to advocate specific medical changes. He used ideas of revolution and reform to give voice to a powerful utopian vision of a medical future, a vision that was shared by many of his colleagues and friends. Certainly, sectional interests were at work here, even if they were sometimes expressed in an indirect form. At other times Cabanis quite openly proclaimed his hostility towards unlicensed medical practice using a politically charged language of conflict.

Cabanis was able to present a convincing, yet unthreatening view of revolution and reform. His historical sketch was of enormous help in conveying the panoramic vision of medicine he originally intended the *Coup d'Œuil* would give full expression to.[31] An awareness of the past was one aspect of a general reflexiveness which I believe characterized Enlightenment medicine. Cabanis subjected the history of his profession to critical scrutiny, just as he did its methodology, its pedagogic practices, its relations with other disciplines and its clinical practice.

It is possible to interpret the *Coup d'Œuil* as an attempt to bring together a number of the major strands of Enlightenment thought, and to weave them into a convincing picture depicting both a coherent overview of medicine and a persuasive account of its social and political importance. Cabanis repeatedly insisted on the importance of observation and on organizing the resulting knowledge in a coherent fashion. He thereby paid tribute to the primacy of first-hand experience and to classificatory techniques as a way of systematically managing the results of experience. He also espoused a form of the analytical method, which was so successfully popularized by his fellow *idéologues,* just as he absorbed prevailing ideas about language. While he stressed the need for literary studies, he was equally insistent that the 'art' peculiar to medicine required special development. In these respects Cabanis was typical of those medical practitioners most closely associated with the Enlightenment.

The fact that his work was written during the Revolution gives it added interest. However we interpret the relations between the Enlightenment and the French Revolution, there is no doubt that the latter offered men such as Cabanis a chance to think afresh, to put, or rather attempt to put into practice the spirit of renewal evident in earlier medical writings.[32] If the realities of the revolution made the implementation of reform a difficult process, at least in his writings Cabanis tasted a kind of mastery. In constructing the *Coup d'Œuille* he set himself an ambitious programme that he failed to bring to fruition, but, even in the version he did complete, it is possible to follow the intricate negotiations he undertook. The revolution carried dangers for writers too, but Cabanis seems to have felt relatively at ease thinking and writing medicine afresh.

There was a powerful vision of medicine in his text – a vision that included most of the claims Enlightenment medicine held most dear; revolutions in the service of progress and rational reform, medicine for the common good, medicine that is systematic, well organized – both intellectually and institutionally – and properly taught, a medicine integrated with polite culture and sensitive to the needs of all patients. Cabanis could write such medicine if he could not practise it, and in writing it he used and promoted history as an enterprise akin to medicine. In his writing he empowered both domains. His sense, not just of medicine in its historical *circonstances,* but of history as a rich source of insight and reform, permits us to understand Cabanis as an assiduous student of the enlightenment ideas and as an important medical reformer of the late Enlightenment.

Notes

Acknowledgements: this is a revised and shortened version of papers presented at the University of California, Los Angeles, the Annual Meeting of the Canadian Society for Eighteenth-century Studies (1990), and the Wellcome Unit for the History of Medicine, University of Oxford. My thanks to all concerned.

1. On Enlightenment medicine see W. F. Bynum, 'Health, Disease and Medical Care' in G. Roussesau and R. Porter (eds), *The Ferment of Knowledge: Studies in the Historiography of Eighteenth-Century Science* (Cambridge: Cambridge University Press, 1980), 211–53; A. Cunningham and R. French (eds), *The Medical Enlightenment of the Eighteenth Century* (Cambridge: Cambridge University Press, 1990); G. Risse, 'Medicine in the Age of Enlightenment' in A. Wear (ed.), *Medicine in Society: Historical Essays* (Cambridge, Cambridge University Press, 1992), 149–95; P. Gay, *The Enlightenment An Interpretation: The Science of Freedom* (New York: Knopf, 1969), ch. 1; R. Forster and 0. Ranum (eds), *Medicine and Society in France* (Baltimore: Johns Hopkins University Press, 1980).
2. The standard work on Cabanis remains M. S. Staum, *Cabanis: Enlightenment and Medical Philosophy in the French Revolution* (Princeton: Princeton University Press, 1980). On medicine in the French Revolution see also D. Vess, *Medical Revolution in France 1789–1796* (Gainesville: University Presses of Florida, 1975); D. Outram, *The Body and the French Revolution: Sex. Class and Political Culture* (New Haven: Yale University Press, 1989); E. Ackerknecht, *Medicine at the Paris Hospital. 1794–1848* (Baltimore: Johns Hopkins University Press, 1967). For Cabanis' writings see C. Lehec and J. Cazeneuve (eds), *Oeuvres Philosophiques de Cabanis* (Paris: Presses Universitaires de France, 1956), 2 vols. All quotations from Cabanis are my own translation from this edition, hereafter *O.P.C.*
3. I. B. Cohen, 'The Eighteenth-Century Origins of the Concept of Scientific Revolution', *Journal of the History of Ideas,* xxxvii (1976), 257–88 and *Revolution in Science* (Cambridge: Harvard University

Press, 1985); A. Levin, 'Venel, Lavoisier, Fourcroy, Cabanis and the Idea of Scientific Revolution: The French Political Context and the General Patterns of Conceptualization of Scientific Change', *History of Science,* xxii (1984), 303–20.

4. For example, J. C. Lettsom, *History of the Origins of Medicine* (London, 1778); William Black, *An Historical Sketch of Medicine and Surgery* (London, 1782); K. P. J. Sprengel, *Beitrage sur Geschichte der Medicin* (Halle, 1794–6).
5. R. J. J. Martin, 'Explaining John Freind's *History of Physick*', *Studies in History and Philosophy of Science,* xix (1988), 399–418.
6. C. Webster, 'The Historiography of Medicine', in P. Corsi and P. Weindling (eds), *Information Sources in the History of Science and Medicine* (London: Butterworth Scientific, 1983), 29–43.
7. On the *idéologues* see F. Picavet, *Les Idéologues* (New York: Burt Franklin, 1971, first published 1891); S. Moravia, *Les Pensiero degli Idéologues* (Florence: La Nuova Italia, 1974); G. Gusdorf, *La Conscience Révolutionnaire, les Idéologues* (Paris: Payot, 1978); E. Kennedy, *A Philosophe in the Age of Revolution: Destutt de Tracy and the Origins of 'Ideology'* (Philadelphia: American Philosophical Society, 1978); G. Rosen, 'The Philosophy of Ideology and the Emergence of Modern Medicine in France', *Bulletin of the History of Medicine,* xx (1946), 328–39.
8. Biographical details may be found in Staum, *op. cit.* (note 2), while *O.P.C.* contains full bibliographical details of his published work.
9. In her recent study of La Mettrie, Wellman stresses just these points in order to place him at the centre of the medical Enlightenment: K. Wellman, *La Mettrie: Medicine. Philosophy and Enlightenment* (Durham: Duke University Press, 1992).
10. *O.P.C.,* Vol. 2, 68.
11. *Ibid., 69.*
12. *lbid.,* 70, 68.
13. *Ibid.,* 249–50.
14. In her excellent study of attitudes to medical education in Edinburgh, Rosner discusses the question of literary skills, the classics and polite culture: L. Rosner, *Medical Education in the Age of Improvement: Edinburgh Students and Apprentices 1760-1826* (Edinburgh: Edinburgh University Press, 1991).
15. On hygiene see T. Ogawa, (ed.), *Public Health* (Tokyo: Saikon, 1981).
16. *O.P.C.,* Vol. 2, 250. The French reads: '... la culture des lettres et des art d'agrément, peut se lier aux travaux sévères de l'art de guérir'.
17. A recent discussion that bears on this question is B. Stafford, *Body Criticism. Imaging the Unseen in Enlightenment Art and Medicine* (Cambridge: MIT Press, 1991), see also *Art History,* xv (1992), 537–42, for a critical assessment of this approach to visual epistemology.
18. R. Williams, *Keywords: A Vocabulary of Culture and Society* (London:

Fontana, 1983, 2nd edn), 40–3.

19. William Hunter is an excellent example of a medical practitioner whose cultural activities were of paramount importance: W. F. Bynum and Roy Porter (eds), *William Hunter and the Eighteenth-Century Medical World* (Cambridge: Cambridge University Press, 1985). Also I. Pears, *The Discovery of Painting: The Growth of Interest in the Arts in England 1680–1768* (New Haven: Yale University Press, 1988).
20. On the *Décade Philosophique* see J. Kitchen, *Un Journal 'Philosophique': La Décade 1794–1807* (Paris: M. J. Minard, 1966).
21. *O.P.C.*, Vol. 2, 214–21.
22. *Ibid.*, 218.
23. *Ibid.*, 221–5.
24. *Ibid.*, 225.
25. *Ibid.*, 147. W. F. Church (ed.), *The Influence of the Enlightenment on the French Revolution. Creative, Disastrous or Non-Existent?* (Lexington: Heath, 1964) and P. Hulme and L. Jordanova (eds), *The Enlightenment and its Shadows* (London: Routledge, 1990).
26. *O.P.C.*, Vol. 2, 253–4.
27. *Ibid.*, 254.
28. *Ibid.*, 71.
29. On the use of the classics in relation to science and medicine, see Outram, *op. cit.* (note 2).
30. *O.P.C.*, Vol. 2, 71.
31. *Ibid.*, 66–7.
32. It might be fruitful to compare Cabanis with Thomas Beddoes (1760–1808), his almost exact contemporary and a practitioner also committed to medical reform: R. Porter, *Doctor of Society: Thomas Beddoes and the Sick Trade in Late-Enlightenment England* (London: Routledge, 1992).

7

The Enlightenment Encountered: The German Physicus and His World, 1750–1820

Mary Lindemann

No one in the eighteenth century could have suspected that the short, almost rhetorical query, 'What is Enlightenment?' would generate an historical industry, nor have anticipated that some two hundred years later the answer would continue to elude us. Historians' questions about the influence of the Enlightenment on medicine have tended to focus rather narrowly on medical education, medical theory, and the intertwined processes of professionalization and medicalization. We still have far to go before closing the book on the relationship between medicine and the Enlightenment.[1] Despite an avid pursuit of the social history of medicine over almost two decades, it is not unfair to say that the historian's gaze in this respect (with some clear exceptions) still tends to fix on the upper levels of medical practice, on the professors and physicians who staffed medical faculties, served at court, and contributed to the medical press. The 'enlightened proletariat' among physicians, the 'private' practitioners, the state or town physician in an outlying or backward region, those medical equivalents of Robert Darnton's Grub-Street hacks, have received scant scholarly attention. We know something about their education, but much less about their personal lives and beliefs. We also know little about how the realities of medical practice both shaped and were shaped by the ideals and objectives of Enlightenment. Did some physicians closely identify themselves with the programmatic goals of Enlightenment? If so, how did they define Enlightenment in their own minds, or through their own actions? What role did they allot it in their lives and in their medical practice?

To answer these questions we must probe the day-to-day experiences of physicians, the *Alltag* of medical practice. This article focuses on state-salaried physicians (the *Physici*) in Protestant, northern

Germany from about 1750 to 1820, in terms of the above query. If we are indeed curious about the extent to which the Enlightenment penetrated the lower echelons of medical practice – a practice far removed from universities and cities – then this is where we must dig. Here we can likewise best gauge the extent to which the Enlightenment might have percolated up from a substratum of petty officials and ordinary practitioners as well as diffusing down from a highly-educated medical élite. In addition, it is at this level that we can learn about the reception of the Enlightenment and about how people encountered the Enlightenment in their daily lives.

In the second half of the eighteenth century the Enlightenment in Germany was intricately woven into older principles of cameralism. It had also become what one historian refers to as 'a Protestant lay theology'.[2] That is, it represented a set of ideas and goals generally subscribed to by wide sections of civil and political society. Enlightened policies, conflated with cameralism and populationism, had permeated most circles of government by the 1750s and 1760s, and the goals of Enlightenment often braided themselves nicely into the larger ambitions of rulers and their ministers. Moreover, an older view of the intrusive territorial state, that is, a state that had literally to muscle its way into communities, to be met there by the stiff opposition of customs and privileges defined (almost) since time immemorial, is a false one. Resistance to state encroachment was by no means uniform; the state was often courted and welcomed, or called in to support the machinations of one party against another.[3] This insight proves extremely useful for grasping how eighteenth-century German society and public health worked, as well as for prying open the paradoxes of Enlightenment at the level of the everyday.

If the eighteenth-century state cannot unrealistically be perceived as one standard-bearer of the Enlightenment, what role did the Physicus – the officer of health – play in its day-to-day reality? By the middle of the eighteenth century, numerous German territories regularly named Physici to serve in small cities and rural districts, where they acted not only as forensic experts: they also gathered and interpreted information, monitored public health, tracked diseases, prepared an increasing number of reports, and supervised the surgeons, midwives and apothecaries in their districts.[4] The position of the Physicus is thus a nodal point, but one situated in something of a geographical and cultural limbo. A Physicus was in bureaucratic terms the sensitive finger-tip placed on the pulse of public health. Yet the Physicus cannot be cast exclusively in the role of bureaucrat: that locates him far too firmly in an administrative hierarchy and isolates him from the richer and more complex milieux which enveloped and sometimes suffocated him. It is also easy to overlook the fact that he fulfilled multiple roles in a community, roles that had little – often nothing – to do with medicine directly. These extra-official and extra-medical aspects of his life – his position as property owner and *paterfamilias*, as debtor and creditor, his propriety, his piety, his bearing, and even his clothes and manner of speech – determined to a large extent his acceptability to a wider public. The behaviour of a medical officer in these several roles conveyed potent social and cultural messages about his fitness to join the community, as well as ultimately determining his qualifications as a healer in a world that did not, yet, finely separate the social and the medical and where medical decision-making turned overwhelmingly on non-medical principles. Because medical practice lay deeply embedded in everyday routines and was poorly distinguished from other aspects of life, the relationship between patients and practitioners was as sharply contoured by perceptions of probity, commonsense, and piety, as by any objective weighing and measuring of an ability to cure or by the careful calculation of costs.

And even if we accept the vision of a vigorous enlightened state in action, there is no compelling reason to dress every physician willy-nilly in the garb of enlightenment. The characteristics of enlightened medical practice might be expressed in many ways. The dense archival information available on the hundred or so men who assumed the duties of Physicus in the duchy of Braunschweig-Wolfenbüttel between 1750 and 1820, makes it rather difficult to argue that their medical practice and position in the community can best be appreciated or categorized as 'enlightened' or 'unenlightened'. This observation does not deny, however, the prevalence of a certain strain of thought and action, rhetoric and representation that might at least heuristically – if crudely – be defined as enlightened. One could, for example, select certain templates of enlightenment in medical practice: a general, if not unanimous, enthusiasm for smallpox inoculation, and later vaccination; a growing tendency to unlink conditions of health and illness from sheer environmental determinism; a propensity to assign individuals responsibility for their own health; an outspoken assault on 'quackery'; and, finally but not incidentally, a veritable passion for publicity that begot a whole generation of physician-scribblers.

Yet these congruities do not unequivocally define a medical enlightenment in action. Nor do they speak conclusively for a conscious adoption of the enlightenment by physicians or for one that deeply permeated their lives. Clearly most Physici in official reports and in their other writings fulminated against superstition, and sketched out plans for the improvement of medical care. But it proves very difficult to disengage this language and this rhetoric from a cameralist-tinged discourse. It is even trickier to determine – if it can be determined at all – to what extent words mirrored beliefs or merely signalled an astute ability to present, or represent, actions and motivations in ways calculated to further modest careers and gain public or occupational recognition. If language, then, remains an uncertain guide to the impact of the enlightenment on the average physician, perhaps we should seek evidence in other places: in the lifestyles and repeated actions that testify how the enlightenment revealed itself in daily life as well as illuminate the reaction the enlightenment evoked among the unenlightened. This circles us back to our point of departure: a reflection on the day-to-day operation of communities and the multiple roles the Physicus and the physician played in them.

Lifestyle in this world was never a matter safely left to individual volition. Personal traits were immediately and irrevocably situated in broader social, cultural and moral frameworks. Villages and neighbourhoods functioned to a large extent on face-to-face politics, and a community still judged its members on a contingency of roles, rarely filtering out, for example, the doctor from the father, from the property-owner, from the church-goer, from the debtor or creditor. I present this point with some trepidation. One can play the game of 'community' in many ways: community is not, of course, invariably holistic, nurturing, monolithic. Early modern communities were less static and more fluid, less caring and more cruel, and less insular and more open to the outside world than we once believed. Certainly by 1750 it would be foolish to portray them as havens in a heartless world. Most – even the smallest – were linked to, and rapidly becoming dependent on, regional and international trade networks, and thus should not be seen as tight, homogenous, and suspicious little knots of implacable resistance to external pressures or innovations.[5] Yet a degree of 'closedness' persisted, although it was slowly dissolving. This gradual 'opening', a growing suppleness in what remained a fairly stiff communal system is what characterizes eighteenth-century rural life. Still, in this world, medical decision-making continued to rest heavily on broader judgements about the personal characteristics of healers, inclinations that seldom turned – and perhaps even today, rarely turn – on medical variables alone. This comes perilously close to arguing that 'medicine didn't matter' in the early modern world, or (at least) that it was not terribly important. That is not quite my intent. Rather I stress that medical practice in the eighteenth century was one element of many, was locked into complex series of relationships, and cannot be comprehended if we limit ourselves to a simple oppositional taxonomy of 'good' and 'bad' or 'enlightened' and 'unenlightened' medicines.

The documentation on the Physici shows how poorly many Physici fit into their communities. There were notable exceptions, men who had won the trust and even the affection of their clients and fellow-villagers, perhaps quickly, perhaps only after long years of struggle. Moreover, the rejection of outsiders and innovative practices by peasants has long been overstated. The true story of the interaction between state and village, between the enlightened and the unenlightened, and between insiders and outsiders, is far more complex than dichtomous terms imply. For example, despite the frequent, bitter complaints of physicians about the benightedness of peasants in respect to all aspects of health and medicine, there seems in fact to have been remarkably little concentrated resistance to the introduction of a whole series of what have traditionally been considered enlightened reforms. There was, for example, no widespread popular outcry against the introduction of smallpox inoculation, although some individuals, of course, protested. Paradoxically, many *physicians* remained sceptical. Communal officials cautiously calculated the costs of projects to improve water supplies, drain swamps, and introduce new crops, but seldom rejected them out of hand as either undesirable or pointless. They did, however, carefully assess advantages and disadvantages, often coming to conclusions that differed from those of more distant planners. Finally, villagers and the 'common folk' never avoided physicians with the practically rabid fear and intense distrust that medical pamphleteers and professional medical publicists were so fond of describing (and which some historians have swallowed as reflecting true conditions), although admittedly patterns of serial or simultaneous consultation which often sandwiched visits to a physician between trips to the cowherd and the apothecary did not exactly correspond to the physician's ideal.[6] By and large, annoyance with any one Physicus, or a pronounced dislike for the office of Physicus in general, grew out of personal experiences, and usually stemmed from a perception of the Physicus's inability to adapt to a specific community. Complaints clustered overwhelmingly on lifestyle and behaviour. Dissatisfaction with cures may have been common, but it was not often remarked, and malpractice charges were so rare as to be almost non-existent.

One story, that of Dr Christian Joseph Loeber, highlights how medical practice, even in the closing decades of the eighteenth century, remained firmly implanted in routines of life and cannot be detached from them historically. Loeber's case is by no means typical, but it does demonstrate, if in a perhaps exaggerated way, how a certain lifestyle could generate tensions and initiate proceedings against a Physicus. Yet if Loeber is not the norm, his story dramatizes one kind of Enlightenment as a lived and observed experience.

Nothing in the five short lines that make up the official biography of Christian Joseph Loeber hints at scandal.[7] The brief, almost perfunctory entry suggests a modestly utilitarian, modestly successful, and totally unexceptional, if perhaps boring, life. Born in 1743 in Saxony, Loeber studied medicine in Erfurt, receiving his doctorate with a dissertation on the anatomy and physiology of the heart. Although he never published much, just three works in an entire lifetime, he did participate in a small way in a medical republic of letters dominated by a far more prolific group of physician–writers.[8] Loeber ended his days as Physicus in the small town of Vorsfelde. All in all his career would seem nothing more than a footnote to history, if not for the other, darker side, of this eighteenth-century Dr Jekyll. For behind his prosaic facade lurked a monster, at least if contemporary reports can be credited. The rumours swirling around Loeber were shocking. Contemporaries portrayed his behaviour as mad, macabre, and perhaps even criminal: he robbed graves, defiled corpses, blasphemed, and frittered away his wife's fortune. These suppositions and others – about his enormous debts, his vindictive behaviour, his bizarre actions, his insufferable posturing and arrogance – conveyed negative messages about his qualifications as a physician and about his suitability as a member of the community.

In February 1790 a group of concerned citizens in the small market town of Vorsfelde communicated with the duchy's Collegium medicum in Braunschweig on the matter of the selection of a new Physicus. Vorsfelde's Physicus had died a few months earlier, and the Collegium medicum was deep in the midst of deliberations concerning a replacement. 'It has come to our attention', the letter began,

> that Dr Loeber who previously resided in Schöppenstedt, and who now lives in Gommern near Magdeburg is to receive the post of Physicus here in Vorsfelde. We have learned that this man in the last few years has lived in Hornburg, Schöppenstedt, and Heßen, and that he left all these places in haste, and then took up residence in Gommern. Hearsay does not allow us to expect much good from him, as he had not conducted himself very well [in the past] especially in Heßen and Schöppenstedt.[9]

Rumours of misconduct, of impiety, of unpaid debts; these were the things that disturbed the good citizens of Vorsfelde.

> One hears that in Heßen he used coffins to mock religion and led the youth there astray; in Schöppenstedt, he is said to have dug up his own child and painted him blue; and it is also whispered about that he ran up debts and did not pay them.[10]

This archival spoor leads to a series of 'odd and troubling' incidents connected with Loeber, incidents that repeatedly awakened the suspicions and aroused the mistrust of the members of the communities in which he resided. For example, in Schöppenstedt in April 1785, the magistrates had conducted a hearing into the strange circumstances of Loeber's exhumation of his own, recently deceased child. The nightwatchman and gravedigger, a simple soul named Beekl, testified that early on the morning after the funeral, Loeber had appeared through the mist at the cemetery and requested that he open the grave. Thinking that Loeber wished to place a remembrance in the coffin with the child, Beekl complied and dug a small opening 'about the width of a spade' in the ground. 'But', he went on,

> Professor Dr Loeber was not satisfied, and asked me to enlarge the hole; which I did, not suspecting any mischief. Finally I hit the coffin ... as I climbed out of the grave, Dr Loeber sprang in, loosened the lid ... lifted out the corpse, wrapped it in a sheet ... and without another word hurried away.[11]

That was a peculiar and disturbing tale, but the stories did not stop there. Loeber's 'excesses' continued, and the displeasure his actions evoked drove him from one place to another. The whole story is rather too long to recount in detail here, but from 1780 until the move to Vorsfelde in 1790, Loeber wandered restlessly from Hornburg, to Schöppenstedt, to Gommern, seeking but apparently never finding his niche.

In Hornburg, Loeber had stepped on the toes of the resident physician there and left, or was driven out.[12] He went to Heßen, where he served as Physicus for a time. The magistrates there admitted that 'at first [he] was well-liked' and probably could have earned a decent living 'if he had pursued an upright and prudent life and if he had not drawn upon himself the distrust and scorn of almost everyone because of his immoral lifestyle and his uncouth behaviour'.[13] Thus, despite a good start, and despite the important support of friends and relatives in Heßen, he was soon in deep trouble, personally and occupationally. His behaviour continued to excite attention, but hardly approval. For example, it was reported that

> in the garden he rented . . . he erected a number of graves painted with large crosses as monuments to the deceased [poet Christian

> Fürchtegott] Gellert and to an old man named Hubert [or Herbek] who, according to Loeber, attained the age of 108; [moreover] he built a so-called 'Schneckenberg' [a maze] and a linden-tree loggia, which he called his hermitage and had the roof tiled and put in a ventilator and four large windows although the entire leaf-work was open [to the air].

Through this and similar 'useless and laughable' experiments he had wasted his money and was soon driven to pawn what possessions remained to him and borrow heavily from others.

He then took in the 11-year-old son of an impoverished locksmith as his servant and 'dressed him in a ridiculous garb just like his own' – a long, loose robe decorated with stars. He persuaded a young vagrant, who had made his living by harp-playing and begging, to come lodge with him 'for what purposes we can only guess at and fear'. To these 'pupils' he added a day-labourer's son and a lad from nearby Veltheim; the four formed the first class in his self-styled 'Philanthropie', the educational institute he founded to train poor boys as surgeons. At the same time, the report maintained, Dr Loeber 'charged excessively' for his services and, quite illegally, dispensed his own 'concoctions' thereby hurting the local apothecary's trade greatly.

He persisted in his 'wild and disorderly' lifestyle. His neighbours held against him that 'he paraded up and down the streets with a burning pipe [in his mouth] and even went into the barns with it'. Thereupon, he forfeited 'all the trust, esteem, and credit' he might have enjoyed as a physician and Physicus. At the same time, one pupil 'proved the results of *his* pious education', by stealing money from his teacher. Now, Loeber was in serious financial difficulties. To recoup his losses, he organized a subscription to finance his school. To no avail. Those he persuaded to contribute soon renounced their pledges when they realized that 'he was a hypocrite and dissembler' and that the instruction he provided would only produce 'lazybones and scamps'. Deprived of even this hope of support, students soon fled his 'starvation school' and 'plagued our citizens with their insistent pleas for alms'. Loeber sank into the deepest financial distress, his creditors hounded him, his landlord took away his bed and held it as security against unpaid rent.

Everyone viewed his Philanthropie as a farce. They judged his plan to educate his pupils in religion as 'drivel'. He had been raised a Lutheran, although he later converted to Catholicism to please his first wife. When she died, he returned to the Lutheran fold. But, the report pointed out, 'he can only have been very poorly instructed in his own creed, as he denies the miracles of Christ and seeks to make them suspect'. He had apparently told two apprentice barbers that the gospel story of how Christ restored sight to the blind man was no miracle at all, but the work of a natural physician. Where the purported miracle had occurred, there was slate [*Schieferstein*], which, Loeber insisted, 'can cure all eye diseases'. Christ knew this and his miracle was therefore nothing more than to spit on the stone shavings, making a salve of them. He then smeared the blind man's eyes with this natural unguent. The report commented drily '[it] was a good thing for his young pupils that their "instruction" lasted only a few days!'

Loeber's purposed educational curriculum was elaborate, and included instruction in reading and writing, as well as in mathematics, natural science, anatomy and languages.[14] These were great expectations, but close observers saw only a fully misconceived and even lunatic scheme. Indeed, the report positively sneered: 'It seems pretty odd [to us] that Dr Loeber proposes to instruct his pupils in Latin and Greek . . . when these ragamuffins can barely read German'. Although the school quickly folded, its failure did not diminish Loeber's enthusiasm for new ventures. He took into his home a young, blind woman in order to restore her sight. When this attempt failed, Loeber attributed his lack of success 'to her inability to remain still enough' during the operation. The report concluded with the note that Loeber had been forced to leave Heßen 'for lack of substance' but before he went 'he pressed his clients – who had already paid their bills in full – for more money'.

In many ways it is not relevant whether these stories about Loeber were true or false, vastly exaggerated or basically accurate, or whether a series of enemies wove a web of lies around him. Decisive is that the flaws and faults listed by the citizens of Heßen and elsewhere were ones that were credible and meant something to the community that raised them.[15] That is, the crimes which the notables of Heßen accused Loeber of perpetrating were ones that they themselves found suspicious and loathsome, and which they felt would unfailingly arouse the same feelings of abhorrence and repulsion in others.

Each charge, each accusation, therefore, cannot be dislodged from its historical matrix, from a contextual world that rendered actions meaningful. A few incidents from the long chronicle of Loeber's malefactions – the exhumation of his child, his Philanthropie, his veneration for the ancient Hubert, and, finally, his blasphemy – illustrate this essentiality of context.

When Loeber went to the graveyard and had his child dug up, he violated one of the oldest communal taboos – that separating the living from the dead. Touching a corpse, or dissecting it, remained moments of tension, of liminality in early modern societies. Only slowly did people conquer their cultural horror of corpses, especially of those who perished by drowning.[16] The numerous life-saving and resuscitation institutes founded in the late eighteenth century worked hard to root out an ancient dread of contact with a drowned corpse, and sought to instil a humanitarian responsibility for saving lives. Equally great was the horror of being buried alive.[17] Fear of dissection was just as vivid and Loeber's actions seemed monstrous: to exhume his own child, dismember it, and in the words of one man to 'turn it into a mummy' deeply disgusted the average observer in a way that we can only imperfectly comprehend today. What Loeber did, in fact, was, with the assistance of a surgeon, perform an autopsy: he examined the oesophagus, glands of the neck, the tongue, and the cerebrum, and separated out these parts to preserve them as anatomical 'Praeparate'.[18] If his neighbours and the magistrates, as well as churchmen (Loeber was fined by church authorities for desecrating a grave) found Loeber's behaviour bizarre, unacceptable, and even blasphemous, Loeber, the Collegium medicum, the ducal Privy Council, the medical faculty at the University of Helmstedt, and an enlightened public could think differently.[19] These men could – and did – interpret Loeber's actions (at least to some extent) as the laudable efforts of an enlightened man, and a true father, seeking to lay bare the cause of death of his own child, to pursue science in the face of superstition, and to promote the welfare of others in the future.

Similar apprehensions and misapprehensions surfaced in regard to other incidents in Loeber's life. He was foolish as well as ghoulish. One cannot miss the sarcasm notables used in describing Loeber's many projects: his Philanthropie, his monuments to Gellert, to 'that old man of 108', his garden-house and hermitage, were uniformly labelled 'absurd'. If in other circles all these found a more sympathetic reception, and even excited admiration, that was not the reaction elicited in the small towns and villages dotting the eighteenth-century German countryside.

For instance, one of Loeber's pet projects was the establishment of an educational institute for pauper children. Faith in the ability of education to improve the human race, and the educational reforms that accompanied it – the establishment of schools and training centres – formed one of the most cherished goals of the Enlightenment. Education was not only supposed to alleviate poverty, it was also expected to promote the florescence of state and society.[20] In 1782 Loeber had unsuccessfully petitioned the ducal government for financial assistance in setting up his Philanthropie.[21] Despite lacking official sanction or funds, he went ahead, inaugurating his school with a handful of pupils. The conditions at this 'starvation school', if the report of the magistrates is to be believed, rivalled Dickensian horrors. Students were neglected and languished in ignorance. It was not merely Loeber's inefficiency that his contemporaries scorned, rather they regarded the entire enterprise in conception as well as in execution with the greatest possible scepticism and revulsion. His choice of pupils – a wandering harp-player and three poor boys – added to the general impression that little good would come of the school. The underlying criticism implied that all four would have been better off left in their true station in life rather than having their heads stuffed with potentially harmful nonsense. Little could come of this sort of training, locals insisted, except to breed up burdensome bands of cutpurses and beggars.

Equally ostracizing was his blasphemous and sacrilegious behaviour. His conversion to Catholicism (even to please his wife) and his subsequent return to the Protestantism of his youth, left good citizens suspicious of the fixity and orthodoxy of his beliefs. His naturalistic interpretation of a miracle of Christ – Christ restoring the blind man's sight – which Loeber explained as medical rather than supernatural and providential only heightened a sense of the religious and social decay that his presence in a community could cause.

Loeber, like many other enthusiasts of a pre-Romantic age, virtually quivered in the presence of unspoiled nature. Like them, he built a maze and a garden house to bring him closer to the natural world. All this elicited the vast amusement and unmitigated contempt of other less enlightened but perhaps more practical souls who dismissed such efforts as a waste of good land, valuable time, and much money. Those who still conceived of nature as an enemy to be conquered rather than a goddess to be worshipped, saw little sense in venerating a harsh environment that circumscribed rather than enlarged the possibilities of their lives. This was not, however, merely another clash between the forces of light and knowledge on the one hand, and the troops of darkness and superstition on the other. Rather it represented the resistance of an older style of life, one rooted in the precepts of prudent husbandry and, for that matter, reinforced by cameralist-informed initiatives and modern agronomy, against the artifice and artificiality of show and sentimentality. Likewise, Loeber's monument to the poet Gellert, whose fanciful tales profoundly stirred imaginations and jerked tears from hundreds of eighteenth-century readers, could only appear inane to the residents of a tiny town in Germany. Once again, the clash of cultures rings out, but it is a clash of values as well, and not merely the cacophony raised when the spears of Enlightenment clattered noisily (if ineffectually) against the hard bulwarks of superstition. Much of the Enlightenment had its underside, and here at the level of Grub-Street, its triviality, gimcrackery, and sheer looniness.

Most of all it is necessary to see how one group might judge certain behaviours as perfectly sane, even laudable (or at the worst, idiosyncrasies that presented no dangers to society), while another group regarded them with derision, but also consternation. Loeber's 'worship' of an old man who 'knew how to stretch his life to 108 years' certainly evoked these responses. Loeber's neighbours in Schöppenstedt were more than amused: they were disdainful of a man who would waste his substance on anything so asinine as a monument to such an absurd object of veneration. The aged were rarely valued in an early modern world of limited resources, and one chronically plagued by a short supply of arable land. If Loeber's admiration for this modern Methuselah caused his neighbours to shake their heads (and us to smile somewhat condescendingly), other contemporaries partook of his enthusiasm for macrobiotics, that is, for the science of longevity. Macrobiotics flowed easily out of the mainstream of medical thought in the eighteenth century, attracting the attention of extremely reputable figures such as the famous Berlin physician and publicist, Christoph Hufeland.[22]

Thus while Loeber's neighbours and the local notability regarded his actions with a scepticism bordering on abhorrence, others regarded his sins as less besetting and his flaws as nothing more than minor personality quirks. The Collegium medicum, for example, while its members were quite concerned about Loeber's seeming propensity to attract debts (a matter which bothered locals even more!), regarded as mere foibles the very behaviours that so deeply distressed his neighbours and which formed the basis for their overwhelmingly negative judgements on his suitability as a fellow-citizen and physician. Yet there was enough in the Vorsfelde petition to impel the Collegium medicum to probe a bit more deeply before confirming Loeber's appointment. The evidence from Heßen and Schöppenstedt was somewhat disturbing, but from his current residence in Gommern came a reassuring report on his conduct.[23] As members of the Collegium medicum deliberated on Loeber's appointment, they agreed that while he was perhaps not the best imaginable candidate, little could be held against him as a physician. They all judged him 'knowledgeable'. One member pointed out that the man who posted the damning report from Heßen was indeed 'no friend of Dr Loeber's'. Moreover, as the report contained only 'simple calumnies' and proof rested 'merely on gossip', the real question in his mind was: 'Can Dr Loeber be faulted as a physician?' To which he answered unequivocally, 'no'. Another concluded 'that what the [magistrates in] Heßen bring up, only concerns his *moral* behaviour [of] eight years ago and [it] was [then] not well substantiated. . . . In respect to his education as a physician, nothing in the report indicates any vice, but rather virtue'.[24]

Yet the opinions voiced by the Collegium medicum and of Loeber's peers ignored a crucial point: medical decisions and medical decision-making for the vast majority of people rarely turned (and perhaps even today rarely turn) solely or even principally on *medical* issues. As Loeber's case demonstrates, we need to depict the medical world of the eighteenth-century physician (or the Physicus) in the softer terminology of matrix and milieux, while avoiding the more uncompromising nomenclature of knowledge and ignorance.

And Loeber's case is only illustrative of the clash of consciousness that characterized relationships between physicians/ Physici and their clients, neighbours, and fellow-villagers. Of course, not all quarrels between individual Physici and their communities can be interpreted as a clash of consciousness, nor were deep-seated issues of ideology and *mentalité* always at stake. Community protests were usually directed against individuals (not against the office *per se*), and objections were based overwhelmingly on the personalities and personal conduct of particular men in question. The flaws most often remarked were those of character. Drunkenness, impiety and a vaguer, but equally disconcerting 'ill repute', numbered highest among the objections communities raised to the Physici in their midst. For example, in 1776, the magistrates in Schöningen reported the death of their Physicus, Dr Georg Christoph Scheibner, and asked for a replacement, hoping to be given a man, in their words, 'better' than Scheibner who offended by 'his religiously and morally reprehensible conduct'.[25] In 1791 public opinion in Schöppenstedt blocked the appointment of Dr Carl Heinrich Spohr to the position of Physicus. The magistrates there cited rumours of 'his [suspect] character and morals' as their principal objection.[26] Drunkenness, too, was offensive, although it seemed less worrisome to locals than 'bad character' or 'irreligiosity'. Locals frequently forgave 'understandable' lapses. For instance, Dr Pini's notorious, persistent inebriety in the late 1760s disquieted both local magistrates and the Collegium medicum greatly. For almost a decade they had been dealing with the problem. But Pini was not without reputable advocates who excused his drunkenness by arguing that he had good reason to turn to the bottle: they hinted at a sordid affair between his wife and a lodger.[27]

While we might dismiss imperfections of character and personality as ubiquitous and timeless, and thus not historically relevant, they assume greater weight when placed in specific contexts. Cases like Loeber's reveal the contest between two ways of thinking and acting, an encounter that often pitted an obscurantist and cranky enlightened figure against his commensensical and unimaginative neighbours.[28] The eccentric was not merely odd: he was dangerous, and could be identified by his character defects and by his inability to conduct himself in a seemly manner. Such a man could not, by common definition, be a successful healer. The history of these tussles between the Physicus and his neighbours sharpens the focus on differing perceptions of proper behaviour and their meanings. Two cases provide particularly nice illustrations. For example, in 1765 a battle broke out between the Physicus in Gandersheim, Lct. Conrad Hartwig Blum, and a forceful, even imperious, ducal official, Ludolf Granzien. The conflict had several important dimensions: it was clearly a battle over prerogatives and the exercise of authority. What helped win supporters to Granzien's side was the peculiar behaviour of Blum. Blum had taken up gemstone grinding, making an infernal din at all hours of the day and night with his grindstones, irritating his neighbours, and thereby helping convince them of his unsuitability as a physician. The Privy Council and the Collegium medicum viewed Blum's various weaknesses, in particular his hobbies, as less egregious sins or completely harmless fancies.[29]

In the early 1780s, Dr Müller in Seesen assumed in the minds of his neighbours an almost Faustian stature. He had already had a series of run-ins with the Collegium medicum over dilatory reports and sloppy bookkeeping. And not only the Collegium medicum was displeased with Müller. An anonymous denunciation related how Müller neglected his duties, while lavishing attention on his 'giddy whims'. He had, for example, built and exhibited a 'clever mechanism', and displayed 'peep-shows, like those the Italians carry around . . . in which one was allowed to look for a few pennies'. In addition, he had constructed a 'solar microscope' and transformed his study into a workshop 'more becoming a locksmith ... [than] a man responsible for supervising health in our district'. He squandered his time cutting glass. Several other witnesses confirmed these rumours of his odd behaviour, while the Collegium medicum refused to attribute any greater significance to it.[30]

Thus the problems that divided the Physici from their communities were not disputes over medical practice, or rather not over medical practice as we understand it. Because most people rarely separated medical practice from other activities, it was hard for them to accept that men like Loeber, Pini, and Müller, with their oddities and quirks, their peculiar notions and curious deeds, could function as effective physicians. While the healer's skill was still perceived as emanating from his ability to offer care and support as much as to cure, and to be good neighbours more than clever inventors and erudite scholars, such men could never fulfil the expectations the public had of them.

Notes

1. See the other essays in this volume. Cf. A. Cunningham and R. French (eds), *The Medical Enlightenment of the Eighteenth Century* (Cambridge: Cambridge University Press, 1990).
2. J. Whaley, 'The Protestant Enlightenment', in R. Porter and M. Teich (eds), *The Enlightenment in National Context* (Cambridge: Cambridge University Press, 1981), 108.
3. Thomas Robisheaux observes that '[s]tate power did not simply expand in the sixteenth and seventeenth centuries; it was very often drawn into the village by the villagers themselves. State power was also checked, frustrated, often turned to purposes no ruler completely controlled'. *Rural Society and the Search for Order in Early Modern Germany* (Cambridge and New York: Cambridge University Press, 1989), 258.
4. On the Physicus in Germany, see M. Stürzbecher, 'The Physici in German-speaking Countries from the Middle Ages to the Enlightenment', in A. Russell (ed.), *The Town and State Physician in Europe from the Middle Ages to the Enlightenment* (Wolfenbüttel: Herzog August Bibliothek, 1981); *idem*, 'Über die medizinische Versorgung der Berliner Bevölkerung im 18. Jahrhundert', in *idem*, *Beiträge zur Berliner Medizingeschichte. Quellen und Studien zur Geschichte des Gesundheitswesens vom 17. bis 19. Jahrhundert* (Berlin: de Gruyter, 1966), 1–66; *idem*, 'Vom Physikus zum Amtsarzt', *Öffentliches Gesundheitswesen*, xxxv [Sonderheft 3] (1973), 119–23; A. Fischer, 'Die kulturhistorische Wirksamkeit der Landphysici Gustav Viktor und Gustav Friedrich Jägerschmidt', in *idem*, *Beiträge zur Kulturhygiene des 18. und zu Beginn des 19. Jahrhunderts im deutschen Reiches* (Leipzig: J. A. Barth, 1928); W. Kaiser and A. Völker, *Universität und Physikat in der Frühgeschichte des Amtsarztwesens*, *Wissenschaftliche Beiträge der Martin-Luther-Universitäts Halle-Wittenberg*, liii (Halle, 1980); M. Wessling, 'Official Medicine and Customary Medicine in Early Modern

Württemberg: The Career of Christoph Friedrich Pichler', *Medizin, Gesellschaft und Geschichte*, ix (1990), 21–44.

5. Robisheaux, *op. cit.* (note 3), 258.
6. This argument cannot be fully developed here. Evidence gathered from the extensive documentation available on investigations of 'quackery' in Braunschweig-Wolfenbüttel from 1648–1820 shows that peasants and 'ordinary people' often consulted physicians as well as other medical practitioners.
7. S.v. Christian Joseph Loeber in A. Hirsch, E. Gurlt, and A. Werner (eds), *Biographisches Lexikon der hervorragenden Ärzte aller Zeiten und Völker* (2nd edn, 5 vols; Berlin and Vienna: Urban & Schwarzenberg, 1929–34).
8. 'De cordis fabricia et functione, etc.', (Erfurt: 1767); *Sendschreiben von widergekommenden Pocken nach der Einpfropfung* (Jena: 1767); *Anfangsgründe der Wundarztneykunst* (Langensalza: 1770); *Sendschreiben von einer glücklich geheilten Lungenentzündung* (Friedrichsstadt: 1771).
9. From 6 February, 1790, Niedersächsisches Staatsarchiv Wolfenbüttel [hereafter: StAWf] 111 Neu 1133, 3.
10. Petition from 'Die Bürgermeister und Geschworne in Vorsfelde, wegen Besetzung des Physicats daselbst', *ibid.*, 4.
11. From 1 April, 1785, StAWf, 1N Schöppenstedt I Nr. 460 (unpaginated file).
12. Ratsarchiv der Stadt Hornburg, 37.G. 'Prof. Dr Loeber (1780)'.
13. See two reports from Heßen, 1 March, 1790, StAWf, 111 Neu 1133, 7–11 and, earlier, 31 January, *ibid.*, 2 Alt 11363, 30–31.
14. 'Plan zum Kinder und Armen Institut', 24 June, 1782, StAWf, 2 Alt 11405, 8–11.
15. As N. Z. Davis points out, the fictional aspects of tales and stories are important. People constructed stories they felt were believable and would be believed. *Fiction in the Archives: Pardon Tales and Their Tellers in Sixteenth-Century France* (Stanford: Stanford University Press, 1987), 1–6.
16. R. Richardson, *Death, Dissection and the Destitute* (London and New York: Routledge & Kegan Paul, 1987), 3–29; O. Beneke, *Von unehrlichen Leute: Culturhistorische Studien und Geschichte aus vergangenen Tagen deutscher Gewerbe und Dienste* (2nd rev edn, Berlin: W. Hertz, 1889); W. Dankert, *Unehrliche Leute: Die verfemten Berufe* (Bern and Munich: Francke, 1963).
17. A. Fischer, *Geschichte des deutschen Gesundheitswesens*, Vol. ii, *Von den Anfängen der hygienischen Ortsbeschreibungen bis zur Gründung des Reichsgesundheitsamtes (Das 18. und 19. Jahrhunderts)* (Berlin: Kommissionsverlag F. A. Herbig, 1933), 226–9.
18. Loeber's explanation to the magistrates in Schöppenstedt, 13 [?] April, 1785, StAWf, 1N Schöppenstedt I Nr. 460.
19. See the decision of the Privy Council to allow Loeber to retain the

'Praeparate', 15 April, 1785, in *ibid.*

20. See H. Chisick, *The Limits of Reform in the Enlightenment: Attitudes toward the Education of the Lower Classes in Eighteenth-Century France* (Princeton, N.J.: Princeton University Press, 1982); J. Van Horn Melton, *Absolutism and the Eighteenth-Century Origins of Compulsory Schooling in Prussia and Austria* (Cambridge and New York: Cambridge University Press, 1988); U. Herrmann (ed.), *'Das pädagogische Jahrhundert': Volksaufklärung und Erziehung zur Armut im 18. Jahrhundert in Deutschland* (Weinheim: Beltz, 1981).
21. 'Plan zum Kinder und Armen Institut', 24 June, 1782, in StAWf, 2 Alt 11405, 8–11.
22. C. W. Hufeland, *Die Kunst das menschliche Leben zu verlängern* (Jena: 1797).
23. 25 February, 1790, StAWf, 111 Neu 1133, 16.
24. 21 March, 1790, StAWf, 111 Neu 1133, 15.
25. 21 March, 1776, StAWf, 111 Neu 1114, 3–4.
26. 14 February, 1791, StAWf, 2 Alt 11355, 22–4.
27. 'Untergenannte Einwohner der Stadt Scheppenstedt bitten unterthänigst: dem cassirten Doctoren Pini das Stadtphysicat gnädigst wieder zu schencken', 19 July, 1775, StAWf, 2 Alt 11396, 47–51; letter of support from widow of Colonel Bötticher, 7 February, 1776, *ibid.*, 67–8.
28. A perceptive observation by Colin Jones at the conference on 'Medicine and Enlightenment' (London, May 1992) prompted me to develop this interpretation more fully.
29. Granzien's report, 30 August, 1756, StAWf, 2 Alt 11471, 48–52; from Privy Council to Granzien, 2 September, 1756, *ibid.*, 54–5.
30. The denunciation was signed 'M.C.' and was not dated. StAWf, 111 Neu 1095, 135–6; for more on Müller's eccentricities see 2 Alt 11381, 56 and 2 Alt 11382, *passim.*

8

Conflicting Attitudes Towards Inoculation in Enlightenment Germany

Andreas-Holger Maehle

Man macht Gesunde krank, die Krankheit zu vertreiben,
Gibt ihnen Gift, daß sie vom Gift verschonet bleiben,
Und pfropfet durch die Kunst mit Zwang die Blattern ein,
Damit die Blattern einst dadurch verhütet seyn.
Daniel Wilhelm Triller, *Geprüfte Pockeninoculation (1766)*

Introduction

Traditional historiography has seen smallpox inoculation as an important, progressive element of eighteenth-century medicine and as a precursor of the successful practice of Jennerian cowpox inoculation or vaccination.[1] In fact the older practice of smallpox inoculation, i.e. the intra- or subcutaneous application of pus or crusts from actual human smallpox, bears marks of that rationality which is usually associated with the term 'Enlightenment'. Essentially it meant to give one's children deliberately a somewhat milder form of genuine smallpox, with a lesser, though not inconsiderable, risk of death, in order to protect them against the rather high risk of death that was connected with a natural infection with the same disease. It is well-known, for instance, that Voltaire became a passionate advocate of inoculation, having learned about it during his stay in London in the late 1720s.[2] Enlightened absolutist rulers, such as Catherine II of Russia and Joseph II of Austria, promoted its practice.[3] Contemporary opposition to this preventive measure, on the other hand, has been described as linked with conservatism or an inability to overcome traditional ways of thinking.[4] Yet, if we look at Immanuel Kant, for example, whose encouragement to use one's own rationality – the famous *sapere aude* – has become inseparable from our ideas of the Enlightenment, we find very cautious remarks. In his *Metaphysik der Sitten* (1797) he raised the question 'Is the inoculation of smallpox allowed?' without giving a definitive answer. Someone who decides to have the smallpox inoculated (wrote Kant) risks his life in uncertainty. And though he does it in order to *preserve his life*, his case is morally much more questionable than that of the sailor who entrusts himself to the storm. The sailor at least has not *made* the storm, whereas the former has (intentionally) contracted the disease which endangers his life.[5] From one of the notes that Kant used to make to aid his memory it is known more precisely where he saw the problem here. Inoculation of smallpox is allowed, he stated, if the government makes it obligatory, because then it would be inevitable for every individual, and thus permitted.[6] In other words, Kant wanted the state to assume responsibility for inoculation, since this responsibility was too heavy a burden for the individual.

Attitudes towards inoculation were not only subtly diversified, as illustrated by these comments of Kant. Adrian Wilson and Francis M. Lobo have recently suggested that pro- or anti-inoculationist commitment in England correlated with spçcific politico-religious allegiances.[7] The inoculation controversy, it seems, was more complex than a simple clash of enlightened advocates of the practice on one side and fatalistic or prejudiced adversaries on the other side.

Chiefly thanks to the classic study by Geneviève Miller and the more recent works by Peter Razzell, J. R. Smith, Deborah C. Brunton, Jean-François de Raymond, and Pierre Darmon we are quite well informed about the ways in which the originally Oriental practice of smallpox inoculation was introduced into European medicine in the early eighteenth century, how it was adopted in England, Scotland, and France, and about the debates that were connected with this process.[8] The use of statistics and quantitative arguments within the English and French debates has recently been studied in detail by Andrea A. Rusnock.[9] Very little is known, however, on the practice of inoculation – and on attitudes towards it – in the German states.[10] This chapter firstly provides some insights into the little-known discourse on inoculation in Germany. The second part of this contribution discusses examples of the actual activities of German inoculators. A third part looks into concepts and plans to eradicate smallpox totally, which were propagated by German physicians and others inspired by Enlightenment optimism towards the end of the eighteenth century; and the last part pays attention to ethical judgements of contemporary philosophers, who commented on inoculation as such and as a means of smallpox eradication.

The Discourse

A convenient measure for the varying intensity of the debate on inoculation is the number of publications per year on this subject. *Figure 1* shows the numbers of such publications in the German states, France, and Britain during the period 1714 to 1790, compiled from two special bibliographies that were edited by the German doctors Johann Georg Krünitz (1728–96) and Franz Olberg (1767–1840) in 1768 and 1791, respectively.[11] Not surprisingly, there is a first peak for Britain in the early 1720s, reflecting the introduction of inoculation in England by Lady Mary Wortley Montagu, Sir Hans Sloane and the Royal Society, and others.[12] These events had some repercussions in Germany, which seem to have been stronger than in France. As a whole, however, the German inoculation debate followed more the pattern of the French discussions. A first flood of publications started in Germany only after 1755, as a reaction to Charles Marie de La Condamine's campaign to introduce inoculation in France, and another one came in response to the ban of inoculation by the Paris *Parlement* in 1763 and the ensuing French controversies.[13] The debate on inoculation continued in Germany after 1770 with a fluctuating output of publications, while it seemed to run out in France and Britain. This continuation of the German discourse on inoculation was probably a reflection of sustained opposition to the practice (see below). The following paragraphs refer to this late phase of the German debate, which clearly profited from the earlier exchanges of arguments in Britain and France. An evident indicator for this are the comparatively high numbers of translations (mostly from French and English) among the German publications (see *Figure 1*).

Generally, the debate centred around a choice: either to trust medicine and to give one's child (or oneself) the smallpox in the artificial way by inoculation, or to wait for the natural smallpox, trusting nature and hoping that the child (or oneself) survives the disease. In the second half of the eighteenth century the risks and chances expressed in numbers were well-known from the English and French debates, and they were frequently quoted and confirmed by German data. Even strong advocates of inoculation admitted that one out of one hundred inoculated persons might die. On the other hand the lethality of smallpox contracted by natural infection was known to be between 10 and 20 per cent. Smallpox was endemic in the cities, and smaller towns expected an epidemic every five or six years. According to contemporary estimates, only five per cent of the population was never infected.[14] Late eighteenth-century German statistics showed that nearly a fifth of the total mortality was due to smallpox.[15]

Figure 1

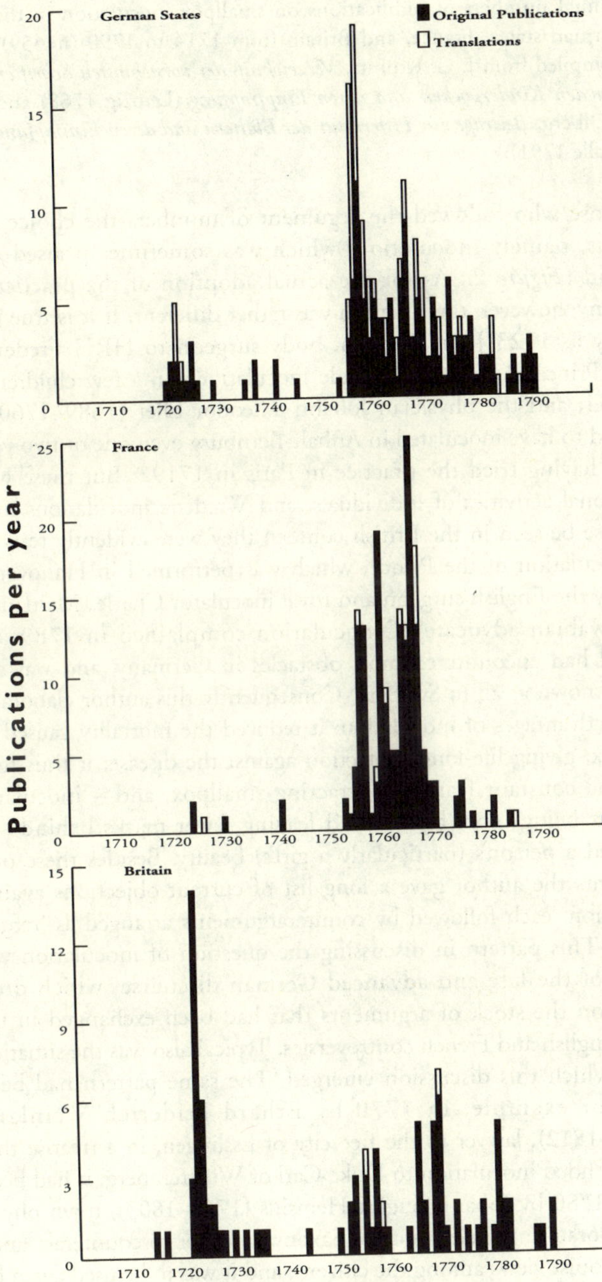
German States
Original Publications
Translations
France
Britain
Publications per year
1710
1720
1730
1740
1750
1760
1770
1780
1790

Figure 1

Annual numbers of publications on smallpox inoculation in the German states, France, and Britain from 1714 to 1790 (n=459). Compiled from J. G. Krünitz, *Verzeichniß der vornehmsten Schriften von den Kinderpocken und deren Einpfropfung* (Leipzig 1768) and F. Olberg, *Beiträge zur Littertatur der Blattern und deren Einimpfung* (Halle 1791).

For those who followed the argument of numbers the choice was obvious, namely inoculation, which was sometimes praised as a godsend (*Figure 2*). As for the actual adoption of the practice in Germany, however, the situation was rather different. It it is true that as early as 1723 John Wreden, body-surgeon to HRH Frederick Lewis, Prince of Wales, had made inoculations on a few children in Hanover; and the physician Johann Theodor Eller (1689–1760) is reported to have inoculated in Anhalt-Bernburg even one or two years earlier, having tried the practice in Paris in 1719.[16] But these were exceptional activities of individuals, and Wreden's inoculations must of course be seen in the British context: they were evidently tests for the inoculation of the Prince, which was performed in Hanover in 1724 by the English surgeon and royal inoculator Charles Maitland.[17] As a Swabian advocate of inoculation complained in 1789, the method had encountered most obstacles in Germany, and was still hardly known at all in Swabia.[18] Consequently this author elaborated on the advantages of inoculation: it reduced the mortality caused by smallpox, giving life-long protection against the disease; it thus took away the constant fear of contracting smallpox; and – inoculated smallpox being more benign and leaving fewer marks behind – it preserved a person's (particularly a girl's) beauty. Besides these pro-arguments the author gave a long list of current objections against inoculation, each followed by counterarguments arranged as 'refutations'.[19] This pattern in discussing the question of inoculation was typical of the late and advanced German discourse, which drew heavily on the stock of arguments that had been exchanged in the earlier English and French controversies. Typical also was the situation out of which this discussion emerged. The same pattern had been used, for example, in 1770 by Erhard Friderich Weinland (*c.*1745–1812), lawyer to the free city of Esslingen, in a treatise that recommended inoculation to Duke Carl of Württemberg; it had been used in 1780 by Johann August Heinsius (1745–1803), town physician of Sorau in the electorate of Saxony, in order to counteract anti-inoculationist views among the citizens; and it was to be used again by

Johann Christian Wilhelm Juncker (1761–1800), professor of medicine in Halle, Prussia-Brandenburg, in a campaign to introduce inoculation as a general practice.[20] So, what were the objections that German advocates of inoculation faced, or which were thought to be behind public resistance?

Figure 2

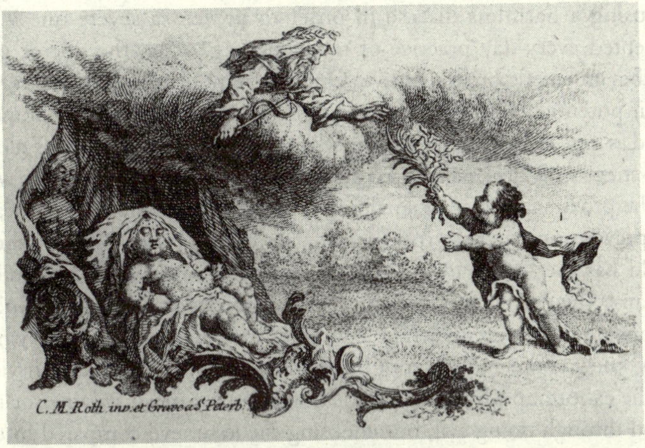

An inoculated child thanks a figure that is partly Aesculapius, partly God the Father. In contrast to this the child in the left foreground, who has not been entrusted to art, but to nature (multibreasted figure in the back), and has contracted smallpox in the natural way, suffers severely. Title vignette of J. H. Jänisch, *Kurze Geschichte und Beschreibung der vortheilhaftesten Art, die Pocken einzuimpfen* (St Petersburg 1768), reporting on inoculation trials made at the request of Johann von Betzkoy, chamberlain of Empress Catherine II, on 80 children in custody of the Kayserliche Academie der Künste and the Kayserliches Fräuleinstift.

Objections were usually categorized as (1) 'religious or moral' and (2) 'medical or physical'. The central argument within the first group was that inoculation interfered with divine providence. Human beings, and particularly Christians, ran the argument, are not masters of their lives; they are not allowed deliberately to inflict a disease which endangers their own (or their children's) existence. Diseases are inflicted only by God, as punishment or as a test of faith. Therefore it is better to await the natural smallpox. If it brings death, this was God's will. How, on the other hand, can parents console themselves, if their child has died from inoculated smallpox, i.e. has virtually been killed by their own hands? And, after all, was it not taught by the apostle Paul that one should not do something evil in the hope of producing something good?

The counterarguments brought forward by the advocates of inoculation ran like this: Inoculation, with its capacity to save human lives, is really a gift of God, since He wants human beings to use their rationality to protect their lives. It is presumptuous to reject that gift. Causing a harmless disease in order to prevent a severe one is an accepted every-day practice of medicine, e.g. when the doctor prescribes an emetic or a purgative. Only the remote cause of diseases, i.e. their potentiality, is of divine origin; the proximate causes are human. God is not directly responsible, when a mischievous boy runs along the street with his smallpox crusts, infecting his playmates in this way. If the proximate cause of smallpox is human, however, human means of prevention, such as inoculation, are appropriate. Parents whose child has died from inoculated smallpox do not have to feel guilty, because they acted to the best of their knowledge and belief. Guilty rather are those parents whose child dies from natural smallpox, when they knew about inoculation, but refused to apply it. Finally, in view of the exhortation by Paul, inoculation does not mean striving for the good through doing evil, but choosing the lesser evil compared to the greater evil of the natural disease. Such a choice, however, is acceptable for the Christian.[21]

In an attempt to characterize these two lines of argument, one might say that the former (i.e. the anti-inoculationist) reflected a traditional, fatalistic attitude, whereas the latter (i.e. the pro-inoculationist) showed features of an enlightened, rational faith, which gave man a more active and independent role in his life. Yet it would be rash to identify the two sides in the inoculation controversy wholly with these two different basic attitudes. The second group of objections, i.e. the 'medical or physical', contained purely rational arguments, such as the following:

Inoculation causes no true smallpox, or it can fail, so that the individual may still get the natural disease later. Some persons never contract smallpox in their whole life and are thus put to the risk of inoculation in vain. The lethality of inoculation only seems to be smaller than that of natural smallpox, because only healthy children are inoculated, and these are also looked after with special care. Total mortality is not reduced by the practice. Other diseases, such as syphilis, may be transmitted by way of inoculation. Artificial smallpox is unable to 'exhaust' completely that 'matter' within the body, which makes a person susceptible to natural smallpox. Therefore inoculated individuals are liable to other diseases and have a shorter life expectancy. Finally, freshly inoculated persons are dangerous, because they may infect others in the natural way and thus become starting points of epidemics.[22]

All these rational objections were of course answered by equally rational and detailed arguments in favour of inoculation. The general point which can be made of the late eighteenth-century German discourse is that not only the pro-inoculationist, but also the anti-inoculationist side used to a great extent enlightened, rational arguments. Contemporary opposition was not merely a consequence of a traditional attitude toward health and disease. It was also, and perhaps even more, the result of conscious benefit-risk weighing.

Another differentiation has to be made concerning the motives of the advocates of inoculation. There is no reason to doubt that Enlightenment philanthropy played a major role. Yet two other considerations came in as well. Firstly, the saving of human lives from death by smallpox was sometimes explicitly put in relation to mercantilist and cameralist concepts. For the Esslingen lawyer Weinland, mentioned above, this was even the central aspect. He based his case on the works of cameralists, such as Johann Heinrich Gottlob von Justi (1720–71), and elaborated on the connections between total population and economic and political power of a nation. Weinland put particular emphasis on the economic importance of factories, which required a large population. The rise of Prussia with its general policy of increasing its population was quoted as a proof for the correctness of such a concept.[23] Secondly, it was sometimes hardly concealed that inoculation could be financially attractive for physicians. The Halle professor Juncker particularly emphasized that its practice should be kept limited to physicians, with the exception of specially instructed and bound surgeons. Though he chiefly pointed out that this would guarantee competent, safe, and responsible inoculation, he did not neglect the financial aspects. He made it clear that from well-to-do clients considerable fees could be expected, affirming simultaneously that he – personally – would never make a profit out of the practice.[24] Despite this affirmation, however, he did not escape later suspicions that his commitment to inoculation was actually based on mercenary motives.[25]

Practice

Some physicians, who tried to introduce inoculation in their towns and principalities, documented their efforts by publishing the histories of their inoculation cases. Such detailed information exists, for instance, for the small principality of Quedlinburg, which in the second half of the eighteenth century was a Lutheran ecclesiastical territory belonging to Brandenburg, and for the counties of Tecklenburg and Lingen, north of Münster, that had both been acquired by Prussia earlier in the century. Christoph Jakob August Ziegler (1735–95), town physician of Quedlinburg, reported on 37 children, whom he had inoculated during a smallpox epidemic in 1775; Leonhard Ludwig Finke (1747–1837), town physician and teacher of midwifery, first in Tecklenburg, then in Lingen, communicated 63 inoculations, which he had performed in both counties between 1776 and 1792.[26] Both physicians inoculated children of a wide range of ages, from about three months up to 15 years, the average age being in both groups approximately five years. The ratio of male to female inoculated children was both times about 3 to 2, a fact which might cautiously be interpreted to suggest that inoculation was rather used to protect the life of a male heir than the life and beauty of a daughter. Considering the average age of the children, it can be assumed that the natural excess of male births had already been balanced by the higher mortality of male new-born babies.

Each of the two physicians experienced one lethal case, which they attributed to other, unexpected disorders complicating the course of inoculated smallpox. There was some tendency towards self-exculpation here, which must be seen in the context of the generally hostile environment in which both physicians carried out their inoculations. Ziegler wrote that he encountered very strong resistance in the population, including 'scholars' and 'persons knowledgeable in the art'. Counterarguments were – as he noted – either of a religious or a medical nature – a statement that corresponds to the findings regarding the general discourse.[27] Similarly Finke reported that most of his fellow-citizens, including several medical colleagues, were very hostile to the practice.[28]

In consideration of these remarks it is interesting to look at the social origins of the inoculated children, which in most cases can be identified from the histories (*Table 1*). The numbers are too small here for statistical analysis, since some fathers had several or all of their children inoculated. Still it can be seen that the more eminent, respectable members of these small communities were well represented, who of course would also have been the patients of an academic physician at that time. It was also those one would expect to have been receptive to Enlightenment ideas. The lower social strata were evidently under-represented. This finding matches only in part, however, the statements of other inoculating physicians. The district physician of Gumbinnen in East Prussia, for example, reported in 1798 that 'the more wealthy part of the local inhabitants' had its children frequently inoculated, and added that he had performed himself 140 inoculations, each time at the request of the parents, within the 16 years of his medical practice.[29] But his colleague in Züllichau, Brandenburg, reporting on 285 own inoculations in the years 1771 to 1796, emphasized that his inoculated were 'by far not all of noble class or birth, or of great wealth, but for the most part children of common artisans, also some children of farmers'. He added that among the latter much more could have been inoculated, had he not been so busy in his practice with other tasks.[30]

Table 1

	Ziegler	Finke
nobleman	1	3
civil servant	2	14
officer	–	3
clergyman	2	3
cantor	1	–
physician	1	1
other academic	–	1
surgeon	2	2
apothecary	–	1
landlord	–	1
trader	2	1
farmer	1	1
unidentified	3	4

Fathers of 37 children inoculated by C. J. A. Ziegler in Quedlinburg in 1775, and of 63 children inoculated by L. L. Finke in Tecklenburg and Lingen from 1776 to 1792. Compiled from the case histories in Ziegler, *Wahrnehmungen bey der Einimpfung der Blattern* (Quedlinburg, 1776) and Finke, *Specimen medicum historiam sistens insitionis variolarum in comitatibus Tecklaburgensi atque Lingensi exercitae* (Lingen, 1792).

This somewhat contradictory evidence seems to indicate that there was actually an upper class bias for the practice of inoculation in Germany, which is not surprising in view of the fact that in other countries, such as England, France and Russia, royals and other members of the nobility had propagated it by their own example.[31] Still, the number and social composition of inoculated children obviously depended also on the commitment of the individual physician in charge.

Easy generalizations cannot be made either concerning religious resistance. Franz Olberg, physician in Dessau (Anhalt), reported in 1792 about negative attitudes towards inoculation among the local Jewish population, whose rabbi argued like Christian opponents that it interfered with 'God's rights'.[32] The above-mentioned town and district physician of Züllichau, C. S. Ungnad, however, noted only six years later that in his area the Jews had 'no prejudice' against this practice and that he had inoculated Jewish children in South Prussia as well.[33]

Figure 3

Zeit, Ort und Zeugen.	Zahl der Einge=impften die wirkl blatter=ten.	Zahl der Ver=stor=be=nen.
In der Grafschaft Essex 1767 nach Gatti über	9000	0
Sloane = = =	200	1
Die beyden Gebrüder Suttons =	20000	3
Dimsdale = = =	11000	1
London 1779 = = =	3444	10
In der Einimpfungsanstalt zu Petersburg, 1773 = = =	106	1
Eben daselbst 1773 bis 1779 =	328	0
Moskau 1773 bis 1780 nach Jänisch	694	3
In Rußland in Irkurzkischen Gouvernement 1781 = = =	3082	16
Eben daselbst in der neuerrichteten Kolywanischen Herrschaft 1781 (Rahn Magazin II. 75.) = =	1442	13
In den Pockenhäusern 1782 hinter Zarkoe=Selo an Flusse Issora in einem kleinen finnischen Dorfe und nahe dabey, auch in Illika hinter Oranienbaum und in Kracknoe=Selo = =	580	3
Philadelphia. = =	700	1
Hadeln 1770 ꝛc. (Gründe für und gegen die Blattereinpfropfungen. Memmingen, 1789. S. 61.) =	60	1
Müllhausen 1782 (nach B. Tabellen über die Bevölkerung der Stadt Müllhausen. Basel, 1783.) =	94	0
Zu Painswick in Glocestershire 1785 sogar während einer bösartigen Epidemie nach J. E. Jenner =	738	12
Thilenius zu Lauterbach, 1782 =	126	3
Hufeland zu Weimar 1788 =	54	0
Halle, seit 1766 = =	58*)	1

Part of an international compilation made by the Halle professor of medicine Johann Christian Wilhelm Juncker (1761–1800). It shows numbers of successful inoculations (left column) and of deaths following these inoculations (right column). From: J. Ch. W. Juncker, *Gemeinnützige Vorschläge u. Nachrichten über das beste Verhalten der Menschen in Rücksicht der Pockenkrankheit* (Halle and Leipzig 1792), p. 114.

It is known that in England parishes in the second half of the eighteenth century paid for general inoculations of the poor in view of approaching epidemics.[34] Evidence of such measures has not yet been found, either for the two selected territories Quedlinburg and Tecklenburg/Lingen, or for other German territories. This negative finding is also supported by contemporary descriptions of smallpox epidemics in German towns. Such reports have been published, for example, on Weimar for the year 1788 (by the renowned Christoph Wilhelm Hufeland), on Erlangen for 1790, on Halle for 1791 (by Juncker), and on Göttingen for 1792.[35] It can be gathered from these reports that inoculation was practised to some small extent as soon as the epidemic approached the town, or after the first smallpox cases had actually appeared within town. But organized, free inoculation for the general public was not mentioned. Moreover, as Peter Albrecht has recently shown for the City of Braunschweig, even if the local authorities were ready to finance inoculation, and in spite of the support of the local press, the practice did not gain ground: in the years 1767 to 1787 nearly 18,000 births were registered in Braunschweig, but approximately only 350 inoculations were performed in this period, which saw five major smallpox epidemics.[36]

A similar picture is given by local and regional reports on the smallpox situation in the year 1796, which had been collected by Juncker from physicians and clergymen in many parts of Germany.[37] For Prussia such reports had been made obligatory through an order of King Friedrich Wilhelm (issued 30 August, 1796, following a request of Juncker). They provided detailed numbers for smallpox morbidity and mortality, the latter often being put in relation to total mortality. Only exceptionally, however, numbers for inoculations and their success were included (e.g. in the reports for Wernigerode and Regensburg)[39], and these numbers were small.

A more complete picture of the extent of inoculation in the German states would of course require more local and regional studies. At any rate, the impression that the practice was rather limited corresponds to the contemporary complaints by its advocates (such as that of the Swabian mentioned above). It also seems to match with contemporary lists of numbers of inoculations in certain years and at different places in England, Russia, Germany, and other countries, which were compiled by Juncker in 1792 (*Figure 3*). The numbers of inoculations reported from Germany were small compared to those reported from England and Russia. Apart from the obvious disadvantage that these numbers lack references to population sizes or birth rates, such historical compilations are too incomplete and unreliable, however, to allow further conclusions. Furthermore, two principal *caveats* must be made. Any attempt to estimate the extent of inoculation faces the problem of unknown numbers of inoculations performed by medical laymen and parents;[40] and for Germany the situation is particularly obscure, because the extent of the activities of foreign travelling inoculators (trained in France and England)[41] is not clear. Complaints about foreign competitors, however, do not seem to have been voiced.

Figure 4

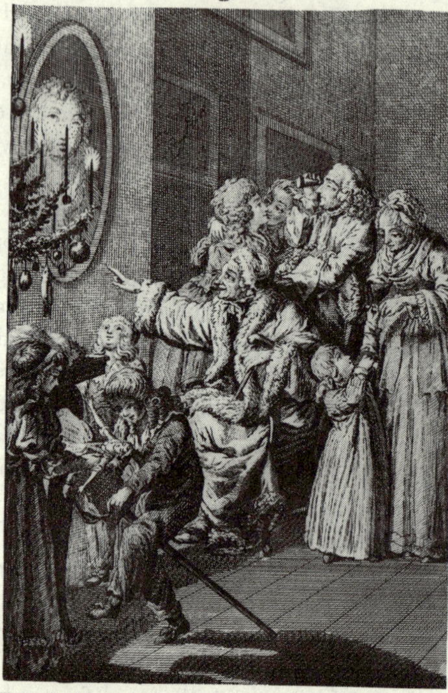

Frontispiece of Juncker's *Gemeinnützige Vorschläge* (1792), illustrating his 'dream': in 1840, or maybe in 1940, smallpox would have been almost eradicated, and at Christmas people would commemorate those of their ancestors who had died from that nearly forgotten disease. Surrounded by a healthy family the great-grandfather would point to a picture of his deceased wife, who had still been so unlucky to contract smallpox.

Concepts for Smallpox Eradication

The evidence discussed above, suggesting as a whole a rather limited practice of inoculation in the German states, contrasts in part with contemporary hopes to eradicate smallpox once and for all (*Figure 4*). Characterized by strong Enlightenment optimism, these hopes manifested themselves partly in very vague concepts, partly in concrete programmes and projects. An example of the former type is that of the Mannheim physician Friedrich Casimir Medicus (1736–1808). In 1763 he published his view that smallpox was an unspecific 'inflammatory fever', which was dangerous only because of the fearfulness of people. Once people would have been enlightened about the nature of the disease and educated that it had to be treated at an early stage with 'a rational cure' (using cold water), it could be eradicated.[42] More realistic and concrete concepts were propagated in the early 1790s by F. L. von Pufendorf, a lieutenant of the Royal British and Electoral Brunswick-Lüneburg infantry regiment at Wunstorf, and by Bernhard Christoph Faust (1755–1842), a popular Enlightenment physician and philanthropist at Bückeburg.[43] Both were directly influenced by the Chester physician John Haygarth (1740–1827), who had published in 1784 a detailed plan to eliminate smallpox. Haygarth had suggested a 'two-pronged attack on the disease': 1. general, free inoculation of the poor and 2. compliance with special 'Rules of Prevention', which included chiefly isolation of smallpox patients from persons who had not yet had the disease as well as from the general public, and strict cleanliness and several hygienic measures in the infected household.[44] These suggestions were taken up selectively by Pufendorf and Faust.

Pufendorf thought that general inoculation could hardly be introduced into the European states, because of 'the prejudices and the hostility of the great mass' towards the method. He was not ready to advocate legal force here, though such a suggestion had already been made in the 1760s, but was generally rejected. Pufendorf adopted, however, Haygarth's 'Rules of Prevention' and moreover proposed to set up special 'smallpox houses' outside the towns to facilitate isolation and treatment of smallpox patients. In addition he recommended those preventive measures that were known from the fight against the plague, i.e. cordons around infected areas and quarantine for susceptible persons who might have been infected.[45] These latter proposals were rejected by Faust, because they interfered with 'doings and dealings'. Otherwise his eradication concept corresponded to that of Pufendorf. He particularly shared the latter's rather negative attitude towards the plan of general inoculation. According to Faust, the idea of inoculating *all* human beings was not only impracticable, but – since it meant deliberately causing a disease – 'horrible'. Pufendorf and Faust agreed that inoculation would become superfluous anyway, if only the other preventive measures were properly organized and implemented.[46]

Figure 5

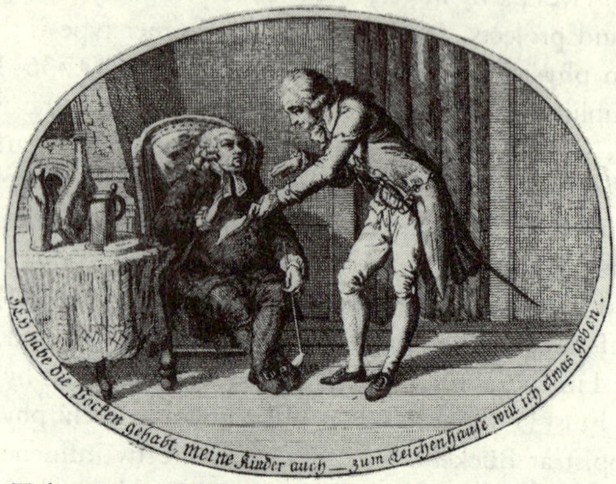
Ich habe die Pocken gehabt, meine Kinder auch — zum Leichenhause will ich etwas geben.

Title vignette of Juncker's *Gemeinnützige Vorschläge* (1792), illustrating his campaign for the eradication of smallpox. Juncker complained that those who themselves, or whose children, had survived the disease were often reluctant to support this campaign, though they were ready to pay for other philanthropical projects, such as the building of mortuaries to prevent burying alive. Accordingly the caption runs: 'I have had the smallpox, and so have my children - I will give something for the mortuary.' As Juncker emphasized in the preface, the depiction of the man in the chair as a preacher was merely due to artistic freedom.

This view contrasted, however, with that of Juncker, who – after the Halle epidemic of 1791 – propagated the most extensive and detailed plan for smallpox eradication in these years (*Figure 5*). In three volumes (one for the educated general public, two for physicians), published between 1792 and 1796, he explained his programme.[47] While including isolation of smallpox patients and hygienic measures, it strongly emphasized the value of widespread inoculation. As many people as possible should be encouraged to use it. For the poor and for the children of 'the husbandman and the common soldier' it should be free. In order to avoid natural infection of others through inoculated persons, the operation should be performed only in so-called 'inoculation houses'. These could simultaneously be used for the treatment and isolation of patients with natural smallpox. Juncker noted that such 'inoculation houses' had already been set up in a few cities, mentioning as an example the Smallpox and Inoculation Hospital of London, which had been founded in 1746. But he critizised the fact that inoculation was practised there only on the side, i.e. not as a strategy for the systematic *eradication* of smallpox.[48]

Juncker was not content with outlining programmes in books, but started a campaign to implement his aims. He founded a society of physicians against smallpox, collected money, and in 1796 created a journal devoted to smallpox eradication, entitled *Archiv der Aerzte und Seelsorger wider die Pockennoth* (Archive of Physicians and Clergymen against the Misery of Smallpox).[49] This journal, which existed until 1799, published reports and statistics on smallpox from many parts of Germany (cf. above), made detailed proposals for smallpox eradication, and tried to convince with pro-inoculationist articles. In 1798 Juncker reported to King Friedrich Wilhelm that Prussia had lost over 26,000 lives to smallpox during the year 1796. In fact the King soon ordered the *Collegia medica et sanitatis* (i.e. the Boards of Health) of Prussia to examine Juncker's proposals. But their report was negative. Eradication of smallpox, they declared in September 1799, was just wishful thinking.[50]

Ethical Considerations

Another of the initiatives of Juncker, however, deserves special attention, because it was unique *vis-à-vis* the English and French efforts to propagate inoculation. In April 1799 he sent out letters to several professors of philosophy, asking them to comment on the moral implications of inoculation as such, and specifically on those of his programme of general inoculation combined with isolation and hygiene, for which he coined the term 'Ausrottungsimpfung' ('eradicating inoculation').[51] Five answers, all from Halle philosophers, which came in up to the summer of the same year, were published in the seventh and last issue of Juncker's *Archiv*.[52] Kant also received an inquiry from Juncker, but only in August 1800, and his answer is not known (apart from the short note mentioned above).[53] Two of the responding Halle professors, however, Ludwig Heinrich Jakob (1759–1827) and Johann Heinrich Tieftrunk (1759–1837), were Kantians; two others, Johann August Eberhard (1739–1809) and Johann Gebhard Ehrenreich Maaß (1766–1823), active Anti-Kantians. The fifth, Johann Christoph Hoffbauer (1766–1827), was initially influenced by the Anti-Kantian Eberhard, but later became a follower of Kant in his ethics.[54] Though ideas of Kant actually figured in the answers of Tieftrunk and Hoffbauer,[55] there was no correlation between a generally Kantian, or Anti-Kantian, orientation of the Halle philosophers and their opinion given on the morality of inoculation. Eberhard, Jakob, and Maaß pronounced themselves in favour of the practice, as did Hoffbauer, albeit with reservations; Tieftrunk came to mainly anti-inoculationist conclusions.

The central argument within the general discourse (see above), i.e. that the risk of dying from inoculated smallpox was clearly smaller than that of dying of the naturally contracted disease, was also decisive in the comments of Eberhard, Jakob, and Hoffbauer. On the basis of this calculus of probability, they argued, inoculation was an individual's moral duty. Hoffbauer, who was chiefly a psychologist, only made the qualification that in cases of 'strong abhorrence' at inoculation it should be dispensed with, because this emotion 'could make the otherwise not dangerous disease deadly'.[56] Eberhard and Jakob emphasized that it was also a duty to prevent infection of others by freshly inoculated persons, thus endorsing Juncker's concept of additional isolation and hygiene. For Eberhard this was a demand following from 'the eternal laws of justice and humanity': the practice of inoculation in the higher strata of society (he stated) must not spread smallpox among the lower classes.[57] That this actually happened had been illustrated by a communication of Olberg (Dessau) to Juncker. When a smallpox epidemic had started in Dessau in 1791, a 'Madame V***' arrived with her two children from Cöthen and had them inoculated by the court surgeon Schwabe. The two children, having been taken back home again immediately afterwards, developed smallpox, infected the neighbours' children in Cöthen and in this way started an epidemic there.[58]

Neither Eberhard and Jakob, nor Hoffbauer, made use of a generic ethical principle in their efforts to determine the morality of inoculation. Such a principle was applied, however, in the answers given by Maaß and Tieftrunk. The former started with the utilitarian demand that 'I shall not hinder anybody's aims at will, but rather promote the aims of all as far as possible, or, since perfection is the aim of all, that I shall not arbitrarily reduce anybody's perfection, but strive to promote the perfection of all'.[59] Applying this to Juncker's concept of 'eradicating inoculation', he could not find any moral objections. In contrast to this, Tieftrunk encountered difficulties with Juncker's plans, when he applied Kant's categorical imperative to them. In doing this he distinguished between a 'maxim of smallpox eradication' ('Ausrottungsmaxime') and a 'maxim of inoculation'

('Impfungsmaxime'). Whereas the former maxim fulfilled the categorical imperative, i.e. could be thought as a 'general law', this was not the case with the latter. If the 'maxim of inoculation' became 'general law', Tieftrunk argued, all human beings would have to practice inoculation, and thus smallpox would deliberately be made ubiquitous and eternal. This was not acceptable, however, because in his view smallpox – being an infectious disease – was *principally* avoidable through isolation and hygienic measures, if only sufficient efforts were made. It was, therefore, immoral to contract smallpox intentionally by inoculation, since 'a self-made disease' was 'a self-made obstacle to moral action and integrity'. Despite this radical conclusion, however, Tieftrunk was not blind to the realities of his time, which taught that it was *practically* nearly impossible to escape an infection with smallpox. Ultimately he was, therefore, ready to accept inoculation as a 'provisional emergency measure': having an inoculation made in view of the acute danger of natural infection was like running through the flames in order to rescue oneself out of a burning house, which had been set alight by others.[60]

Tieftrunk felt unable to see how general inoculation could be a means to eradicate smallpox once and for all.[61] In this he tallied with Hoffbauer, who furthermore stressed that smallpox eradication could work only as an international, world-wide endeavour. Such activities, however, were a mere hope and far from reality. Even worse, a nation that had succeeded in becoming free of smallpox over several generations would be in immense danger: since the population would lack a naturally acquired protection, any accidental introduction of smallpox from another country would cause a disaster. Therefore, Hoffbauer eventually tried to dissuade Juncker from implementing a programme of eradication on the national level.[62]

The End: Vaccination

While these philosophical opinions were published, however, Edward Jenner's method of cowpox inoculation or vaccination became known in Germany. His now famous *Inquiry into the Causes and Effects of the Variolae Vaccinae* of 1798 was reviewed in the same year by Faust in the sixth issue of Juncker's *Archiv*.[63] In the following issue (1799) Juncker himself gave his view on the new method. Though he was open-minded about vaccination, he raised some critical questions, e.g., whether the protection acquired in this way might not be only temporary, and whether the vaccine kept its efficacy, if it had passed through several human beings by inoculation from arm to arm. He also pointed to the still very limited experience with vaccination and therefore suggested to keep up his concept of 'eradicating inoculation' until more practical knowledge was gained.[64] Yet, already in August 1800 Juncker was convinced enough to vaccinate his daughter. In December of the same year he died unexpectedly and with him his campaign.[65] In general, however, the new method of cowpox inoculation quickly created new hopes to solve the smallpox problem. In 1802 a first institute for vaccination was set up in Berlin, which had the task of supplying cowpox lymph and vaccinating adults and children free of charge.[66] Already within the first third of the nineteenth century some German states made vaccination obligatory, e.g. Bavaria, Württemberg, Hesse and Anhalt-Bernburg.[67] Inoculation of smallpox was formally forbidden in Bavaria in 1807 and in Prussia in 1835.[68] Yet, the introduction of cowpox inoculation brought problems and controversies as well. The inoculation debate of the eighteenth century was followed by the vaccination debate of the nineteenth century.[69] Many of the old arguments and difficulties surrounding smallpox inoculation continued to be discussed - just with a new livery and on a different level.

Conclusions

The introduction of smallpox inoculation during the eighteenth century caused considerable medical and moral concern in the German states. In its contents and intensity the German debate on this subject for the most part reflected corresponding controversies in England and France, but it lasted longer through the century, probably due to sustained opposition to the practice. Though the pro-inoculationist position can be linked with Enlightenment rationality, and the anti-inoculationist view with a more fatalistic attitude, many purely rational arguments were used by adversaries of inoculation as well. Enlightenment philanthropy was certainly a motive for this preventive measure, yet cameralist ideas and mercenary considerations also played a role.

Qualitative and quantitative evidence points to the conclusion that inoculation was practised only to a limited extent in the German states, probably most among the higher social classes. The attitude of the public towards it being generally critical, if not hostile, it was mainly seen as a risky emergency measure during smallpox epidemics. The argument that the intentional contraction of the disease interfered with divine providence was voiced both among the Christian and Jewish population.

Unique to the German inoculation debate were the elaborate comments of professors of philosophy on the ethical implications. The pro-inoculationist view that the practice was justified, because it had a clearly lower risk of death than smallpox contracted in the natural way, was shared by several philosophers. Inoculation was thought to be compatible with utilitarian principles, but not with Kant's categorical imperative. Kant himself regarded smallpox inoculation as morally questionable, though he was apparently ready to accept it, if it was made obligatory by the state. The efforts of Juncker, however, to acquire the sanction of the Prussian king for a programme of smallpox eradication, which combined general inoculation with isolation of patients and hygienic measures, had no success. In contrast, Jenner's safer new method of cowpox inoculation (vaccination) very soon gained official support in several German states. Though not without controversies, it was put much more easily into general practice. One might speculate, therefore, that smallpox inoculation would have become more widespread in the German territories, had it been vigorously promoted and supported by state authorities – instead of leaving it chiefly to the personal initiative of some enlightened physicians.

Acknowledgements

I gratefully acknowledge the support of the Wellcome Trust whilst I worked on this essay. Moreover I would like to thank Dr Andrea Rusnock and Professor Roy Porter, London, for their valuable comments on an earlier draft, and Christiane Bartels, M.A., and Axel Wolf, Dipl.-Bibl., Göttingen, for their kind bibliographical and technical assistance.

Notes

1. A. C. Klebs, *Die Variolation im achtzehnten Jahrhundert: Ein historischer Beitrag zur Immunitätsforschung* (Gießen: Töpelmann, 1914); W. Kaiser, 'Impfärzte des 18. Jahrhunderts', *Zahn-, Mund- und Kieferheilkunde*, lxiv (1976), 385–96.
2. Voltaire, 'Letter XI. On Inoculation', in *Letters Concerning the English Nation*, with an introduction by Ch. Whibley (London: P. Davies, 1926), 57–64; A. H. Rowbotham, 'The "Philosophes" and the Propaganda for Inoculation of Smallpox in Eighteenth-Century France', *University of California Publications in Modern Philology*, xviii (1935), 265–90; P. Gay, *The Enlightenment: An Interpretation* (2 vols, New York: A. A. Knopf, 1967–9), i, 16.
3. Klebs, *op. cit.* (note 1), 56; Ph. H. Clendenning, 'Dr Thomas Dimsdale and Smallpox Inoculation in Russia', *Journal of the History of Medicine and Allied Sciences*, xxviii (1973), 109–25; J. Wimmer, *Gesundheit, Krankheit und Tod im Zeitalter der Aufklärung: Fallstudien aus den habsburgischen Erbländern* (Vienna and Cologne: Böhlau, 1991), 116–21.

4. Rowbotham, *op. cit.* (note 2), 281; Kaiser, *op. cit.* (note 1), 392; A. Völker, 'Johann Christian Wilhelm Juncker (1761–1800) und die Dessauer Impfpropagandisten', in W. Kaiser and H. Hübner (eds), *Johann Juncker (1679–1759) und seine Zeit (I): Hallesches Juncker-Symposion 1979* (*Wissenschaftliche Beiträge der Martin-Luther-Universität Halle-Wittenberg*, 1979/29, T 31, Halle), 86--96, on 90.
5. I. Kant, *Metaphysik der Sitten*, edited by K. Vorländer (Hamburg: Meiner, 1966), 271. For a mathematical analysis of the risks and benefits of inoculation see the controversy between Daniel Bernoulli and Jean d'Alembert in the 1760s, translated and edited by L. Bradley, *Smallpox Inoculation: An Eighteenth Century Mathematical Controversy* (University of Nottingham: Adult Education Department, 1971). See also A. S. Emch-Dériaz, 'L'inoculation justifiée ... vraiment?', *Canadian Bulletin of Medical History*, ii (1985), 237–63.
6. H. Bohn, 'Ueber Kant's Beziehungen zur Medizin', *Altpreussische Monatsschrift*, ix (1872), 609–27, on 624.
7. A. Wilson, 'The Politics of Medical Improvement in Early Hanoverian London', in A. Cunningham and R. French (eds), *The Medical Enlightenment of the Eighteenth Century* (Cambridge, New York, Port Chester: Cambridge University Press, 1990), 4–39; F. M. Lobo, 'John Haygarth, Smallpox and Religious Dissent in Eighteenth-Century England', *ibid.*, 217–53.
8. G. Miller, *The Adoption of Inoculation for Smallpox in England and France* (Philadelphia: University of Pennsylvania Press, 1957); P. Razzell, *The Conquest of Smallpox: The Impact of Inoculation on Smallpox Mortality in Eighteenth Century Britain* (Firle, Sussex: Caliban Books, 1977); J. R. Smith, *The Speckled Monster: Smallpox in England, 1670–1970, with particular reference to Essex* (Chelmsford: Essex Record Office, 1987); D. C. Brunton, 'Pox Britannica: Smallpox Inoculation in Britain, 1721–1830' (Ph.D. thesis, University of Pennsylvania, 1990); *eadem*, 'Smallpox Inoculation and Demographic Trends in Eighteenth-Century Scotland', *Medical History*, xxxvi (1992), 403–29; J.-F. de Raymond, *Querelle de l'Inoculation ou Préhistoire de la Vaccination* (Paris, Librairie Philosophique J. Vrin, 1982); P. Darmon, *La Variole, les Nobles et les Princes. La petite vérole mortelle de Louis XV* (Brussels: Editions Complexe, 1989). See also D. van Zwanenberg, 'The Suttons and the Business of Inoculation', *Medical History*, xxii (1978), 71–82; A. M. Moulin, 'La métaphore vaccine. De l'inoculation à la vaccinologie', *History and Philosophy of the Life Sciences*, xiv (1992), 271–97.
9. A. A. Rusnock, 'The Quantification of Things Human: Medicine and Political Arithmetic in Enlightenment England and France' (Ph.D thesis, Princeton University, 1990).
10. Klebs, *op. cit.* (note 1), 47–9; Miller, *op. cit.* (note 8), 174–9; Kaiser, *op. cit.* (note 1), Völker, *op. cit.* (note 4).
11. J. G. Krünitz, *Verzeichniß der vornehmsten Schriften von den*

Kinderpocken und deren Einpfropfung (Leipzig: Ch. G. Hilscher, 1768); F. Olberg, *Beiträge zur Litteratur der Blattern und deren Einimpfung, vom Jahre 1768 bis 1790* (Halle: J. G. Trampens Wittwe, 1791).

12. See Miller, *op. cit.* (note 8), 70–133.
13. See *ibid.*, 195–240.
14. Cf. e.g. Anonymous, *Darstellung der Gründe für und gegen die Blatterneinpfropfung für Leser aus allen Ständen* (Memmingen: A. Seyler, 1789), 26–7; Ch. W. Hufeland, *Bemerkungen über die natürlichen und künstlichen Blattern zu Weimar im Jahr 1788* (Leipzig: G. J. Göschen, 1789), 1–3; J. Ch. W. Juncker, *Gemeinnützige Vorschläge u. Nachrichten über das beste Verhalten der Menschen in Rücksicht der Pockenkrankheit. Erster Versuch für die mittlern Stände nebst einem Anhange für Aerzte* (Halle and Leipzig: Verfasser and H. Hahn, 1792), 20–2, 130–1.
15. According to a calculation made from the data on total and smallpox mortality in 20 German districts and territories in 1796, that were given in J. Ch. W. Juncker (ed.), *Archiv der Aerzte und Seelsorger wider die Pockennoth*, iii (1797), 1–145.
16. J. Wreden, *An Essay on the Inoculation of the Small Pox. To which are Added, Some Examples of Persons Inoculated with Good Success at Hanover* (London: J. Jackson, 1729), 29–43; Kaiser, *op. cit.* (note 1), 385.
17. Miller, *op. cit.* (note 8), 176.
18. Anonymous, *Darstellung der Gründe*, Einleitung.
19. *Ibid.*, 24–136.
20. E. F. Weinland, *Die Vortheile, welche der Staat durch die Einführung des Blatterbelzes erlangt, aus Staatsgründen betrachtet* (Zelle: G. C. Gsellius, 1770), 55–82; J. A. Heinsius, *Gründe Für und Wider die Pockeninoculation, gesammelt und verglichen* (Leipzig: Ch.G. Hertel, 1780), 7–109; Juncker, *op. cit.* (note 14), 115–32. An obvious model was Samuel Auguste André David Tissot's propagandistic treatise *L'inoculation justifiée* (1754), which was translated by Friedrich Simon Morgenstern: *Tissot's practische Verteidigung des Einpfropfens der Pocken* (Halle: C. Ch. Kümmel, 1756). See also A. S. Emch-Dériaz, 'L'Inoculation Justifiée – or Was I?', *Eighteenth Century Life*, vii (1982), no. 2, 65–72.
21. Cf. the references given in notes 19 and 20 above.
22. Cf. *ibid.*
23. Weinland, *op. cit.* (note 20), 13–33, 83–91; see also F. L. von Pufendorf, *Ausführbare Vorschläge zur gänzlichen Vertilgung der Blattern Regenten, Staatsmännern und Menschenfreunden zu reiflicher Erwägung und Beherzigung empfohlen* (Braunschweig: Schulbuchhandlung,1792), dedication and 1–15.
24. Juncker, *op. cit.* (note 14), 15, 56–7, 95–104; *idem*, *Gemeinnützige Vorschläge wider die Pockenkrankheit. Dritter Versuch: Für möglichst alle Aerzte, die der deutschen Sprache kundig sind; zur Sammlung ihrer Gutachten hierüber* (Halle: Hemmerde und Schwetschke, 1796), 47–56.

25. When Juncker opened a bank account and asked his medical colleagues for payments to support his campaign for inoculation, he was suspected of having contrived a dubious finance operation. Because of this accusation he went to law for libel in 1799 against Christian Gottfried Gruner (1744–1815), professor of medicine in Jena, and Johann Jacob Hartenkeil (1761–1808), personal physician of the archbishop of Salzburg. Cf. F. Schlichtegroll, *Nekrolog* xi/2 (1800), 254–77. See also K. Sprengel, *Versuch einer pragmatischen Geschichte der Arzneykunde* (5 parts, 3rd edn Halle: Gebauersche Buchhandlung, 1821–28), v/2, 928, who spoke of 'undignified quarellings' ('unwürdige Zänkereyen') caused by Juncker and his ideas on smallpox eradication.
26. Ch. J. A. Ziegler, *Wahrnehmungen bey der Einimpfung der Blattern* (Quedlinburg: Ch. A. Reußner, 1776); L. L. Finke, *Specimen medicum historiam sistens insitionis variolarum in comitatibus Tecklaburgensi atque Lingensi exercitae* (Lingen: F. A. Jülicher, 1792).
27. Ziegler, *op. cit.* (note 26), 5.
28. Finke, *op. cit.* (note 26), 3–4, 28.
29. Report by Dr Melhorn in Juncker, *op. cit.* (note 15), v (1798), 30–48, on 38.
30. Report by Dr C. S. Ungnad, *ibid.*, 2–24, on 8.
31. See Klebs, *op. cit.* (note 1), and Miller, *op. cit.* (note 8).
32. Extract of a letter by F. Olberg, dated 27.3.1792, in Juncker, *op. cit.* (note 14), Anhang, 83–5, on 84. See also A. Völker, *Die Entwicklung von Medizinalorganisation und Bevölkerunsversorgung am territorialen Beispiel von Anhalt* (*Wissenschaftliche Beiträge der Martin-Luther-Universität Halle-Wittenberg*, 1985/18, E 65, Halle), 101–2.
33. Ungnad in Juncker, *op. cit.* (note 15), v (1798), 8.
34. Razzell, *op. cit.* (note 8), 44–7.
35. Hufeland, *op. cit.* (note 14); *idem, Anhang zu den Bemerkungen über die natürlichen und geimpften Blattern zu Weimar im Jahr 1788* (Leipzig: G. J. Göschen, 1792), 83–5; J. M. Plinta, *Historia epidemiae variolosae Erlangensis anni 1790* (Erlangen: J. J. Palm, 1792); Juncker, *op. cit.* (note 14), 18–22, 32–41; C. G. H. Erxleben, *Dissertatio inauguralis medica sistens epidemiae variolosae, Gottingae 1792 grassatae, brevem descriptionem* (Göttingen: H. M. Grape, 1792).
36. P. Albrecht, 'Versuche zur Popularisierung der Blatterninokulation in der Stadt Braunschweig von 1754 bis 1780' (unpubl. typescript). I thank Dr Albrecht for making a copy of this study at my disposal.
37. 'Der Pockenzustand im Jahre 1796' in Juncker, *op. cit.* (note 15), iii (1797), 1–145.
38. See *ibid.*, i (1796), 293–6.
39. *Ibid.*, iii (1797), 60–2, and iv (1798), 208–12.
40. See Juncker's criticism of this 'Layenimpfung' in *op. cit.* (note 24), 47–56.
41. Klebs, *op. cit.* (note 1), 48; Kaiser, *op. cit.* (note 1), 388.

42. F. C. Medicus, *Send-Schreiben Von der Ausrottung derer Kinder-Blattern* (Frankfurt and Leipzig: no publisher stated, 1763).
43. I. Sahmland, 'Bernhard Christoph Faust (1755–1842)', *Medizinhistorisches Journal*, xxvii (1992), 373–9.
44. Cf. Lobo, *op. cit.* (note 7).
45. F. L. von Pufendorf, *op. cit.* (note 23). An 'interposition of government' to put through general inoculation had been suggested by Johann Friedrich Closs in his *Nova variolis medendi methodus, cum specimine observationum* (Utrecht: 1766); cf. 'A New Method of Curing the Small-Pox...From the Latin of John Frederic Closs...By a Member of the College of Physicians' in *A Collection of Pieces Relative to Inoculation for the Small-pox...Given for Publication, by a Member of the Faculty* (Dublin: J. Exshaw, 1768), 65, and the short summary of the German translation (1769) of Closs's work in F. Olberg, *op. cit.* (note 11), 2. Even staunch advocates of inoculation, however, rejected such an idea, e.g. Weinland, *op. cit.* (note 20), 152–5, and Juncker, *op. cit.* (note 15), vii (1799), 96 ('Jede erzwungene Impfung ist uns eine Abscheulichkeit.') Still, indirect force was occasionally used: Prince Leopold Friedrich Franz (1740–1817) of Anhalt-Dessau made inoculation a requirement for admission to the famous school 'Philanthropinum'; cf. J. Konert, 'S.A. Tissot und sein Einfluß auf den "Dessau-Wörlitzer Kulturkreis"', *Gesnerus*, il (1992), 39–44.
46. B. Ch. Faust, *Versuch über die Pflicht der Menschen, Jeden Blatternkranken von der Gemeinschaft der Gesunden abzusondern: und dadurch zugleich in Städten und Ländern und in Europa die Ausrottung der Blatternpest zu bewirken* (Bückeburg and Leipzig: J. A. Grimme and P. G. Kummer, 1794); *idem*, *An den Congreß zu Rastadt über die Ausrottung der Blattern* (Bückeburg: 1798).
47. Juncker, *op. cit.* (note 14); *idem*, *Gemeinnützige Vorschläge und Nachrichten über die Pockenkrankheit. Für Deutschland's Aerzte. Ein Vorschlag aus der Volksarzneywissenschaft* (Halle: Hemmerde und Schwetschke, 1795); *idem*, *op. cit.* (note 1).
48. Cf. *ibid.*, 473–6.
49. See also Kaiser, *op. cit.* (note 1), 394–6; *idem* and Karl-Heinz Krosch, 'Zur Geschichte der Medizinischen Fakultät der Universität Halle im 18. Jahrhundert (IX,X)', *Wissenschaftliche Zeitschrift der Martin-Luther Universität Halle-Wittenberg*, Mathematisch-Naturwissenschaftliche Reihe, xiv (1965), 357–432, on 422–7.
50. M. Pistor, 'Geschichte der preussischen Medizinalverwaltung', *Deutsche Vierteljahrsschrift für öffentliche Gesundheitspflege*, xl (1908), 225–50, 500–54, 749–810, on 781. Kurt Sprengel – though clearly pro-inoculationist – called Juncker, as well as Faust, a 'visionary' ('Schwärmer') and their concepts for smallpox eradication 'effusions' ('Schwärmereyen'); cf. Sprengel, *op. cit.* (note 25), v/2, 928.
51. Cf. Juncker, 'Ueber die Sittlichkeit der Impfung', *op. cit.* (note 15), vii (1799), 38–96, on 38–47.

52. *Ibid.*, 48–96.
53. Bohn, *op. cit.* (note 6), 624.
54. For the philosophical profiles of Erhard and Jakob see the entries on them in the *Neue Deutsche Biographie* and for those of Maaß, Tieftrunk, and Hoffbauer in the *Allgemeine Deutsche Biographie*.
55. Hoffbauer criticized Kant's view that the case of the sailor who entrusts himself to the storm was morally less questionable than inoculation: though the sailor was of course not responsible for the storm, he still put himself deliberately in danger, just as someone who had himself inoculated. Cf. Juncker, *op. cit.* (note 15), vii (1799), 87–8.
56. Cf. *ibid.*, 88–9.
57. Cf. *ibid.*, 56–7.
58. Cf. Juncker, *op. cit.* (note 14), Anhang, 83–4. See also Völker, *op. cit.* (note 4), 86. – Ungnad admitted to have caused the smallpox epidemics of 1795 and 1796 in Züllichau through inoculations, which he had performed with matter obtained from Frankfurt/Oder. Cf. Juncker, *op. cit.* (note 15), v (1798), 8–9.
59. Cf. *ibid.*, vii (1799), 66.
60. Cf. *ibid.*, 70–85.
61. *Ibid.*, 83.
62. *Ibid.*, 92–4.
63. Faust, 'Von den *variolis vaccinis*, die den Menschen vor den Pocken schützen sollen; nach Edward Jenner', *ibid.*, vi (1798), 278–80.
64. Juncker, 'Wären sogar die gepriesenen Vorzüge der Kuhpockenimpfung eben so gewiß gegründet, als zuverlässig sie zum Theil ungegründet sind, zum Theil aber noch mehrjährige Bestätigung fordern: so würden wir des Gesetzes der Pockentafel dennoch bedürfen', *ibid.*, vii (1799), 159–89.
65. Cf. Kaiser and Krosch, *op. cit.* (note 49), 426.
66. Pistor, *op. cit.* (note 50), 782.
67. See P. Kübler, *Geschichte der Pocken und der Impfung* (Berlin: Hirschwald, 1901), 179; J.-P. Rupp, 'Die Entwicklung der Impfgesetzgebung in Hessen', *Medizinhistorisches Journal*, x (1975), 103–20.
68. Yves-Marie Bercé, *Le chaudron et la lancette: Croyances populaires et médecine préventive (1798–1830)* (Paris: Presses de la Renaissance, 1984), 75.
69. See A.-H. Maehle, 'Präventivmedizin als wissenschaftliches und gesellschaftliches Problem: Der Streit über das Reichsimpfgesetz von 1874', *Medizin, Gesellschaft und Geschichte*, ix (1990), 127–48. For the English debate see D. Porter and R. Porter, 'The Politics of Prevention: Anti-Vaccinationism and Public Health in Nineteenth-Century England', *Medical History*, xxxii (1988), 231–52, and for the French Bercé, *op. cit.* (note 68).

9

Honeyed Words: Bernard Mandeville and Medical Discourse

Francis McKee

In 1711 Bernard Mandeville published the first edition of one of his best known works, *A Treatise of the Hypochondriack and Hysterick Passions.* The book aims to teach patients suffering from hypochondria how to question medical rhetoric and it is woven together from a combination of a wide variety of disparate texts – recipes, stories, quotations, diagnosis, case histories, articles, cited authorities etc. The cumulative effect of this mixture is a questioning of the origins of medical discourse and, indeed, the origin of an illness such as hypochondria or hysteria – pointing out how an illness may be no more than the sum of the texts describing it.

The question of origins is raised immediately in the Preface where Mandeville places the work in the context of the Fall of Man saying,

> When the crafty Tempter of Mankind meditating their ruine, attacked our first Sire in his Pride, he shew'd himself profoundly skill'd in Humane Nature; from which the vice I named is so inseparable that it is impossible the latter should be ever entirely destroy'd, as long as the first remains. I have no design, Reader, to tire you, with the Catalogue of irretrievable Calamities, it has been the occasion of, both before and since the Creation; but shall only observe to you, that as it was destructive to unexperienced Adam, by bringing Sickness and Death upon him, so it has still continued to be no less pernicious to his forewarn'd Posterity, by principally obstructing the progress of the glorious Art that should teach the Recovery as well as Preservation of Health.[1]

Here, the Fall is seen as the putative origin of all sickness and the source of the vice of pride. Before the curse of knowledge, Adam is 'unexperienc'd' and in a state of healthy grace. With 'original' sin he gains knowledge, pride and illness.

For the modern physician the Fall creates two problems. The first is the difficulty of curing an illness and restoring a patient to the state of grace. The second is overcoming the temptation of pride which persuades doctors to speculate and to propound theories as if they were derived from true knowledge:

> Tis Pride that makes the Physician abandon the solid Observation of never erring Nature to take up with the loose conjectures of his own wandering Invention ... and it is pride in the Patient, that makes him in love with the reasoning Physician, to have an opportunity of shewing the depth of his Penetration.[2]

Overcoming these temptations becomes even more difficult as medical discourse assumes the proportions of a crisis comparable to the Tower of Babel,

> to advance this Doctrine is swimmimg against the Stream in our sprightly talkative Age, in which the silent Experience of Painstaking Practitioners is ridicul'd, and nothing cried up but the witty Speculations of Hypothetical Doctors.[3]

Mandeville's silent practitioner is immediately recognizable as a follower of Iapis, the physician alluded to in the motto on the title page,

> *Scire potestates herbarum, usumque medendi Maluit, & Mutas agitare inglorius artes*

The motto is taken from Book 12 of Virgil's Aeneid and refers to the doctor who comes forward to treat Aeneas when he is wounded in battle with Turnus. Iapis, like Mandeville, had artistic talents but chose instead to practice medicine.

The dialogue form, then, provides Mandeville with a mask which allows him to voice the personal, emotional elements that permeate his scientific outlook. It would be unwise, however, to assume that Mandeville has simply chosen to state his current views on hypochondria through the persona of Philopirio. Typically, his apparently innocent statement of intent raises the immediate suspicions of his readers. He claims that

> In these Dialogues, I have done the same as Seneca did in his Octavia, and brought my self upon the Stage; with this difference, that he kept his own Name, and I changed mine for that of Philopirio, a Lover of Experience, which I shall always profess to be: Wherefore I desire my Reader to take whatever is spoke by the Person I named last, as said by myself; which I entreat him not to do with the Part of Misomedon ...[5]

Such a statement would present the reader with no problems if Seneca was ratified as the author of Octavia. However, while Seneca's tragedies have been reluctantly accepted as 'authentic', Octavia has remained doubtful. Assessing the status of the tragedies, E. F. Watling concludes that

> it is clear that the authenticity of Octavia is a matter of considerable doubt... The play could evidently not have appeared in its final form ... before the death of Nero, three years after that of Seneca. One is strongly tempted to assume that Seneca knew more than nothing about it.[6]

Mandeville as Philopirio cannot be taken at face value. Nor can his assertion that Misomedon is free of Mandevillian opinion – the hypochondriacal patient often proves to be an even more effective mask to voice the unsayable against apothecaries and rival physicians. All origins are under scrutiny in the *Treatise*, whether they be the origins of Senecan drama, medical discourse, the author's father or Adam in the Garden of Eden.

The Preface, itself, underlines this subversion of origins in several ways. Derrida has pointed out the philosophical quandaries induced by the pretence that a preface introduces a 'main' text and yet must be written after that text:

> From the viewpoint of the foreword, which recreates an intention-to-say after the fact, the text exists as something written – a past – which, under the false appearance of a present, a hidden omnipotent author (in full mastery of his product) is presenting to the reader as his future. Here is what I wrote, then read, and what I am writing that you are going to read. After which you will again be able to take possession of this preface which in sum you have not yet begun to read, even though, once having read it, you will already have anticipated everything that follows and thus you might just as well dispense with reading the rest.[7]

In the *Treatise*, Mandeville highlights this issue as his preface constantly apologizes for specific passages in the main text which implies that the whole work must be read before the preface can be understood. At the same time the preface masquerades as an introduction, preparing readers for an unknown text and warning them to slough off bad reading habits. Tackling nothing less than the consequences of the Fall and the works of the 'Crafty Tempter of Mankind', Mandeville demands that his readers approach the main text alert and critically.

The playfulness of the preface, for instance, not only sharpens the reader's wits for the following dialogues but demonstrates one of the possible therapies for hypochondria or 'the hyp'. Humour was a well known palliative for sufferers of this disease and many new books of the day catered for this taste.

In the *Treatise,* however, Mandeville begins to extend his exploration of the dialogue form, testing its usefulness as a therapeutic tool in the doctor–patient relationship. In the preface he suggests that the dialogue may be ideally suited to the hypochondriac (Mandeville assumes a reader must be a hypochondriac). Conventional medical prose is 'far from diverting' and prone to 'tedious Enumeration of Signs and Causes'. Such a text is more likely to induce hypochondria and at the least must be 'tiresome and disagreeable to People that seek relief in a Distemper of which Impatience is one of the surest Symptoms'.

By using the dialogue, Mandeville draws the reader into a dramatic world focusing on the relationship between doctor and patient. The actual discussion of the illness reveals the tensions and desires which characterize this relationship, and the later scenes between the husband and wife illustrate the links between personal relationships and illnesses. By dramatizing the medical discourse, Mandeville attempts to produce a cathartic effect on the reader and patient. The dialogues 'divert' and 'entertain', thus combating hypochondria to some degree. More importantly, they dramatize the analysis of medical discourse, creating a polyphony of texts which finally persuade the reader to accept ignorance as a therapeutic state of grace, an aim implied early on in the preface,

> The emphatical Truth is lost upon the Times, and he must not expect to be believed by our acute Philosophers, whose Pride won't allow that it is possible Nature should have recesses beyond the reach of their Sagacity, and reckons the injurious assertion an Affront to human Understanding.[8]

Logotherapy, in the *Treatise,* is designed to not only cure by words but to cure you of the disease of words, theories, tracts, medical journals, countless case histories and medical texts. Recalling his favourite metaphor of reading as a process of digestion, Mandeville claims that the *Treatise* will be a healthy meal,

> I resolv'd to deviate from the usual method, and make what I had to say as palatable as I could to those I had in view for my Readers...I pitch'd upon the Physical Remarks, which you shall find interwoven with the main matter. *Acriora orexim excitant enbammata.*[9]

This meal is presented within the context of a society glutted on a surfeit of luxury. Mandeville's patients, revelling in the profits of the rising British Empire, are suffering from various forms of indigestion, having consumed too many texts, too many consumer goods and too many exotic foods that are new to the British diet. In *The English Malady,* a treatise on hypochondria, George Cheyne describes this society succinctly, saying

> When I behold...such Scenes of Misery and Woe, and see them happen only to the Rich, the Lazy, the Luxurious, and the Unactive ... those who are furnished with the rarest Delicacies, the richest Foods, and the most generous Wines ... I ... conclude, that it must be something received into the Body, that can produce such terrible Appearances in it, some flagrant and notable Difference in the Food...And that it is the miserable Man himself that creates his Miseries, and begets his Torture...[10]

In the first dialogue of the *Treatise* Mandeville outlines this society in more detail through the case history of Misomedon. In a speech that runs for 16 pages, Misomedon recalls the main events of a life divided equally between total idleness and a study of medicine and hypochondria. The speech incorporates portraits of two physicians who diagnose and treat Misomedon's illness. The patient's life itself is divided into two parts – his early life in which profligacy is his main occupation and his later years in which his only occupation is the study of his own illness.

Misomedon's early life is described in a style reminiscent of the hero of a restoration comedy,

> I wanted but two Months of being One and Twenty, when my Father Died and left me Three Hundred a Year ... upon this I left the University... I quickly became Extravagant ... and minded nothing but my Pleasures; of which some were very Expensive ... half of my Estate was hardly sufficient to Pay my Debts, and clear the remainder. At Five and Twenty I Married; my Wife's Fortune paid off some Scores... Love and Pastime was all our Employment, from Morning till Night ... Neither of us could be call'd Extravagant, yet both desired to live handsomly; my Wife admired Cloaths, and I loved good Eating, and our necessary Expences, exceeded twice my Income....[11]

Misomedon is rescued from inevitable bankruptcy at this stage by an inheritance from a distant relation and he prudently trims his lifestyle to attain financial stability. Having inherited a library too, he turns to the study of classical literature though he remains 'rei Uxoriae addictissimus'. This, his first lapse into Latin, marks the beginning of a constant series of classical allusions revealing an element of pretentiousness on the part of Misomedon. For Philopirio it is the sign of badly digested texts and he swaps classical banter with his patient only to humour him until he can be cured.

Having reached thirty-seven, Misomedon's body begins to suffer the consequences of his earlier lifestyle,

> I began to be troubled with the Heart-burning, which in a little time became a constant Companion to me.[12]

He responds with some small remedies but finds that the problems are growing more serious,

> Hitherto I had only Quack'd with my self ... I perceived, that all the Remedies, I had taken, were only Palliatives, and none of them had touch'd the Cause, but to the contrary I grew daily worse, and the Heart-burning was no more the only Symptom that disturb'd me. After every Meal I had flushings in my Face; all Day long I was troubled with Wind and sowre Belches, and every Morning as long as I was Fasting, I had my Mouth continually fill'd with a clear insipid Water, which without any straining came off my Stomach....[13]

The narrative of the Restoration rake has disappeared, to be replaced by the eighteenth-century hypochondriac in this account of Misomedon's sufferings. This new discourse is replaced as quickly, however, by the arrival of an 'Eminent Physician' who gives his account of the patient's illness in true Galenist jargon,

> I was inform'd that the heat and burning all along the Oesophagus, from which the Distemper seem'd to have deriv'd the Name of Heart-burning, as well as the Flushings in my Face after Meals, were certo certius, occasion'd by an Interperies hepatis calide, which in my Case happen'd to be accompanied with an Intemperies Stomachi frigida, as was manifest from the cold Pituita, which I voided every Morning, as well as the Wind, sowre Belches, and other signs of Indigestion.[14]

The suggested cure reinforces this smokescreen of medical verbiage,

> As to the Cure...repeated bleeding from the left Salvatella would satisfie both Indications, and to use his own terms, utramque fere paginam absolveret; for that by this means the Fountain of heat, the Blood of which my Liver had too much, would by way of Antipasis or revulsion be drawn from the Right side.[15]

The physician continues in this style for several more pages, outlining a course of bleeding and purging to be followed by a visit to Epsom Spa. Misomedon follows the prescription and finds himself drained and exhausted by the time he reaches Epsom. There he is saved by an 'honest Gentleman' staying in the same lodgings. He dismisses all suggestions of purging and instead applies traditional common sense:

> he ... call'd for a Bottle of French Claret, which he order'd to be burnt with good store of Cinnamon, Cloves and Mace, and a pretty deal of Orange-Peel; whilst this was a-boiling he sent for some Syrup of Quinces to sweeten it, and when it was ready, made me take half a Pint of it, with a very brown Toast well rubb'd with Nutmeg, and sup it off as hot as I was able to bear it.[16]

Having abandoned the rhetoric of a Galenist for that of a cookery book Misomedon finds his strength beginning to return. He is, in fact, sufficiently healthy to avoid doctors for nearly two years. When he finally succumbs to medicine again in the shape of a physician 'of the Modern Opinion'. This doctor bears a striking resemblance to the young Mandeville of *De Chylosi Vitiata* and his account of Misomedon's illness is a neat précis of that Latin treatise,

> He told me, that the part affected was indeed the Stomach; but that it was a vulgar Error, to think, that there was a great heat required for the Concoction of our Food, since in some Creatures it was altogether perform'd without, as was evident in Fishes, in whom there was not so much as any perceptible warmth; yet, said he, be feeding on their own Species, and swallowing one another, it is plain, that, Bones and all, they digest whole Bodies, sometimes half as big as themselves, without the help of chewing, and consequently are endued with a stronger Concoction than other Animals: He made me sensible; first, that the Aliment in every Creature was digested, and dissolv'd by means of a certain adapted Menstruum, that by insinuating it self into the Pores was able to break the contexture of it: Secondly, that this Menstruum did not act by any Muscular or other Organick Force, but an Intestine motion not unlike that of Yest, or Leaven in Dough, from which Analogy in the Operation it had received the same name in Latin, and was call'd a Ferment: Thirdly, that on the various faults of this Ferment all manner of Indigestion depended...
>
> The first I was to do, was to take an Emetick Potion or two, to discharge the Viscid Saburra, that oppress'd my Stomach; then with Chalybeats and other powerful Alcalicks to subdue the fix'd Acid Salts, and with Carminatives and Specifick Stomachicks mix'd with Volatile Salts, endeavour to Meliorate, and if possible restore the Ferment to its Pristine State.[17]

Thus young Mandeville succeeds in easing Misomedon's suffering and remains in favour. Even after he has gone his recipes continue to provide ease and are the only successful remedy before the appearance of Philopirio. The recipes, however, only ease pain and even then Misomedon becomes immune to their palliative effects. Mandeville is admitting, through this, that his earlier work on chylification was not effective enough, though it had sure foundations. Later in the *Treatise* he will argue that the true cure must go far beyond the simple fact of prescribing drugs. Misomedon's recitation of his case history is already an example of this belief. His long speech is essentially a history of textual digestion as he imitates and absorbs the styles of restoration rake, Galenist physician, classical authors etc. What Philopirio perceives in this case history is that Misomedon has not yet learned to select texts judiciously and maintain a spare and healthy diet.

This is confirmed by Misomedon as he completes his case history. From the Epsom incident onwards he became interested in medical theory and begins to study it in earnest:

> For above two Years together I read Hippocrates, Celius Aurelianus, Aretaeus, Galen, Celsus and several other Volumes of Greek and Roman Authors without any great advancement as to Knowledge, till being acquainted with the Physician, I lately mention'd, I was put in a better way, went first thro' two of three Modern Anatomists, and slipt no opportunity of seeing publick Dissections, not forgetting in the mean time Harvaeus *de Generatione* and Borellus *de motu Animalium*... Having laid this foundation, I read with great avidity the inventive Sylvius de la Boe, and faithful Etmuller, and of our own Nation the speculative Willis, and practical Sydenham.[18]

Not content with a study of medical systems, Misomedon then decides to explore medical theories of hypochondria,

> Having gone through the Practical Authors, with which as I told you, I began, I went over to Fernelius, Sennertus, Jacotius, Salius, Varandaeus, Zecchius, Thomas a Veiga, Riverius, Forestus, and several others of the first rank among the Learned: After them I consulted ... Cardan, Sanctorius, the Voluminous Mercatus, Ferrerius, &c. not forgetting the excellent Cautions of Ballonius, or ...Septalius ... Claudinus Agricola, Martini, Wedelius, Hartmannus, Matthiolus, Doringius, Rhodius, Petraeus, Fisherus, and both those lower shelves.[19]

Having gorged on physicians Misomedon ends by consuming their words on the basis of quantity alone, making room for a short but 'voluminous' list of pharmacopoeias. At this point, the reader begins to suffer from the same indigestion that afflicts Philopirio's patient.

Mandeville has deliberately constructed a medical Tower of Babel where theories of digestion jostle for attention. It is within this context that he turns the dialogue towards an analysis of medical training and the propagation of medical theories. Beginning with the notion of a young medical student graduating from university he argues that

> such a one is no more capable of discharging the weighty Office of Physician, than a Man, that should Study Opticks, Proportions, and read of Painting and mixing of Colours for as many Years, would without having ever touch'd a Pencil, be able to perform the part of a good History Painter.[20]

Despite this, a young doctor can quickly earn himself a reputation by contributing to the babble of medical discourse,

> Physicians ... have found more Compendious ways to Renown and Riches ... writing of, or performing something with accuracy in any one of the shallow auxiliary Arts, that all together Compose the Theory of Physick, they ... insinuate themselves into the publick Favour...The witty Philosopher ... Cures all Diseases by Hypothesis, frightens away the Gout with a fine Simile, but oftener reasons a trifling Distemper into a Consumption.[21]

Through language and the dramatizing of a disease by metaphor a physician can quickly gain recognition. Philopirio is attempting to make Misomedon aware of the dangers inherent in the application of language and metaphor to the human body and illness. If the rhetoric of medical discourse is dominated by self-interest then the gap between the actuality of bodily illness and its verbal definition will inevitably increase. In the case of hypochondria the disease eventually exists more as a linguistic construction than as a verifiable physical phenomenon. But, paradoxically, the power of language and metaphor can have a tangible influence on the body. Reading, therefore, is a physical act and a reader can read himself into hypochondria.

Philopirio recommends instead that doctors should follow a more silent course based on the quiet observation of patient and their illness:

> The Tedious, the Difficult, but the only useful, in regard of others, the Practical part which is not attempted by many, is only attain'd by an almost everlasting attendance on the Sick, unwearied Patience, and Judicious as well as Diligent Observation.[22]

The model and precedent for such a course of study is Hippocrates who is linked by Philopirio to the claim that

> Tis Observation, plain Observation without discanting or reasoning upon it that makes the Art, and all, that neglecting this main point have strove to imbellish it with the Fruits of their Brain, have but

crampt and confounded it.[23]

Philopirio goes on to argue that this long course of observation should be linked to a system of specialized research at universities, a scheme he has adapted from Giorgio Baglivi. This championing of Hippocrates is part of Mandeville's broader strategy in which he aims to question the authority of medical discourse and to analyse the motives behind medical writing. Hippocrates provides him with a useful tool in this analysis. Within the official 'canon' of medical writers Hippocrates is one of the greatest figures, one of the 'origins' of medical discourse. At the same time, the authorship of the Hippocratic texts is more difficult to ascertain. Hippocrates is a shadowy figure, his authorship cannot be definitely proven for any of the texts and if he did exist he probably inspired a school of physicians who contributed many of the works now under his name.[24] Mandeville reads these works as a clear exhortation to practise observation and to reduce medical discourse to a simple record of these observations. This paradoxical figure is then set in opposition to that of Galen, another 'originator' who betrays all the unsavoury motives of the modern physicians who have followed him:

> Galen himself a Man of very great Sense, and no less Pride, having entertain'd the Ambition of raising himself above any of his Contemporaries, foresaw, that to exceed the most skillful of them in real Knowledge, would be a very difficult task, if not impossible, and at best a tedious work of endless labour: He was well acquainted with the state of Physick and the Palate of his Garrulous Age, and found, that nothing would sooner establish his Reputation, than his Wit: Accordingly he left the Observation to them that liked them, and fell a writing, as fast as a Bird could fly ... This was the beginning of People's reasoning about Physick, and that the cause of it all the Hypotheses we have had since, the best of which will be always defective and full of Error.[25]

Medical discourse is revealed to be just another branch of rhetoric, here liable to the same need to be properly 'cooked' to suit the 'Palate of his Garrulous Age'. Galen's motives for constructing medical hypotheses are also seen to be self-serving in contradiction to the traditional image of the 'noble physician'. Mandeville succeeds in undermining both the authority and the scientific objectivity of medical discourse in this discussion of Hippocrates and Galen. Having done so, he then goes on to examine some medical hypotheses in detail in the second Dialogue.

Having begun this section with brief discussions of some of the main issues in digestion theory of that time, Mandeville allows Misomedon to quote a lengthy passage from Thomas Willis's *Of Fermentation.*

In this quotation Willis outlines the commonly used metaphor of the brain as an alembic, saying

> the Brain with Skull over it, and the appending Nerves, represent the little Head of Glass Alembick with a Spunge laid upon it, as we use to do for the highly rectifying of the Spirit of Wine: For truly the Blood when rarified by heat is carried from the Chimney of the Heart to the Head, even as the Spirit of Wine boiling in the Cucurbit, and being resolved into Vapours, elevated into the Alembick; where the Spunge covering all the openings of the hole, only transmits the more penetrating and very subtile Spirits, and carries them to the Snout of the Alembick.[26]

This metaphor is developed by Willis for a further two pages and Philopirio patiently listens as Misomedon quotes it in full. His immediate comment on the passage, however, is cutting:

> The admirable Willis is here as he is every where full of wit; his Speculations are as Sublime, as imagination can carry them, and the contrivance of all he supposes are most Ingenious. These Similes I confess are very diverting for People that have nothing else to do: In some of our Modern Hypotheses there is as much Wit to be discover'd as in a tollerable Play, and the contrivance of them costs as much labour; what pity it is they won't cure Sick People.[27]

The evident frustration and anger in Philopirio's final comment is indicative of a constant problem in medicine as new generations still face the obstacles of metaphor. Susan Sontag, analysing the dangerous acculturation of metaphors for the AIDS virus, recalls how she first became aware of this danger after she was diagnosed as having cancer,

> It was my doleful observation, repeated again and again, that the metaphoric trappings that deform the experience of having cancer have very real consequences: they inhibit people from seeking treatment early enough, or from making a greater effort to get competent treatment. The metaphors and myths, I was convinced, kill. (For instance, they make people irrationally fearful of effective measures such as chemotherapy, and foster credence in thoroughly useless remedies such as diets and psychotherapy.) I wanted to offer other people who were ill and those who care for them an instrument to dissolve these metaphors, these inhibitions...to regard cancer as if it were just a disease...Without 'meaning'..Illness as Metaphor is not just a polemic, it is an exhortation. I was saying: Get the doctors to tell you the truth; be an informed, active patient; find yourself good treatment, because good treatment does exist.[28]

Mandeville, like Sontag, wants to offer his readers and patients 'an instrument to dissolve these metaphors'. His second dialogue between Philopirio and Misomedon attempts just that, as the physician dissects the rhetoric of Willis's metaphor, teaching his patient how to read prudently. At the end of the lesson his pupil will have been taught how to choose critically from the wealth of images and texts available to him. Philopirio's lesson runs as follows:

> *Phil.:* Let us once examine the Simile, and take the Still to Pieces. First, What Comparison is there between the Function of the Heart, the great Treasury of Blood and Life, and the vile Office of a Chimney?
>
> *Misom.:* But you are Captious, Won't you allow of either Trope or Figure? By Chimney he means the Furnace that gives the Heat, the Fire place of the Still.
>
> *Phil.:* No, Misomedon, there is more Artifice in this than ye are aware of: The word Chimney is made use of designedly, to hide, as much as possible, the deformity of the Still: For the Caput Mortuum being in the Spleen, if he had call'd the Heart the Furnace, as he ought to have done, it would have been too plain, that he had made the Fire between the Head and bottom of the Still.[29]

Misomedon's misreading of Willis's metaphor reveals the dangers of using tropes to convey medical information. As a rhetorical device the metaphor will convey a striking image to the reader which will reinforce the theory being put forward. If the metaphor is accepted uncritically, the medical ideas behind it will also be unquestioned and, worse, they may be misrepresented by the metaphor. The dangers of rhetorical seduction are clearly presented to Misomedon.

If, however, metaphor is a localized danger in medical discourse, Philopirio argues that there is a much greater evil – the medical hypothesis. The case for any hypothesis in medicine rests on a claim to knowledge of the body claims Philopirio, and he goes on to demonstrate that it is this original sin of pride which is the flaw of all hypotheses:

> *Misom.:* You say the Hypothesis is ingeniously contriv'd, and may be easily defended; but yet you seem to dislike something in it ... what have you to object against it?
>
> *Phil.:* Nothing, but what I have against all Hypotheses in general; I can't endure a Man should make a formal Description with so many Circumstances to make you believe it is true, and write a

> whole Book upon a thing which he is sure in his Conscience he knows nothing of. We are altogether in the Dark, as to the real use the Liver, the Milt, and Pancreas are of to our Bodies; nay, wholly ignorant of their several Offices otherwise than that they are Organa Colatoria ... and all that has been said of them besides, by the most Sagacious Man has been nothing but Conjectures, in which the best Anatomists could yet never agree.[30]

Philopirio's cure for this rash of conjectures is yet again, observation. This time he refers Misomedon to Baglivi's advice for physicians to model their hypothesizing on that of astronomers who

> ascend into Theories exactly delineated after a Geometrical manner; and when they have Learnedly examin'd, and are thoroughly vers'd in these things, they are able to foretel, and define all the Motions, Sites, Conjunctions &c. of those Bodies with all the certainty imaginable: So that first they take care of having a vast Train of Observations, and then they compose a Theory.[31]

Philopirio goes on to note that the theory devised by such an astronomer will be almost bound to be wrong but that at least a body of accurate observations has been compiled. Comparing a lifetime's study of medicine and astronomy he concludes that

> an exquisite Genius, vers'd in Arithmetick, and every thing else, but the two Arts I named, would not believe the Knowledge, that could be got by observing the different motions of the Celestial Bodies more capable of ever being reduced to an Art of Rules and Certainty, than that which might be acquired by likewise observing the various courses of Distempers incident in our Terrestrial ones.[32]

It is our pride then which blinds us to our true ignorance. Man abuses science by declaring each new system to be infallible, the product of knowledge (the product of the Fall). Instead, Philopirio advocates the acceptance of a shifting, uncertain world filled with contradictions and relative values. The path to any real certainty is deferred for centuries perhaps,

> It is as yet inconceivable, to what prodigious pitch human Knowledge in all things, that fall under the Senses, tho' never so changeable, remote or irregular, may be carried by diligent Observations, when they are faithfully transmitted from one to another, and without intermission continued for several Ages.[33]

For Mandeville this is a particularly important passage as it marks one of the earliest statements of his theory of evolution, to be worked out in much greater detail in his later works. He posits, here, a slow accumulation of observations, facts and information that may one day, far in the future, lead to a moment of certainty. This implies a present-day world of uncertainty and it is the physician's role, therefore, to master the art of uncertainty. Having done so, he can then lead his patients to an understanding of this condition.

For the hypochondriac, it means the learning of a new way of reading and a re-examination of the self. Patients must learn to see themselves surrounded by a network of texts, images, metaphors and theories which attempt to define an illness. The authority centred in medical discourse and the medical establishment tries to present this patient as a passive receiver on which the network is imposed.

Through the dialogues in the *Treatise,* Mandeville hopes to reinvigorate the reader and the patient. Through the dialogic technique of splitting the self, he forces the reader to interrogate medical discourse and to experience, through the patchwork of literary styles, the relative and uncertain nature of medical discourse. By assigning an active role to the patient, he is implying that the dialogue between doctor and patient is a vital part of the therapy. This is underlined by Mandeville's presentation of his own theory of chylification. In his original thesis, his theory was laid out clearly, point by point, beginning with the etymology of terms used in digestion theory and ending with a series of recipes to alleviate patient's distress.

In the second dialogue of the *Treatise,* Philopirio presents Mandeville's thesis to Misomedon. Now, however, the work is placed in a much subtler context. Philopirio introduces the thesis to his patient in the following manner:

> Phil.: It is the custom in all our Foreign Universities for Students in all Faculties ... to compose and defend against all that will oppose a Thesis or Disputation ... Mine was *de Chylosi vitiata,* which I defended at Leyden in the Year 1691, Dr William Senguerdus, Professor of the Aristotelian Philosophy, being then Rector Magnificus.[34]

Philopirio then goes on to outline many of the points raised in the 1691 thesis. This is not, however, a simple insertion of an earlier work by Mandeville and the reworking of his thesis can only be appreciated fully by an examination of the structure of the entire second dialogue of the *Treatise.*

The dialogue is based on the structure of Mandeville's original thesis on chylification but with one major change. Rather than beginning with the ancients, Philopirio opens the dialogue with a statement of the contemporary theory of fermentation and its role in digestion.

He then runs through a brief examination of the physicians who contributed to the formation of this theory – Sylvius de la Boe, Van Helmont and Thomas Willis. His discussion of Willis's metaphors leads to his criticism of the authority invested in medical hypotheses and this creates the context in which he presents the main arguments of his thesis. Having just stressed the relativity of hypotheses he launches his own with typical Mandevillian humour – the contents page for this section states unequivocally that this section outlines 'The Chief Cause of the Hypochondriack and Hysterick Passions.' He continues to toy with the reader in his presentation of the thesis as he combines it with ideas from his earlier work, *Disputatio Philosophica de Brutorum Operationibus.*[35]

The most radical change to his thesis is found, however, in Mandeville's use of the dialogue format to expand various points and to interrogate his earlier theories. The looseness and informality of dialogue style permits him to heighten descriptions of medical 'facts' dramatically. In his thesis, for example, he refers to an observation of Platerus on perverted appetites,

> Platerus, in an observation, refers to a girl who ate an onion which had previously been applied to a plague swelling, also without any harm: although it can't be doubted that the onion was plainly infected with poison.[36]

In the *Treatise,* this description has been digested and absorbed into a livelier text where it reads as follows,

> Platerus ... relates, that a Girl of about Seventeen, had so depraved and perverse an Appetite, as not only to fancy but likewise to eat an Onion, that in the time of a raging Plague, having been applied to a Pestilential Boil, and being blacken'd and putrified by the Poisonous exhalations was thrown down by the Fire-side. The Girl, says he, received no hurt, and remain'd free from a Disease otherwise so Contagious.[37]

Philopirio continues by recalling his use of a quotation by Hippocrates and here uses it to introduce the notion that the stomach's ferment is composed partly of chyle and partly of animal spirits from the brain. However, the role of these animal spirits has now become much more central to the whole process of digestion and to the disorders of hypochondria:

> Next to Experience, I shall make use of what is the result of it, the Testimony of Hippocrates, who in one of his Aphorisms tells us, the Aliments, which our Appetite stands enclined to, are far better digested, than those we don't fansie. From these Anatomical and

> Practical Observations I conclude first, that if the Animal Spirits, which continually trickle down into the Stomach through the innumerable little Nerves, that discharge themselves there, do not wholly compose ... the Stomachick ferment, Menstruum ... by virtue of which our Aliments are digested, they at least make a considerable, and the most essential part of it. Secondly that some of the Spirits, that help to Constitute the Ferment are of a greater subtilty, and more refin'd than the rest that serve only for Muscularly motions, and other actions of force.[38]

These spirits of 'greater subtilty' create the stomach's ferment and are also 'the Spirits, which are immediately employ'd in the act of thinking'. With this statement, Mandeville links the brain and the stomach in an intimate dialogue. Food can, he implies, influence the brain and hence the mind's thoughts. Likewise, the mind can influence the stomach and, by implication, the rest of the physical functions. The Cartesian problems of the mind's relationship to the body have resurfaced in this discussion of chylification, and Mandeville's earlier thesis on the operation of animals is being revisited.

In 1689 he rejected the strict Cartesian division of body and the soul which gave man the power of self-reflexive thought. However, he found nothing more substantial to replace it and admitted his conclusions were highly subjective,

> I preferred to persuade myself that 'Animals are endowed with no thought and all their actions are automatic'. And after I adapted this idea I noticed that many functions of their lives could be explained by mechanics, which previously I thought must be controlled by thought. That many, however, remain which I cannot explain from their structure, I freely confess.[39]

Now Mandeville feels that the concept of subtle animal spirits can provide a new image of the relationship between the mind and the body which is more satisfactory than that of Descartes. He admits that 'The Metaphysical Principle of Monsieur Des Cartes, Cogito ergo sum' is 'the first truth' and furthermore that 'matter it self can never think'. Beyond this, however, the relationship between soul and body is 'Mysterious to us'.[40]

Certain things can be asserted, however, such as the claim that 'there must be an immediate Commerce between the Body and the Soul'. As the soul is immaterial there must be a link between the two (a subject of intense philosophical debate after Descartes). For Mandeville, the link is the subtler animal spirits – 'exquisitely small Particles, that are the Internuncii ... the intermediate Officers between the Soul and the grosser parts of the Body'. This is a vital image in the *Treatise.* The description of the animal spirits as 'intermediate officers' conjures up the metaphor of the body as a commonwealth, with the soul as ruler and the stomach as the mass of the population. Mandeville plays on this allusion but complicates it further by going on to refer to the soul as 'an Artificer, whilst the Organs of the Body are her tools'.[41] To accuse the soul of artifice immediately raises interesting questions about thought and the 'true' nature of the soul. In an exchange between Philopirio and Misomedon, Mandeville outlines the implications of his claims on the issue of thought. It is worth quoting this passage in full as it is not only central to an understanding of Mandeville's views on the body and hypochondria but also a key element in his aesthetics. Discussing the 'mixture' of the body and soul Philopirio concludes,

> For tho' our thoughts be never so elevated or Metaphysical, we cannot form them without Idea's of Words, Things, or joint Notions and Thinking only consists in a various disposition of Images received before.
>
> *Misom.:* Then you would have this variously disposing of the Images to be the work of the Spirits, that act under the Soul as so many Labourers under some great Architect.
>
> *Phil.:* I would so: And reflecting on what is transacted within us, it seems to me a very diverting Scene to think, when we strive to recollect something that does not then occur; how nimbly those volatil Messengers of ours will beat through all the Paths, and hunt every Enclosure of the Organ set aside for thinking, in quest of the Images we want, and when we have forgot a word or Sentence, which yet we are sure the great Treasury of Images received our Memory has once been charged with, we may almost feel how some of the Spirits flying through all the Mazes and Meanders rommage the whole substance of the Brain; whilst others ferret themselves into the inmost recesses of it with so much eagerness and labour, that the difficulty they meet with some times makes us uneasie, and they often bewilder themselves in their search, till at last they light by chance on the Image that contains what they look'd for, or else dragging it, as it were, by piece-meals from the dark Caverns of oblivion, represent what they can find of it to our Imagination.[42]

Mandeville is arguing here against the Platonic, benevolent vision of the soul. He is at pains to stress that thoughts depend on the arrangement of observations and images from the material world, even if they are 'elevated or Metaphysical'. Furthermore, thought relies on the images presented to the retina and is shaped by the disposition of those images. The soul, the ruler, has now become the 'great

Architect', which arranges these images. The brain, as centre of the commonwealth of the body has a 'Treasury of Images' and Mandeville continues by describing the animal spirits as 'airy velocious Agents ... Ministers of Thought' working in 'this Volatile Oeconomy of the Brain'. At the same time, there are darker notes in the description as the soul, once the 'Artificer', now becomes the 'great Architect'. Echoes of the Daedalus myth are multiplied as the animal spirits 'quest ... through all the Mazes and Meanders of the Brain'. The image they seek finally begins to reasemble the Minotaur as they drag it 'by piece-meals from the dark Caverns of oblivion'. This confounding of the soul with artifice and the image of a beast argues violently against any Platonic, idealized image of the soul.

Mandeville has mixed motives for creating this image of the human brain and the process of thought. Within the immediate context of *A Treatise of the Hypochondriack and Hysterick Passions,* he is advocating a new awareness of the importance of observation in medicine and encouraging both doctors and patients to examine the relationship between the mind, the body and health. On a wider level, Mandeville is developing the view of human nature he first propounded in his earlier works such as *The Grumbling Hive* and *The Virgin Unmask'd* in which he attempted to explain the ways in which we can reveal or mask images of ourselves.[43] Having highlighted the need for sharp observation in a social context, he is now attempting to examine the nature of representation and perception.

The Dutch tradition of portraiture provides a valuable model for Mandeville in his description of physicians who must compose a case history of each patient based on observations of the symptoms. Philopirio, as an active example of Mandeville's therapy, has attempted to build up a series of observations on Misomedon's illness in order to compose a case history, or portrait, of his patient. Central to this portrait is the issue of Misomedon's identity. His greedy, untrammelled absorption of so many medical texts and theories has had a weakening effect on his health. His equally unregulated consumption of worldly goods and the joys of venery have contributed to this steady deterioration in health. For Mandeville, such a life is the consequence of a poor understanding of digestion. The consuming and digesting of ideas, goods, or sexual acts should be judicious. Every digestion should be made in the awareness that it is simultaneously a process of imitation and absorption. Misomedon has to be made aware that his identity is ultimately composed of the materials he has digested and synthesized in the creation of his own self. 'Tell me what you eat: I will tell you what you are', as Brillat-Savarin phrased it a century later.[44]

As the culmination of this argument, Mandeville has Philopirio retell the life of Misomedon in the context of all the discussions that have occurred between them. The patient, having absorbed the doctor's well-regulated diet of advice is now ready to accept such a portrait and sets the mood for it when he thanks Philopirio for leading him 'to a noble Prospect of Miracles in the composure of our Frame'.[45] Philopirio's portrait recalls every aspect of his patient's life and at every opportunity he stresses Misomedon's lack of moderation in consumption. Each detail of excess is examined in a portrait which runs to several pages. Finally, Philopirio concludes that it was luxury which permitted the onset of his patient's disease:

> Immoderate Grief, Cares, Troubles, and Disappointments are likewise often Concomitant Causes of this Disease; but most commonly in such, as either by Estate, Benefices, or Employments have a sufficient Revenue to make themselves easie: Men that are already provided for, or else have a livelyhood by their Callings amply secured, are never exempt from Sollicitudes, and the keeping not only of Riches, but even moderate Possessions is always attended with Care. Those that enjoy em are more at leisure to reflect, besides that their Wishes and Desires being larger, themselves are more likely to be offended at a great many passages of Life, than People of lower Fortune, who have seldom higher Ends, than what they are continually employ'd about, the getting of their Daily Bread.[46]

In this passage Mandeville broadens the portrait of Misomedon to view him in his social context. The intense focus of the first two dialogues on the personal life and identity of the patient gives way to a wider world view. Through money, Misomedon had access to the consumer world of the fast-expanding British empire, and the leisure to consume constantly. It was Misomedon's imprudent and excessive consumerism which led to the onset of his hypochondria. It was the luxury of leisure time which then allowed this disease to thrive.

By drawing such a portrait of Misomedon, Mandeville prepares the reader for the third and final dialogue which is more outward looking. Polytheca, the wife of Misomedon, is introduced and there are detailed portraits of their daughter and of Pharmenio, an apothecary. The allusions in the earlier dialogues to the plays of Terence and Plautus now find an echo in the family and social life por-trayed here. As the dialogue in which Philopirio presents his cures for hypochondria, it is dominated by recipes, nostrums and apothecaries bills. Related to this is the underlying theme of wine and fermentation which pervades every aspect of the discussion.

The third dialogue begins after the physician and patient have both dined and the reader is aware that all the participants are digesting their dinner as they speak. The conversation opens with a further discussion of the animal spirits in which Philopirio defines wit:

> Thinking consists in a various Disposition of the Images received; so what we call Wit is nothing but an aptitude of the Spirits by which they nimbly turn to, and dexterously dispose the Images that may serve our purpose.[47]

He goes on to argue that if witty men study too much and ignore exercise, they will also become victims of hypochondria by exhausting the animal spirits. This explanation only raises more questions for Misomedon, however, as it seems to exclude women:

> what equivalent .. wasts the spirits in Women, and is likewise able to make them subject to the Hysterick Passion: for studying and intense thinking are not to be alledged as a cause in Women .. and yet the number of Hysterick Women for exceeds that of Hypochondriack Men.[48]

Philopirio replies that in young girls, at least, a poor diet caused by 'Agues, Green-Sickness, or other Cachexies' produces weakened animal spirits. As he digests his own dinner, the doctor proceeds to outline his view of the digestive process and its centrality to the 'Oeconomy' of the human body,

> We can ask no more of the Stomachick Ferment, than that insinuating it self into the Pores of our Aliments it dissolves the Contexture of them, and makes them into such a Pulp, as being afterwards mix'd with the Gall and Pancreatick Juice, shall suffer its finest parts by the Peristaltick motion to be transcolated through the Glandules of the Intestines into the Lacteal Vessels: This is all what belongs to a good Chylification, which may be done, and yet the Chyle be unfit to make good Blood, if the Aliments are improper; the Stomach is only to be consider'd as a good Cook who may dress every thing to the best advantage, but cannot make the Flesh of a Starv'd Old Cow so Nutritious, as that of a Young well fed Heifer. If the Food when we Eat it, is not endued with a great many Balsamick, Spirituous, or what we call nourishing Parts, the Blood cannot receive them from it, how well soever it may be assimilated with its Mass.[49]

This ecstatic celebration of the digestion process is at the core of Mandeville's thought. The stomach – 'a good Cook' – is dependent on the materials given to it to work with. In the case of young girls this means that eating 'Trash' will give the stomach poor material and the resulting animal spirits will therefore be weakened.[50] In the wider context, where Mandeville imagines life in a complex consumer society, it means that the wrong choice of consumer goods or an excess of goods, theories, acts of lust etc. will destroy personal identity. Prudent choice of goods, food or models to imitate is imperative to retain a stable sense of the self. As Philopirio moves on to a discussion of children he stresses the value of imitation in providing the animal spirits with suitable images to arrange in the act of thinking:

> the aptitude of the Spirits ... is no more so, than the aptitude of the Organs of Speech, and that both are only to be attain'd by Imitation and Practice, of this we see Thousand instances every Day in Infants ... that striving to imitate the actions of others by degrees they model their manner of Thinking...by what their Senses communicate to them of the Thoughts and Words of those they converse with.[51]

Having restated his belief in imitation Mandeville has set the scene for the examination of Misomedon's family and the society they live in. The world he depicts is one of unfit people tyrannized by fashions, jargons and authoritative con-men. Lacking any understanding of the body and health in this society, most people appear to succumb to the wine-laden drugs of apothecaries and doctors.

This section opens with more than ten pages of Misomedon's recipes and prescriptions, transcribed in the abbreviated Latin that requires a pharmacopoeia for elucidation. The prescriptions are typical of the physician of the 'Modern Opinion' mentioned in the first dialogue and several of them are reminiscent of the recipes found in Mandeville's *De Chylosi Vitiata*. However, their presentation by a patient undermines their medical authority. The obsessive interest and enthusiasm which Misomedon displays while showing off these recipes reveals a life lived by stumbling from one drug to another:

> I never found any thing of greater Efficacy against the Sour, and Wind in my Stomach than what I read to you last, and I would never have left it off, but that I imagin'd it bound me up; after that I remember I made use of this Absorbent Electuary.
>
> *Conch. pp.* ℥iij.
> *Ocular.* ss.
> *Lapid. haemat.* ℥iß.
> *Croci Martis,*
> *Chryst. mont.* ℥i
> *Bol. Armen.*
> *Antimon. diaphor.*
>
> M. & C. S Q Conserv. flor. genist. f. Elect. cuius dos. bis indies.[52]

Misomedon is a connoisseur of drugs, proud of his knowledge and ever alert to the effects of every dose, whether imagined or real. In an orthodox medical text the transcription of these recipes would be read as a serious passage of advice. Delivered by Misomedon they become the deadly arsenal of a medical bore. Just as Philopirio seems about to criticize this performance, however, Misomedon's wife arrives.

Polytheca, a name that literally means 'many drugs', is a suitable culmination of this series of prescriptions. She is plagued not only by hysteria but the pressures of suffering from the 'Vapours' when 'the very name is become a Joke'.[53] Her life revolves around the advice and medication provided by her apothecary, Pharmenio, who has pronounced her to be incurable but enamoured himself to her by his constant ability to listen to her when she describes her problems. After introducing herself she quickly begins to describe her case history to Philopirio and then recounts the history of her daughter who suffers equally from the vapours. Their lives are strikingly summarized by Misomedon when he tries to recall his daughter's medicines:

> I know that she has had several Decoctions of Mugwort, Feverfew, Calaminth, Rue, Peony, Peony (sic), Pennyroyal, and such like, with Baths of the same, sometimes she has taken for a considerable time Testaceous Powders, and others, with Crabs-eyes, Red-Coral, Volatil Salt of Tartar, Diaphoretick Antimony, Bole-Armenick; at other times Uterine and Stomachick Electuaries, with Savin, Nutmeg, Myrrhe, Saffron, Volatile Salts, Foetid Oils, &c. several sorts of Hysterick Pills...I remember she had a Bolus prescrib'd her... This she took twice a Day in Six Ounces of a Decoction of Black-Hellebore and Briony-Roots, Pennyroyal, Rue and Mugwort; and at the same time in Regione Umbilici, she wore a Plaister of Galbanum Caracanna, asa foetida and Oil of Tacamahaca.[54]

Mandeville goes on to make it clear that most of these decoctions are mixed with various wines, creating an image of both Polytheca and her daughter as women living in a constant state of dulled inebriation. As with Misomedon, Philopirio constructs a portrait of Polytheca which places her in a social context and takes every aspect of her life into account. This is, in effect, an holistic view of the patient's illness in which Mandeville is arguing both that such a view of the illness is necessary if it is to be treated properly and that the patient's lifestyle is the main cause of the illness.

The reasons why Polytheca has drifted into this condition are never stated explicitly but Mandeville makes it apparent that it derives from the poor relationship between her and her husband. Her speeches are constantly interrupted by Misomedon who mocks her views, dismisses her illness as a figment of her imagination and derides her apothecary.

Any point Polytheca makes about her condition is immediately taken up by her husband and methodically criticized, every argument being reinforced by a battery of medical information. Misomedon is systematically brutalizing his wife with his knowledge as Mandeville demonstrates in their final exchange. Having again attacked apothecaries, Misomedon concludes with this advice to Polytheca:

> *Misom.:* But if you think I don't do them Justice, pray, my Dear, give your self the trouble of reading this little Book, where the Mystery of Compound Medicines as to their intrinsick Value, is very handsomely unfolded: It is the work of an Eminent Physician, Dr Pit, who for the good of the Publick has shewn the vast difference between the prime Cost, that Simples are bought at from the Druggists, and Herb-Women, and the extravagant rates, they are sold at by the Apothecaries, when they have disguis'd them in mixtures of specious Titles. It is very diverting...
>
> *Polyth.:* It may be so, but I have other things to mind. – Oh the Tormenting and Throbbing Pain I feel in my Head! This Minute my Brains are a boiling, and if there was half a Dozen Trunk-makers at work under my Skull, I don't think I could be sensible of more Noise and Beating than I am. I can stay no longer...I am forc'd to withdraw. Oh! the misery of....[55]

The lack of communication between the couple is obvious. Misomedon only seeks an opportunity to broadcast his views of medical issues while Polytheca's vivid complaints and her withdrawal are symptoms of an ailing relationship. When she has departed Misomedon reveals just how little sympathy is left in the marriage when he declares 'she nothing but thwarts and contradicts me'. Convincing himself of her deliberate malevolence he reacts with equal spite – 'I did expect it would put her in the Vapours, if I spoke more against the Apothecaries than she could answer'.[56] Philopirio gently tries to highlight the problem in their marriage by directing Misomedon to a satire by Horace which argues that man should look for the fault in himself rather than criticize others.[57] He has carefully couched his advice in the classics to humour his patient before adding a more direct comment on the exchanges between husband and wife:

> it could not be to please her, that with so much eagerness you snatch'd at every opportunity of speaking against the Apothecaries; and indeed, in my Opinion, you have been too severe upon them.[58]

This comment not only serves as a criticism of Misomedon's marriage but forces the reader to reassess the harsh attacks on apothecaries in the previous pages. While the attacks give a thorough airing to the contemporary debate on the role of the apothecary they go beyond the feud between doctor and pharmacist. Clearly, Pharmenio, the apothecary to Polytheca, has a role in her life which derives from the difficulties of her marriage.

Misomedon remains wrapped in contemplation of his own self and devotes his time to a minute analysis of his own physical condition. He resents the competition for attention provided by Polytheca's vapours and suspects it is a deliberate attempt to annoy him rather than seeing it as a visible sign of the crisis in their relationship. Pharmenio, however, both listens to Polytheca and acknowledges the suffering involved in her illness:

> *Polyth.:* Pharmenio, whom you are pleas'd to call Judicious in Jest, is a Skilful-Man of great Experience, the understands my Constitution thoroughly; he is of Opinion that I am incurable, I have heard the same of Eminent Physicians; yet he has the Patience to weigh my Complaints, or at least the good manners to hear them, and seldom fails of giving me ease, even when I am at the worst, which is what others that boasted of greater learning either could or would not do; so that I should think myself unwise to leave him.[59]

The reason, then, that Polytheca (and perhaps most women at that time) preferred the services of Pharmenio was that he acknowledged her as a person, taking her problems seriously. A doctor would have paid more attention to the illness without acknowledging the broader context of the patient's life. The danger of Pharmenio, however, is that he is essentially a businessman and his remedies often are designed only to offer a state of inebriation which will lessen the pain of a failed marriage.

In Mandeville's burgeoning consumer society the apothecary appears as an ambivalent figure typical of the new society. As a businessman, he persuades his customers to buy his products and thus understands the market forces of the consumer world. He then persuades the customer to swallow the consumer product, often sweetening the pill with sugar and wine. He achieves both of these objectives by feeding his clients with palatable rhetoric. In a memorable portrait Misomedon reveals the apothecary at work,

> I have known an Apothecary in an idle Afternoon go to a Person of Quality's, where they made use of him: There happen'd to be no body at home but Children and Servants, that from the highest to the lowest were all in perfect Health: If here he came for Business (you'll say) he was disappointed; but you are mistaken, the Courteous Gentleman with an engaging familiarity accosts every Servant in the House, and puts off a Purge to the Cook, a Vomit to the Butler, a

> Box of Pills to one of the Footmen, and a Pot of Lucatellus Balsam to old Nurse. The Children absolutely refusing to take any Physick at least inwardly, he Coaxes the little Master into the use of a charming Dentifrice, and a sweet-scented Collyrium to rinse his Mouth with after it, that shall preserve his Teeth and make them look like Ivory, tho' he was to eat nothing but Sugar and Sweet-Meats all Day long; to pretty Miss he'll send a Lotion for her Hair, and a Paste for her Hands, that shall render the one so bright as Silver, and the other whiter than Snow, with a Beauty-wash for their Maid, that assisted in the perswading of them. The affable Gentleman has every Bodies good word: The Children are pleas'd, the Servants commend him, my Lady is obliged to him; and Ten to One but the first opportunity of driving that way her Coach stops at his Door, and she thanks him for the care he took of her Family in her absence.[60]

This is the rhetoric of consumerism at its best. The apothecary, understanding the true nature of consumerism knows exactly how to arouse the desires needed to offload various products, accurately sizing up the articles that will 'sell' to each customer. He is skilled at reading people and situations, just as Pharmenio is skilled at reading the needs of Polytheca and her daughter. Mandeville stresses the rhetorical nature of the apothecary and his art throughout this section of the *Treatise.* Not only can the apothecary read the world but he can easily deconstruct a prescription:

> *Polyth.:* How then come they to understand the Physicians Bill so readily, that are all writ in Latin?
>
> *Misom.:* The Body of a Bill is only compos'd of Medicines, they have in their Shops, and contains nothing but the Names of what they can Sell.[61]

The doctor's bill is an intersecting series of ingredients, each of which represents a consumer item. The bill is no more than a customized consumer item. Just as hypochondria is an illness constructed from a series of intersecting texts and Misomedon's body is the compound of various foods, remedies and digested readings, so the 'Body of a Bill' has ingested various ingredients. Moreover, medical receipts, like culinary recipes, are of indeterminate origin as they are usually the product of a long series of imitations of other receipts.

The apothecary is the embodiment of the 'sprightly talkative Age' which Mandeville warns us of in his preface. Through the seduction of his rhetoric consumer goods are transmitted from retailer to customer with the same promiscuity as the pox passed through London society. Mandeville's portrait of the apothecary is not particularly distasteful however. The tone of the description is comic and there is a definite sense of admiration for the apothecary's ability to match people and products. Mandeville's warnings to Misomedon and to the reader of the *Treatise,* then, are not directed at the new consumer culture in Britain but at those who participate in that culture without understanding how it is constructed.

At the heart of this network of ideas lies Mandeville's theories on ways of seeing and the interpretation of an image. His attention to the lengthy quotation of Thomas Willis's metaphor of the brain as an alembic, his championing of the microscope and the Dutch tradition of portraiture and his notion of the animal spirits arranging images received in the brain all relate to this issue. The 'witty Speculations of Hypothetical Doctors' were multiplying as quickly as the range of choices, commodities and temptations available in the British Empire. To deal with such a constant barrage of images, goods and medical theories Mandeville suggests that it is necessary to have reliable interpretative tools with which to examine the usefulness of each consumer choice. By linking the brain and the stomach through the work of the animal spirits Mandeville makes the reader aware of the effect society can have on the physical constitution. Every image is, in effect, digested by the eye, the stomach and the brain. The case histories of Misomedon, Polytheca and their daughter all attest to the dangerous effects of indiscriminate digestion of images, rhetoric, medical theories, food and drugs. Both doctors and patients must therefore learn to assess every morsel and to moderate their consumption accordingly.

When Mandeville republished the *Treatise* in 1730, he elaborated on this theory of medical aesthetics by allowing Philopirio and Misomedon to discuss the two lines of Virgil's *Aeneid* which appear on the title-page of the book itself. Misomedon begins by relating a story of Michelangelo making a new head for a broken statue of a 'Faunus' by means of educated guesswork. Philopirio replies

> Michael Angelo knew his Task; and tho' perhaps no body besides himself could have made a Head answerable to such a Body; yet it was no Secret, which Part of the Statue it was that was wanting: but in the latent Causes of Diseases we can form no Idea of what we are ignorant of; that is, we don't know the Figures nor the Properties of the things that are hid from us, and we are obliged to make Sounds for, and adapt Words to things that are inexpressible.[62]

Through experience gained by years of observation, Michelangelo can skilfully complete a work of art. Philopirio argues that doctors must approach disease and illness in the same way. Observation will lead to an educated guess at the cause for an illness but there is a gap between reality and language. Misomedon quotes Virgil's lines on the silent arts of Iapis, acknowledging their authority, but admitting that he still desires more:

> There is a Gap between the Observations made on the Symptoms of a disease, and the Cure of it: I want to have that Gap fill'd up; and the most airy Speculations are more satisfactory, than a Man's saying that he knows nothing of it. To consider the Nerves as the Snouts of an alembick, and make the Brain serve for a Spunge, requires at least as much Capacity, as to be altogether silent concerning the Operations of either.[63]

Misomedon has acknowledged the uncertainty of medical theory and the flaws in Willis's metaphor – Philopirio's lesson in the second dialogue. He now agrees with his physician that medical discourse has a strong fictional dimension and has pointed out the exploratory nature of Willis's metaphor. When it is recognized as a possible fiction it can then have an experimental value, probing the gap between observation and language.

As Philopirio presents his cures for Misomedon and his family, relativity becomes the dominating feature of the dialogue. Medical and literary origins again become uncertain as Mandeville cites sources such as Thomas Sydenham, Thomas Fuller, Mercurialis, Suetonius, Terence, Herodicus, Plato and Hippocrates. Many of these figures appear are distanced by appearing indirectly in anecdotes related by other writers cited by Mandeville and Daniel Le Clerc's *Histoire de la Médicine* is a constant secondary source.[64] The other dominant voice is that of Horace the Roman poet, who himself imitated Greek poetic styles. As this ferment of writers is absorbed into the text and digested by Misomedon and the reader, Philopirio outlines a dietary cure for tis patients' illness. Diet supplemented by plenty of exercise is recommended for all three patients. Wine is also discussed through the medium of Horace's poetry, allowing Mandeville to create a ferment of literary images around a discussion of wine's influence on the vapours.

Mandeville's recommendation of diet attempts to present itself with as few traces of medical jargon as possible. His introduction of the cure states that

> Diet, says Le Clerc, was the first, the principal, and sometimes the only remedy that Hippocrates made use of. And shall we lay no more stress upon it, as if it did not belong to the Art of Physick?[65]

Even this simple statement mediates the authority of Hippocrates through the prose translation of Le Clerc and reduces medicine to the simple basics transmitted through the centuries. More emphasis is placed on knowledge of the dietary worth of various foods and the art of cooking than any technical skill in medicine. Philopirio's advice is as follows:

> Let your Diet be Nutritious and inoffensive, and your Cookery be simple, natural, and I won't say unartful, but not operose. As for Example, Let your Fish be neither stew'd or fried, or your Flesh be otherwise than Broil'd or roasted; and neither of them previously Salted...make use of no manner of Sauces (Salt and Pepper only excepted) but plain Butter for the first, and the natural Gravy for the latter.[66]

The austerity of this cookery is reminiscent of the Dutch desire to control what they termed 'overvloed' – conspicuous over-consumption in the kitchen. In *The Embarrassment of Riches* Simon Schama describes the general context of such an approach to diet in Holland:

> The control of overvloed through a dam of pious manners became a standard refrain of Dutch family manuals as it already had been in Renaissance Italy and humanist Flanders. The prolific and immensely popular physician-author, Jan van Beverwijck, in his *Schat de Gezontheyt* (Treasure of Health) followed moralists all the way back to Seneca in urging moderation in diet as the best way of avoiding plague, flux, pox, rheum, ague, and insomnia. The standard cookery book designed for households of the middling sort, *De Verstandige Kok of Zorgvuldige Huyshouder* (The Wise Cook or the Painstaking Householder) similarly connected an orderly, regular and balanced dietary regime ... with a morally wholesome and thriving family life.[67]

Schama goes on to show that the best example of the Dutch idea of a balanced diet could be found in the galleys of the navy where meals were regulated by a republican bureaucracy.

Mandeville appears to have agreed with such a reading of the naval diet as Philopirio recommends it as the basis of his own cure for Misomedon:

> I can advise you to a Dish, which tho' cheap, and in England unregarded, is for goodness of inestimable value: What I mean is stockfish, a kind of Cod that is dried without being Salted...the Fish I speak of, and Grout or Burgoe, make up almost the whole Diet of the Dutch Sailers, who are fully as Robust, and for the generality more Healthy at sea, than those of other Nations that are fed at dearer rates.[68]

Misomedon's objections that there are far more nutritious fish are countered by the argument that his constitution is not able to cope with richer food. Behind this excuse, however, there is a desire on Mandeville's part to recommend a fish which will deliberately remind Misomedon of the need for austerity and a sense of balance in diet. The crude simplicity of the meal will be a therapy in itself as it removes the patient from the seductions of over-specialized medical or culinary vocabulary.

Philopirio's reluctant use of drugs is also couched in the same austerity, emphasizing their simplicity and demystifying their use by prescribing in English:

> I have no Opinion of Syrups, or Simple Waters; the Medicines I give are either always taken in Coffee, Tea, Wine, Fair-water, or other Liquors that are familiar to the Patients, and generally to be had at their Houses or near hand; or if any particular Vehicle be required, I prescribe a Decoction, or Infusion of a few Simples, in plain English, which every body may make at home, or have done where he pleases.[69]

In the 1730 edition of the *Treatise* Mandeville adds one other suggestion as to the necessary skills of the physician claiming that 'all physicians should be good Cooks, at least in Theory'. The deliberate simplicity of his description of the physician's role is reinforced in the closing pages of the *Treatise* where Mandeville focuses on one of the oldest medicinal cures – wine. Philopirio calls it 'the Greatest Remedy in the World' and stresses how its use must be regulated by the relative needs of each drinker. All his comments are mediated by the poetry of Horace which Mandeville has carefully selected to suggest the complex social nature of eating and drinking. His choice of Horace for this task is significant in itself. While Virgil was seen as a more pastoral figure who represented a highly moral stance, Horace was seen as more worldly. His association with Augustus and his constant mixture of love and politics in an urban setting seemed to compromise the purity of his moral position. Because he frequently wrote of food he was often used as a touchstone in debates on taste – both culinary and aesthetic.[70] By choosing Horace, Mandeville places his discussion on wine and food in a social context and uses this to point out the way in which everyone creates their own fiction of society and their place in it. Philopirio quotes Horace, Epistle V, Book 1:

——— operta recludit,
Spes jubet esse ratas, in prælia trudit inermem
Sollicitis animis onus eximit; addocet artes:
Fæcundi calices quem non fecere disertum?
Contracta quem non in paupertate solutum?

[It opens secrets, /gives heart to our hopes, pushes the cowardly into battle, /lifts the load from anxious minds, and evokes talents. /Thanks to the bottle's prompting no one is lost for words,/no one who's cramped by poverty fails to find release.][71]

Here Horace is stressing the transformative powers of wine, its ability to change man's vision of the world. Philopirio pushes this further with his own description of wine's effect, speaking as if the discussion of wine itself has inspired a ferment of images in his brain:

> it is not only in the power of this Vegetable to make the Slave fancy himself to be free, the Poor to be Rich, the Old Young, and the Miserable Happy; but it likewise actually mends visible Imperfections; renders the Infirm Strong, the Decrepit Nimble, and the Stammerer Eloquent; and what neither Circe's nor Medea's Art could ever perform; turns Vices into Virtues, and by the Charm of it, the Coward, the Covetous, the Proud, and the Morose become Valiant, Generous, Affable, and good Humour'd.[72]

Wine and its power to ferment images in the mind stands as a summary of the main lesson of the *Treatise* that fictions pervade medical discourse, our personal lives and our image of ourselves in society. Mandeville celebrates these fictions but argues that we must understand that we are living among fictions before we benefit from them. The role of the physician is essentially to help his patient understand the nature of these fictions and digest them in a balanced, nutritious manner. As early as the first dialogue Philopirio states that

> every Physician, that would discharge his Conscience, ought as much, as he can in his private Capacity, to supply the neglect of the Publick, and wholly apply himself to the study of one Distemper only.[73]

The physician must make each patient aware of the importance of personal health for the benefit of the commonwealth and each physician must himself be aware of the social responsibility involved in the treatment of patient's private problems. The discourse of public and private will be the subject of Mandeville's next major work, *The Fable of the Bees,* in which he will investigate the relationships between the physical body and the operations of society in much more detail.

Notes

1. Bernard Mandeville, *A Treatise of the Hypochondriack and Hysterick Passions* (London: 1711), iii.
2. *Ibid.,* iii–iv.
3. *Ibid.,* iv.
4. *Ibid.,* title-page.
5. *Ibid.,* xi.
6. Seneca, *Four Tragedies and Octavia,* trans. E. F. Watling

(Harmondsworth: Penguin, 1966), 38–9.

7. Jacques Derrida, *Dissemination,* trans. Barbara Johnson. (London: The Athlone Press, 1981), 7.
8. Mandeville, *op. cit.* (note 1), iv.
9. *Ibid.*, viii.
10. *Ibid.*, 20.
11. *Ibid.*, 3–4.
12. *Ibid.*, 6–7.
13. *Ibid.*, 7.
14. *Ibid.*, 8.
15. *Ibid.*, 8.
16. *Ibid.*, 12–13.
17. *Ibid.*, 15–17. Mandeville's medical treatise was published as *Disputatio Medica Inauguralis de Chylosi Vitiata* (Leiden: Elzevier, 1691).
18. Mandeville, *op. cit.* (note 1), 20.
19. *Ibid.*, 27–8.
20. *Ibid.*, 32.
21. *Ibid.*, 33.
22. *Ibid.*, 32.
23. *Ibid.*, 35.
24. G. E. R. Lloyd, introduction, *Hippocratic Writings,* trans. J. Chadwick and W. N. Mann (Harmondsworth: Penguin, 1978), 9–12.
25. Mandeville, *op. cit.* (note 1), 55–6.
26. *Ibid.*, 83–4.
27. *Ibid.*, 86.
28. Susan Sontag, *AIDS and its Metaphors* (London: Allen Lane, 1989), 14–15.
29. Mandeville, *op. cit.* (note 1), 87–8.
30. *Ibid.*, 103–4.
31. *Ibid.*, 109.
32. *Ibid.*, 111.
33. *Ibid.*, 111.
34. *Ibid.*, 120–1.
35. Bernard Mandeville, *Disputatio Philosophica De Brutorum Operationibus* (Leiden: Elzevier, 1689).
36. Mandeville, *De Chylosi Vitiata* (note 17), A4r. 'Platerus in observat ... coepam veneno plane fuisse infectam'.
37. Mandeville, *op. cit.* (note 1), 123.
38. *Ibid.*, 123–4.
39. Mandeville, *op. cit.* (note 35), A5r. 'Et postquam hanc fovi sententiam ... libenter confiteor'.
40. Mandeville, *op. cit.* (note 1), 124–5.
41. *Ibid.*, 125–6.
42. *Ibid.*, 129–30.
43. Bernard Mandeville, *The Grumbling Hive; or, Knaves Turn'd Honest* (London: 1705) and *The Virgin Unmask'd; or, Female Dialogues*

betwixt an Elderly Maiden Lady and her Niece (London: 1709).

44. Jean-Anthelme Brillat-Savarin, *The Philosopher in the Kitchen,* (Harmondsworth: Penguin, 1970), 13.
45. Mandeville, *op. cit.* (note), 142.
46. *Ibid.*, 150–1.
47. *Ibid.*, 164.
48. *Ibid.*, 165–6.
49. *Ibid.*, 170–1.
50. *Ibid.*, 166–9.
51. *Ibid.*, 170–1.
52. *Ibid.*, 192–3.
53. *Ibid.*, 199.
54. *Ibid.*, 207–8.
55. *Ibid.*, 232–3.
56. *Ibid.*, 234.
57. Horace, *Satires and Epistles,* trans. Niall Rudd, (ed.) Betty Radice (Harmondsworth: Penguin, 1973), 50. The passage Philopirio alludes to is in Satires I, iii, 25–8, 'Before examining your own faults you smear ointment/on your bloodshot eyes, but when it comes to your friends' foibles/your sight is as sharp as an eagle's or the Epidaurian snake's./Unfortunately they in their turn scrutinize your deficiencies.' Mandeville first quotes this passage in his *De Medicina Oratio Scholastica,* 13.
58. Mandeville, *op. cit.* (note 1), 234.
59. *Ibid.*, 200.
60. *Ibid.*, 216–17.
61. *Ibid.*, 229.
62. Bernard Mandeville, *A Treatise of the Hypochondriack and Hysterick Passions* (London, 1730), 228.
63. *Ibid.*, 230.
64. Daniel LeClerc, *Histoire de la Médecine* (Amsterdam, 1696).
65. Mandeville, *Treatise,* 254.
66. Mandeville, *Treatise,* 245.
67. Simon Schama, *The Embarrassment of Riches: An Interpretation of Dutch Culture in the Golden Age* (London: Collins, 1987), 158–9.
68. Mandeville, *Treatise,* 246.
69. Mandeville, *Treatise,* 263.
70. In 1705 Dr William King published *The Art of Cookery,* a riposte to Martin Lister's translation of Apicius' *De Re Coquinaria* published in the same year. King's attack on Lister was modelled on the structure of Horace's *Art of Poetry.*
71. Mandeville, *Treatise,* 272. The English translation is taken from Horace, *Satires and Epistles,* trans. Niall Rudd (ed.), Betty Radice (Harmondsworth: Penguin, 1973), 139.
72. Mandeville, *Treatise,* 272.
73. Mandeville, *Treatise,* 40.

10

Shaping Psychiatric Knowledge: The Role of the Asylum

Roy Porter

Introduction

Fierce battles have been fought amongst academics during the last 20 years concerning explanations of the rise of the asylum, against the backdrop, of course, of the 'anti-psychiatry' and 'decarceration' movements. Was there, as Michel Foucault argued, a 'great confinement'? Why did the distinctive institutional form which we know as the lunatic asylum emerge? – was it the most enlightened attempt to treat a particularly terrible species of human misery, or merely a convenient place for dumping inconvenient people? Should it be viewed as an authentic medical initiative, or merely the institutionalization of social control? Did the asylum successfully cure mental illness? Or did it rather beget new maladies – those of institutionalization – while providing the site and the rationale for the rise of the new profession of the 'psychiatrist'?[1]

These issues have been lengthily and intelligently debated. They form the background to this paper, but I do not wish to shovel over this ground again. Rather, I wish to raise a question that may have been unduly neglected: what impact did the coming of the asylum have upon conceptualizations of insanity, perceptions of the mad, and notions of appropriate therapeutics? It is, I believe, a question comparable to Schaffer and Shapin's inquiry as to how the advent of experimental apparatus such as the air-pump transformed the sort of knowledge acceptable as natural philosophy,[2] or to Latour's examination of how Pasteur's 'invention' of the 'laboratory' transformed the biomedical sciences.[3]

Clearly, the relations between institutions and consciousness cannot be discussed without some sensitivity to chicken-and-egg, or form-and-contents problems. The asylum was not some ideologically neutral assemblage of bricks and mortar, just a way of putting a roof over lunatics' heads. Madhouses were doubtless erected as the embodiment of particular philosophies of the causes and cure of lunacy (at bottom, the belief that it should be *confined*); and it would hardly be surprising if such theoretical underpinnings to the asylum continued to inform, indeed, to dominate – beliefs and practice within asylums themselves. Nevertheless, without entering into theoretical imbroglios about the nature of historical causation – how far did the materiality of the madhouse determine attitudes and actions within, or was the madhouse itself primarily the technological embodiment of an ideological construct? – it seems at least worth investigating the role played by this institution in creating those 'knowledges' of mental disturbance dominant over the last couple of centuries. [4]

I should be prepared to argue, in broad terms, that the phenomenon of mass institutionalization gave a decisive direction to the shaping of modern ideas about insanity and to the 'psychiatric gaze'. Clearly, it facilitated – perhaps necessitated – enterprises such as psychiatric diagnostics, the taxonomic impulse, and the increased incorporation of prognostic assumptions within classifications. Intense and prolonged observation of lunatics *en masse* favoured medical models, and highlighted behavioural patterns that led, *inter alia,* to an emphasis upon psychosexual 'perversions', to surveys of chronicity, and to major neurological investigations. The asylum gave rise to therapeutic movements – e.g., non-restraint – whose rationale derived from its own very existence. It also offered the perfect venue for therapeutic experimentation, in turn feeding back into wider conceptualizations of insanity. Such developments were extremely pronounced in the nineteenth century, as the asylum system came into place.

In this paper, I wish to concentrate on the pre-Victorian history of the asylum. And I shall restrict myself to England. Risking gross oversimplification for brevity's sake, we might say that, with the exception of a relatively small number of rather insignificant private asylums, the history of the confinement of the mad in England up to the mid eighteenth century was dominated by Bethlem.[5] Bethlem was not the house of horrors beloved by historical mythology.[6] But, thanks to its staff-patient ratio, and because it was a charity essentially designed for the poor, the accent was on custodialism, punctuated by highly routinized medical interventions (bleedings, vomits, purgings, etc.).

In the second half of the eighteenth century, an increasing number of men – mainly but by no means exclusively medically trained –

involved themselves in insanity, some connected with various new private and charitable lunatic asylums that were being founded. In the 1750s, the eminent physician, William Battie, had criticized Bethlem's regime, arguing that attention to 'management' would do more good than 'medicine', and contending, within an optimistic, Enlightenment value-system, that humanity, reason and kindness were indispensable to successful psychotherapeutics. [7] Most of Battie's contemporaries and successors active in treating the insane – William Perfect, Francis Willis, Benjamin Faulkner, William Pargeter, Thomas Bakewell, and, one could add, the Tukes at the York Retreat, broadly followed Battie's initiatives in championing 'moral management' or, as refined in the Quaker atmosphere of the Retreat, 'moral therapy'.[8]

Moral Management

In the last decades of the eighteenth century, a fresh therapeutics rose to favour, espousing an intensification of personal contact between physician and patient. It was argued that the precise inflections of the madman's demeanour and disposition, attitudes and address, all had to be grasped and then handled in ways appropriate to the individual case sometimes by soothing, sometimes by shocking, perhaps by repose, maybe by labour. By a nice calculation of means and ends, the practitioner had to achieve supremacy, substituting his control for that of the disease controlling the lunatic.

These initiatives they are at the same time novel, yet also secularized echoes of the procedure customarily used by earlier thaumaturgical healers – are spectacularly exemplified by the techniques of two of the more charismatic mad-doctors of the second half of the century. First, the Revd Dr Francis Willis, 'Doctor Duplicate', a Church of England clergyman turned physician and proprietor of a unique asylum at Greatford in Lincolnshire. Willis's priority was to establish mastery over his charges. Summoned to treat George III in 1788, he was so intrepid as to use a battery of harsh expedients to assert his dominion, exercising a strait-waistcoat and purges as persuasives and punishments. And yet, equally boldly – most thought rashly – he allowed the King a razor to shave himself, so as to demonstrate confidence in his royal patient. Required by Parliamentary committee to explain himself, Willis replied:[9]

> It is necessary for a Physician, especially in such Cases, to be able to judge, at the Moment, whether he can confide in the Professions of his Patient; and I never was disappointed in my Opinion.

The trump card in what John Haslam later called 'this fascinating power which the mad doctor is said to possess over the wayward lunatic',[10] lay in Willis's power to command by fixing patients with the eye. Interestingly it was Edmund Burke – himself expert on the aesthetic terror of the sublime - who quizzed Willis about his 'power ... of instantaneously terrifying (the king) into obedience'. In response, Willis offered a demonstration:[11]

> 'Place the candles between us, Mr. Burke,' replied the Doctor, in an equally authoritative tone – 'and I'll give you an answer. There, Sir! by the EYE! I should have looked at him *thus*, Sir' – thus Burke instantaneously averted his head, and, making no reply evidently acknowledged this *basiliskan* authority.

Willis thereby demonstrated himself a true contemporary of Lavater and Mesmer and a proto-Romantic. [12]

The claims of Willis and his sons to have 'cured the King are, at best, not proven; indeed, if Macalpine and Hunter were right that George was suffering from the hereditary metabolic condition, porphyria, such claims become untenable.[13] What is beyond dispute, however, is that before the Willises' coup at Windsor, court physicians-in-ordinary such as Sir George Baker had disastrously failed to stamp their authority upon the King's chaotic condition. By failing to quell his irritation and hyperactivity, they had perhaps exacerbated his sickness. The Willises took charge, mastered the monarch and, by compelling docility and submission, created a climate congenial to his restoration.

Paralleling Willis as what George Nesse Hill dubbed a 'medical artist', was his younger contemporary, Dr William Pargeter. He too vested his faith in an intensely dramaturgic interplay between mad-doctor and patients. 'When I was a pupil at St Bartholomew's Hospital employed on the subject of Insanity', he reported of one of his cases,[14]

> I was requested ... to visit a poor man ... disordered in his mind ... The maniac was locked in a room, raving and exceedingly turbulent. I took two men with me, and learning that he had no offensive weapons, I planted them at the door, with direction to be silent, and to keep out of sight, unless I should want their assistance. I then suddenly unlocked the door – rushed into the room and caught his eye in an instant. *The business was then done,* he became peacable in a moment – trembled with fear, and was as governable as it was possible for a furious madman to be.

A second case reveals Pargeter's conviction that every person required an individual touch. Called in to deal with a melancholy young lady,[15]

> I was introduced to her room and found her in a thoughtful pos-

ture, her elbow on the table, and resting her cheek upon her hand. She did not, for some time, seem to know that any body was in the room; at length she looked up, and the moment I caught her *eye*, for, till then I had been silent, I told her I was perfectly acquainted with the cause of her complaint, and conversed with her on those topics, I thought most suitable to her case, and at last persuaded her to come down to dinner with the rest of the family, and to drink two or three glasses of wine, and to join in the conversation of the table. I recommended an immediate change of residence – gave directions respecting diet exercise – amusements – reading – conversation – and had soon the pleasing satisfaction to be informed of the lady's perfect recovery.

For Pargeter, gaining supremacy involved not only the *coup d'etat* of a *coup d'œil* but taking a personal and family history as well.

Not every late eighteenth-century mad-doctor, of course, exercised charisma in such a theatrical manner. But common to most was the belief that madness was curable (Willis claimed a nine out of ten recovery rate), and was to be conquered through energetic person-to-person encounters. Illuminating here is Thomas Percival's commendation of the essential importance of keeping detailed casenotes in a 'regular *journal*'. In so elusive a disease, a settled strategy was crucial and no detail was to be missed:[16]

> Though casual success may sometimes be the result of empirical practice, the *medicina mentis* can only be administered with steady eficacy by him, who, to a knowledge of the animal oeconomy, and of the physical causes which regulate or disturb its movements, unites an intimate acquaintance with the laws of association; the controul of fancy over judgment: the force of habit; the direction and comparative strength of opposite passions; and the reciprocal dependences and relations of the moral and intellectual powers of man.

To counter the regrettable fact 'that the various diseases which are classed under the title of insanity, remain less understood than any others with which mankind are visited', Percival urged that full particulars of each patient be registered, including 'age, sex, occupation, mode of life, and if possible hereditary constitution'. Finally, he advised the post mortem: [17]

> When the event proves fatal, the brain, and other organs affected should be carefully examined, and the appearance on dissection minutely inserted in the journal.

The contemporary term for this broad and rather new strategy of 'close encounters' was 'moral management' - 'moral' in the sense of addressing itself to the patient's mind, rather than merely to the body, establishing a consciousness-to-consciousness rapport; 'management' because – and here the parallel with industrial entrepreneurs suggests itself – the mad-doctor had to prove consummately dynamic and resourceful, prolific in initiatives designed to impose discipline and sanity. What made management possible was Locke's doctrine of human malleability: in James Burgh's evocative phrase, 'by management the human species may be moulded into any conceivable shape'.[18] Battie's dictum, asserting that management would do more than medicine, was the gospel for what became a progressive movement.[19] In dealing with mental disturbances, John Ferriar stressed, humanity must replace brutality, and moral treatment had to supplant physical:[20]

> The management of the mind is an object of great consequence, in the treatment of insane persons, and has been much misunderstood. It was formerly supposed that lunatics could only be worked upon by terror; shackles and whips, therefore, became part of the medical apparatus.

But such methods, and outrages, was ceasing, Ferriar insisted, and 'a system of mildness and conciliation is now generally adopted, which, if it does not always facilitate the cure, at least tends to soften the destiny of the sufferer'.[21] The point about Ferriar's remarks is that their cadences were already becoming choruses – they could have been uttered by any of a dozen contemporaries. Already a mythology of the bad old days was being articulated. Developing a similar philosophy of moral discipline, William Pargeter used similar terms:[22]

> The chief reliance in the cure of insanity must be rather on *management* than medicine. The *government* of maniacs is an art, not to be acquired without long experience, and frequent and attentive observation. Although it has been of late years much advanced, it is still capable of improvement.

Pargeter regarded management as involving a battle of wits, a war of nerves.[23] 'As maniacs are extremely subdolous', he argued,

> the physician's first visit should be by surprise. He must employ every moment of his time by mildness or menaces, as circumstances direct, to gain an ascendancy over them, and to obtain their favour and prepossession. If this opportunity be lost, it will be difficult, if not impossible, to effect it afterwards; and more especially, if he should betray any signs of timidity.

By consequence, the mad-doctor needed the acting skills of Garrick and the virtuosity of Machiavelli's prince:[24]

> He should be well acquainted with the *pathology* of the disease – should possess great acumen – a discerning and penetrating eye – much humanity and courtesy – and even disposition, and command of temper. He may be obliged at one moment, according to the exigency of the case, to be placid and accommodating in his manners, and the next, angry and absolute.

The precise tactics of interventionist management were personal, differing from individual to individual. But the newer ranks of mad-doctors also had key strategies in common. To a man, they condemned a 'dark age' when lazy approaches to madness were dominant: those techniques, be they soporific draughts or chains, whose goal was merely custodial. They denounced the cruelty of neglect and violence, endorsing instead what Ferriar called a 'system of mildness'. Except for occasional tactical coups, such *physical* punishments as beatings were to be avoided, as above all were casual brutality and arbitrary fluctuations in treatment, for these mixed 'impolicy and impropriety', confusing the patient and arousing his suspicions. Put yourself in the patient's shoes, it was suggested:[25]

> Sudden changes of situation, and sudden removal from friends and relatives, may be attended with fatal, rather than happy consequences. Suppose the mind to be deranged for a moment, and in that moment this violent and sudden change takes place, what more can be wanting, on the slightest appearance of recovery, than the soothing attentions and assiduous cares of affection? What can so soon calm the troubled spirit, or enliven the gloomy imagination, just on the point, perhaps of regaining its powers.

In a similar vein, Joseph Mason Cox, proprietor of Fishponds Asylum, Bristol, and discussed more fully below, commended a form of empathy with patients. No advantage lay, he believed, in attempting to enter into the delusions of the insane. But it was crucial to gauge their progressive *needs* as part of a long-term strategy of normalization. Sensitivity with strength was required.[26]

> It cannot be too frequently repeated that, even in the medical management of maniacs, the physician should never forget that sympathetic tenderness which the sufferings of humanity claim; he should only take care that this be not so far indulged as to diminish the steadiness and presence of mind, for the furious madman as well as the miserable melancholic is frequently sensible to tender impressions, and gentleness of behaviour makes the approach of a physician be felt like that of guardian angel sent to afford ease and comfort.

Mildness, of course, precluded violence. No 'moral manager' dismissed physical coercion and constraint entirely. Rather, the typical argument was that they were at best necessary evils, commonly overused and abused. 'Here', enthused Benjamin Faulkner about his own private madhouse, 'all unnecessary confinement is avoided'.[27] Whereas but a century earlier Thomas Willis had positively urged 'threatenings, bonds, or strokes, as well as Physick', arguing that 'Furious Mad-men are sooner, and more certainly cured by punishments, and hard usage, in a strait room, than by Physick of Medicines',[28] by contrast moral managers stressed that the target of their treatment was the mind. Wiliam Pargeter thus criticized not merely '*chains* and *cords* ... and other galling manacles', but also '*beating* ... a practice formerly much in use in treating the insane'.[29] Writing in the 1790s, he contended that:[30]

> if maniacs are not to be subdued by *management* ... beating will never effect it ... and therefore, I at once condemn this practice, as altogether erroneous, and not justified upon any principles or pretences whatsoever.

Violence was truly redundant. This was demonstrated in a series of parables proving the power of mind over matter, the moral over the physical, sanity over madness. Maniacs might wear a fearsome appearance, but they would cave when faced with the psychological resourcefulness and agility of the morally astute mad-doctor. William Perfect offered a case to prove this:[31]

> In the year 1776, the parish officers of Friendsbury applied to me for my advice in regard to a maniacal man patient they had confined in their workhouse; this unhappy object had been very desperate and committed many acts of violence; was naturally of strong, muscular shape, and rendered much stronger by his present complaint. He had overpowered almost everyone before they could properly secure him, which was now effected in a very extraordinary manner. He was fastened to the floor by means of a staple and iron ring, which was tied to a pair of fetters about his legs, and he was hand-cuffed. The place of his confinement was a large lower room, occasionally made use of for a kitchen, and which opened into the street; there were wooden bars to the windows, through the spaces of which continual visitors were observing, pointing at, ridiculing, and irritating the poor maniac, who thus became a specimen of public sport and amusement.

Violence and counterviolence had formed a vicious circle. It was broken, Perfect argued, by the astute doctor:[32]

> My advice was to take of his shackles and secure him in a strong strait-waistcoat ... it was also my advice to have a small hovel built for his solitary residence ... and to prohibit all persons from going near enough to converse with him, but those who should be appointed to the charge of attending him. Proper attention being paid to his person and diet, in a few weeks the patient entirely recovered his reason; and begging hard to be released from his confinement, after I had been again consulted, it was granted, when he quietly and regularly returned to his labour and employment; and I have not heard of his having had any relapse.

Yet the leading mad-doctors of George III's reign certainly did not espouse the doctrinaire liberalism of kindness for kindness's sake. Clinical experience showed, they believed, that confinement and coercion were sometimes salutary. 'Where maniacs are outrageous', Erasmus Darwin argued, 'there can be no doubt but coercion is necessary: which may be done by means of a strait waistcoat; which disarms them without hurting them.'[33] The crux was to judge what was appropriate in the particular case. Thus, Darwin argued, in some instances confinement worked, whereas 'in others there can be no doubt, but that confinement retards rather than promotes their cure; which is forwarded by change of ideas in consequence of change of place and of objects, as by travelling or sailing'.[34]

Physical threats were a last resort. Moral fear, however, was constructive, and inducing appropriate terror in a patient could be salutary for securing the calm obedience necessary for effective treatment. Robert Darling Willis described a practice he learned from his father:[35]

> If they are delirious, they are put into a strait-waistcoat in which they can neither hurt themselves nor others. It has the further advantage of inculcating salutary fear so that on later occasions the mere threat of it will make them control themselves.

Fear, it was believed, could provide the initial leverage, a starting point:[36]

> The emotion of fear is the first and often the only one by which they can be governed. By working on it one removes their thoughts from the phantasms occupying them and brings them back to reality, even if this entails inflicting pain and suffering. It is fear too which teaches them to judge their actions rightly and learn the consequences. By such means is their attention brought back to their surroundings.

Thus physical should lead to moral treatment. Initially it secured obedience, in time, attention; thereby it concentrated the disordered mind. Moral managers who, with John Gregory, stressed the necessity of an 'intimate knowledge of the human heart', did not see their charges through sentimental Rousseauvian spectacles, maddened by society, everywhere in chains, but needing only example to be restored to innocence. Rather lunatics were confused souls, at war with themselves, devious, damaged; treatments had to be bold, assertive and strictly tailored to individual needs. The metaphors of therapy were those of the battleground and the theatre. Struggle was involved, rather as in a gladiatorial combat. And for success, inventiveness, imagination and panache were imperative.

Moral Management, the Asylum, and New Knowledges of the Insane

It will be evident from the foregoing discussion that the imputs into moral management were broad and multifarious, arising from Enlightenment meliorism, medicine, pedadogy, Mesmerism, proto-Romanticism and economic entrepreneurship.[37] The ideology of moral management chimed with the new, small, private or charitable asylum. It did not, however, *emerge* from it. Some of its advocates – for example Erasmus Darwin – had nothing to do with asylums; others, like William Pargeter, practised upon the insane outside the asylum context – as, clearly, did Francis Willis in the case of George III. [38]

Once, however, moral management was regularly being practised within the new, small asylum, it altered the face of the treatment of the insane. Discourse about madness and the mad changed, in ways often ignored in a historiography that is extremely preoccupied with demolishing, or defending, the asylum. From early modern times, the vast bulk of writings concerning insanity had traditionally been philosophical (for example Burton's *Anatomy of Melancholy*), spiritual-consolatory (for example the writings of Timothie Rogers), anatomico-medical (for example Thomas Willis's works), classificatory (*for example* Battie's *Treatise on Madness*), or promotional (puffing particular proprietory asylums). In a new genre becoming prominent from around the turn of the nineteenth century, these issues began to be eclipsed. Pride of place was given for the first time to practical experience, to attention to individual cases, and the broader generalizations to be derived therefrom. Observation of the minutiae of the every-day behaviour of the insane became regarded as particularly crucial. Therapeutic strategies were devised and depicted which specifically drew on – indeed, would have been impossible without – the favoured conditions obtaining within the asylum itself, an institution both sequestered and quasi-domestic. And the course of the disorder, under treatment, was surveyed. For the first time, the criterion for proper knowledge about madness became the close encounter with the patient under confinement.

The significance of this transformation may be seen in a number of writings appearing around the turn of the nineteenth century. An instructive example of this new genre is Joseph Mason Cox's *Practical Observations on Insanity: In Which Some Suggestions are Offered Towards an Improved Mode of Treating Diseases of the Mind and Some Rules Proposed Which it is Hoped may Lead to a More Humane and Successful Method of Cure: To Which are Subjoined Remarks on Medical Jurisprudence as Connected with Diseased Intellect* (1804).

Cox was the proprietor of the well-known and respected Fishponds Asylum in Gloucestershire, just outside Bristol (though the name of the asylum is hardly mentioned in the book: surely an attempt by a new 'psychiatry' to purge itself of implications of gross puffery).[39] The institution had been established by his grandfather, Joseph Mason, as early as 1738, removing to Fishponds in 1760; Mason's son had subsequently managed it. Neither of the first two owners of the madhouse was medically educated: the impulse leading them to tend the insane may well have been religious (Mason was a Baptist). Neither published on insanity .

It is thus obviously of great significance that Joseph Mason Cox was sent off to Edinburgh, Paris and Leiden to acquire a medical education (his Edinburgh M D was entitled *De Mania*), before assuming control of the family business in 1787. If want of medical training had perhaps encouraged Cox's predecessors to keep their wisdom about madness to themselves, it seems as if a sense of belonging to and participating within the wider medical world induced Joseph Mason Cox to go into print. The first edition of his work appeared in 1804; the second, expanded edition, in 1806.

Certain features of this work are noteworthy, for they indicate how the experience of running an asylum shaped Cox's notion of a proper science of insanity. Discounting 'abstract reasoning' and 'theory', Cox consistently took 'experience' as his yardstick for science, emphasizing, for instance, in his 'Advertisement', that he had 'devoted himself exclusively and assiduously, for a series of years, to the care and cure of maniacal patients', and that his work was therefore the fruit of 'diligent observation, and an uninterrupted experience of many years'.[40] Though a qualified physician, Cox denied that general medicine or even pathological anatomy (for example, brain dissection) had hitherto contributed very greatly to understanding insanity. He condemned the 'abstruse speculations' of general medical authors such as Boerhaave, and was rather dismissive of the attempts of his old mentor, William Cullen, and the Edinburgh medical school to place insanity within wider taxonomies.[41] Cox did not seek to develop his own classification or nosology, or even to generate a diagnostic grid. In such endeavours there was no value or need. 'Much difficulty would attend the diagnosis between mania and melancholia', he wrote, 'but considering them as only modifications of the same disease, the attempt is unnecessary'.[42] As to aetiology, he employed a rough-and-ready scheme of predisposing and proximate causes. As to the nature and aetiology of derangement, he was neither aggressively somatist nor dogmatically psychological. Common sense and practical experience of the insane together testified to the reciprocity of mind and body (as, perhaps, was evident in his favoured term, 'diseases of the mind').[43]

Aptly, Cox called his book '*practical* observations'. Where later writers might speak of 'psychiatry', Cox referred to 'this department of medical practice'. He did not, of course, see himself as practising just like a mere 'empiric', valuing only results not understanding – though he certainly did give trial-and-error methods their due. But he was concerned to append detailed case histories to all his general discussions – he printed 21 substantial cases – recording failures no less than successes, and insisting that 'nothing is more important and useful than a judicious, well conducted case book, in which the history of every maniac subjected to our care should be minutely detailed, every symptom and peculiarity accurately noticed, as well as the methodus medendi'.[44]

Experience, argued Cox, proves various time-honoured general medical interventions positively harmful. Heroic purging had often been used on maniacs, but faith in such depletive treatments was an error born of *a priori* thought; it failed to take into account the fact that mania was often a disorder born of exhaustion. Further evacuations would only make bad worse, confirming the conclusion that 'it frequently happens that insanity, if not occasioned, is continued by the very means adopted for its removal'.[45] But *a priori* alternatives to traditional medications – such as Battie's rejection of vomits – were equally worthless:[46] authentic experience proved that vomits worked well, as did other physical treatments like cold baths, when managed with great exactitude, paying due attention to the specific needs of each patient.[47] Despite certain critics, the value of pharmaceutical interventions was not to be sniffed at. Opium, Cox believed, is almost always worthless for the insane, but digitalis had been proven highly valuable.[48]

Yet Cox denied that general medicine can tackle madness. For the technique of the 'highest importance' in the 'treatment of maniacs' was 'management', and 'the art of management results from experience, and the natural endowments of the practitioner'.[49] Even, Cox insisted, 'in the medical management of maniacs', 'it cannot be too frequently repeated that ... the physician should never forget' the importance of person-to-person sympathy and control. Doubtless, he allowed, 'it would be extremely useful could we lay down certain rules for the moral management of insane patients of every description'.[50] Truth was, however, that 'it must depend on the existing symptoms and circumstances of each case'.[51] Management knew no fixed rules; proper 'address'[52] was necessarily a habit born of the experience which alone could judge the time for tenderness and the time for terror, when to deploy fear, and when to draw upon any other of the 'whole range of passions'.[53] Maniacs were 'artful'; they had to be outgeneraled.[54] Above all, authority must be imposed:[55]

> A firm, resolute demeanour, stern aspects, an assumption of authority, giving orders and seeing them executed, uniformly decided measures, a scrutinizing look fixed on the patient's eye, will, in general, excite dread or confidence, respect and compliance; and the procuring of these effects is a material point gained, which is seldom lost again.

The art of management, it will be clear, demanded the concentrated atmosphere of the asylum, within which the patient could be utterly segregated from family, friends and all other disturbing influences.[56] But the isolation of the asylum, where the superintendant was omnipotent, also created a theatre for a dramatic therapeutics dear to Cox. Cox required an absolute environmental control shrewdly adapted to outwitting the entrenched delusions of his patients, a stage upon which he could orchestrate that gothic anti-carnival that he termed 'pious frauds'.[57]

Such enactments might often involve realizing and dramatizing the patient's hallucinations, while also rewriting the script for him. Take a patient convinced that he was doomed to die because a living animal had become lodged in his belly and was eating him up. It was useless to try to reason him out of this error. One had to 'humour the insane idea', but then outwit him, for instance by introducing a frog into his chamber pot, thereby demonstrating to him that he had voided it himself.[59]

In other instances, Cox believed in the efficacy of manipulating the 'total environment' to create a theatre of terror. One patient was shaken out of his conviction of being the Holy Ghost by the introduction of a bit-part player who insisted that he alone was.[60] Or Cox would use scenic devices 'contrived to make strong impressions upon the senses, by means of unexpected, unusual, striking or apparently supernatural agents. [61] Thus he would awaken patients 'by imitated thunder or soft music, according to the peculiarity of the case'; or, more sinisterly, he would deploy 'signs executed in phosphorus upon the wall of the bed chamber', or 'make strong impressions on the senses' by 'some tale, assertion, or reasoning'. Sometimes he would make dramatic use of a helper 'in the character of an angel, prophet, or devil' ('but', he adds, 'the actor in this drama must possess much skill, and be very perfect in his part'). Such pyrotechnic pantomimes, Cox admits, may seem 'ludicrous', but they were 'not only admissible, but sometimes indispensably necessary'.[62]

Cox was rather fetched with the management of sound. The strains of distant, hidden music were often soothing.[63] But particularly valuable was the art of 'producing unpleasant impressions through the medium of the other senses, as when screeches and yells were made in an apartment painted black and red, or glaring white, when 'every man must be painfully affected' and 'the maniacal patient, however torpid, must be roused';[64] or if raging, the patient should be set 'in an airy room, surrounded with flowers breathing odours, the walls and furniture coloured green, and the air agitated by undulations of the softest harmony'.[65] All such methods were designed to assault the senses, seize the attention, interrupt the grip of delusions, and wrench the maniac out of his raving self – they were refinements upon the well-established fact that such physical accidents as falls often cured even long established derangement.

Not least, the asylum permitted the introduction and testing of therapeutic technologies which further enlarged understanding of the nature of insanity under experimental conditions. Cox's favourite device was the swing chair. The patient was strapped in, and revolved at up to a hundred gyrations a minute.[66] Cox noted the diverse effects at different velocities: slow speeds proved soothing;[67] faster ones induced violent and disorienting giddiness, which created a salutary shock, a traumatization which would break the hold of a delusory system or vicious stubbornness. High levels of 'vertigo' would 'often contribute to correct the morbid state of the intellect'.[68] For, Cox argued, the 'valuable properties of this remedy are not confined to the body', but 'its powers extend to the mind', especially by inducing fear:[69]

> Conjoined with the passion of fear, the extent of its action has never been accurately ascertained; but I have no doubt it would

afford relief in some very hopeless cases, if employed in the dark, where, from unusual noises, smells, or other powerful agents, acting forcibly on the senses, its efficacy might be amazingly increased.

The lengthy case histories which Cox appended here, as elsewhere, showed swing treatment, accompanied by sensory deprivation and other disorienting tactics, sometimes being extended over many months, often with increased dosages. Such technologies, Cox contended, generally produced beneficial results. Patients hitherto highly refractory, obstinate and deceitful, changed and showed improvement. One of them, after a relapse, was threatened with a repeat of swinging, 'but rather than repeat the ride in the whirligig, as he termed it, he submitted entirely to my wishes, and, with some occasional returns of obstinacy and disinclination to persist in the remedies I prescribed, I had the pleasure to see him gradually improve till he advanced to perfect reason'.[70]

Conclusion

It has not been the boast of this paper so reveal how 'the asylum' created 'psychiatry', perhaps in the manner in which Foucault argued that the Paris Hospital gave birth to the 'clinic' and modern medicine.[71] There have been many sorts of asylums and many stages to psychiatry; and the most I would claim is that the advent of asylums such as Fishponds[72] – relatively small, respectable houses for affluent patients, run by reputable, attentive and ambitious doctors and superintendants – imparted certain new impulses and turns to the kinds of knowledge accumulating around the insane. These were to be knowledges *combining* the medical and the moral, built upon extended experience of the behavioural patterns and psychological dispositions of patients, and focusing above all upon the procedures and progress of courses of therapy. The discourse about insanity became a discourse largely committed to discussing how the mad responded under treatment. And this was precisely because the new psychiatric site, the smallish asylum, became, in effect, a new experimental laboratory for investigating such questions effectively for the first time. It hardly needs to be said that subsequent forms of institutions for the insane notably the vast public asylums housing thousands of patients which were erected in the second half of the nineteenth century – would provide the impulse for different kinds of psychiatric knowledges, for example, the classificatory imperative. When so many of these later patients failed to respond to treatment, the knowledge we call 'degenerationism' was required.[73]

What I have tried to indicate is that the asylum did not create psychiatric discourse *ex nihilo* and *de novo.* The optimistic outlook of 'moral management' was already, to some degree, being mobilized before and independently of such asylums – indeed, it encouraged their foundation. The implementation and elaboration of moral management within the asylum provided, however, the basis for a new mode of understanding; the Pargeterian literature of heroic cures gave way to one of close scrutiny of the course of a disease under panoptic conditions within the total environment.

Notes

1. Lively up-to-date assessments on all these issues are to be found in Andrew Scull, *Social Order/Mental Disorder: Anglo-American Psychiatry in Historical Perspective* (London: Routledge, 1989); see also Michel Foucault, *La Folie et la Déraison: Histoire de la Folie a l'Age Classique* (Paris: Librairie Plon, 1961); trans. and abridged as *Madness and Civilization: A History of Insanity in the Age of Reason,* by Richard Howard (New York: Random House, 1965), and evaluations of Foucault's notion of the 'great confinement', see two issues of *History of the Human Sciences* given over to discussion of Foucault (1990, 1991). For modern developments see Andrew Scull, *Decarceration: Community Treatment and the Deviant —A,Radical View,* 2nd edn (Oxford: Polity Press; New Brunswick, N.J.: Rutgers University Press, 1984).
2. Steven Shapin and Simon Schaffer, *Leviathan and the Air Pump. Hobbes, Boyle. and the Experimental Life* (Princeton: Princeton University Press, 1985); David Gooding, Trevor Pinch and Simon Schaffer (eds), *The Uses of Experiment: Studies in the Natural Sciences* (Cambridge: Cambridge University Press, 1989).
3. Bruno Latour, *Les Microbes. Guerre et Paix, suivi de Irréductions* (Paris: Editions A. M. Métaillié, 1984).
4. Pertinent here is Erving Goffman, *Asylums: Essays on the Social Situation of Mental Patients and Other Inmates* (New York: Anchor Books, 1961), for its programmatic claim that the 'total institution' creates a totally new cognitive world. Eighteenth- and nineteenth-century thinkers were deeply aware of the cognitive importance of hermetically sealed environments and the possibilities of panopticism. See Michel Foucault, *Discipline and Punish: The Birth of the Prison,* trans. by A. Sheridan (London: Allen Lane, 1977); Michael Ignatieff, *A Just Measure of Pain: The Penitentiary in the Industrial Revolution, 1750–1850* (New York: Pantheon, 1978); *idem,* 'Total Institutions and Working Classes: A Review Essay', *History Workshop Journal,* xv (1983), 169–72; John Bender, *Imagining the Penitentiary. Fiction and the Architecture of Mind in Eighteenth Century England* (Chicago: Chicago University Press, 1987).
5. For a survey of early developments in Britain see Roy Porter, *Mind*

Forg'd Manacles: A History of Madness from the Restoration to the Regency (London: Athlone, 1987).

6. For revisionism on Bethlem see Jonathan Andrews, 'A History of Bethlem Hospital c. 1600 – c. 1750' (Ph.D. Dissertation, London University, 1990).
7. See William Battie, *A Treatise on Madness,* and John Monro, *Remarks on Dr Battie's Treatise on Madness,* Introduction by R. Hunter and I. Macalpine (London: Dawsons, 1962; reprint of 1758 edn). For a revisionist view of Battie, see Akihito Suzuki, 'Mind and its Disease in Enlightenment British Medicine' (Ph.D thesis, University of London, 1992).
8. See Roy Porter, 'Was there a Moral Therapy in the Eighteenth Century?', *Lychnos* (1981–2), 12–26. For the Retreat see Anne Digby, *Madness. Morality and Medicine* (Cambridge: Cambridge University Press, 1985); *idem,* 'Moral Treatment at the Retreat, 1796–1846', in W. F. Bynum, Roy Porter and Michael Shepherd (eds), *The Anatomy of Madness,* Vol. 2 (London: Tavistock, 1985), 52–72.
9. Ida Macalpine and Richard Hunter, *George III and the Mad Business* (London: Allen Lane, 1969), 282.
10. John Haslam, *Observations on Madness and Melancholy,* 2nd edn (London: John Callow, 1809), 275.
11. Macalpine & Hunter, *op. cit.* (note 9), 271–2.
12. Roy Porter, 'Making Faces: Physiognomy and Fashion in Eighteenth Century England', *Etudes Anglaises,* xxxviii (1985), 385–96; *idem,* '"Under the Influence": Mesmerism in England', *History Today* (September, 1985), 22–9.
13. Macalpine & Hunter, *op. cit.* (note 9), 172f.
14. W. Pargeter, *Observations on Maniacal Disorders* (Reading: for the author, 1792), 50–1.
15. *Ibid.*, 51–2.
16. Thomas Percival, *Medical Ethics* (Manchester: Johnson & Bickerstaff, 1803), as quoted in Richard Hunter and Ida Macalpine, *Three Hundred Years of Psychiatry: 1535–1860* (London: Oxford University Press, 1963), 585.
17. *Ibid.*
18. Quoted in Michael Ignatieff, *A Just Measure of Pain*; *op. cit.* (note 4), 67.
19. Eric T. Carlson and Norman Dain, 'The Psychotherapy which was Moral Treatment', *American Journal of Psychiatry,* cxvii (1960), 519–24.
20. John Ferriar, *Medical Histories and Reflections,* 3 vols (London: Cadell & Davies, 1792–8), ii, 136–7.
21. *Ibid.*
22. Pargeter, *op. cit.* (note 14), 52.
23. *Ibid.*
24. *Ibid.*
25. Benjamin Faulkner, *Observations on the General and Improper*

Treatment of Insanity (London: for the author, 1789), 15.
26. Joseph Mason Cox, *Practical Observations on Insanity: In Which Some Suggestions Are Offered Towards an Improved Mode of Treating Diseases of the Mind ... to Which are Subjoined, Remarks on Medical Jurisprudence as Connected with Diseased Intellect,* 2nd edn (London: Baldwin and Murray, 1806), 42–3.
27. Faulkner, *op. cit.* (note 25), 22.
28. T. Willis, *The Practice of Physick* (London: Dring, 1684), quoted in Hunter & Macalpine, *op. cit.* (note 16), 191.
29. Pargeter, *op. cit.* (note 14), 129–30.
30. *Ibid.*
31. W. Perfect, *Select Cases in the Different Species of Insanity* (Rochester: Gillman, 1787), 131.
32. *Ibid.*
33. Erasmus Darwin, *Zoonomia; or, The Laws of Organic Life,* 2 vols (London: J. Johnson, 1794 & 1796), i, 352. For strait-waistcoats see D. MacBride, *A Methodical Introduction on the Theory and Practices of Physick* (London: Strahan, 1772), 591–2.
34. Darwin, *op. cit.* (note 33), i, 352.
35. Quoted in Hunter & Macalpine, *op. cit.* (note 16), 275.
36. *Ibid.*
37. The parallels between industrial and moral entrepreneurship are worth drawing out. See S. Pollard, *The Genesis of Modern Management* (London: Edward Arnold, 1965).
38. Pargeter's *Observations on Maniacal Disorders, op. cit.* (note 14), in this respect forms an admirable contrast to the work of Cox to be discussed below. They form reasonably contemporary discussions of mania. They are, however, quite distinct, Pargeter's being the product of essentially *medical* experience, Cox's being based upon asylum management. Stanley Jackson's introduction to the 1988 Routledge reprint of Pargeter is invaluable.
39. The following biographical details about Cox are taken from Hunter & Macalpine, *op. cit.* (note 16), 594–6; H. Temple Phillips, 'The Old Private Lunatic Asylum at Fishponds', *Bristol Medico– Chirurgical Journal,* lxxxv (1970), 41–4; *idem,* 'The History of the Old Private Lunatic Asylum at Fishponds Bristol, 1740–1859' (M.Sc. Dissertation, University of Bristol, 1973).
40. Cox, *op. cit.* (note 26), 'Advertisement'.
41. *Ibid.,* 5, vii, 122..
42. *Ibid.,* 38.
43. *Ibid.,* title page.
44. *Ibid.,* ix.
45. *Ibid.,* 40.
46. *Ibid.,* 102.
47. *Ibid.,* 120.
48. *Ibid.,* 129, 112..

49. *Ibid.*, 42.
50. *Ibid.*, 65.
51. *Ibid.*, 65.
52. *Ibid.*, 68.
53. *Ibid.*, 42.
54. *Ibid.*, 69.
55. *Ibid.*, 76.
56. *Ibid.*, 44.
57. *Ibid.*, 47.
58. *Ibid.*, 49.
59. *Ibid.*, 55.
60. *Ibid.*, 66
61. *Ibid.*, 47.
62. *Ibid.*, 48.
63. *Ibid.*, 87.
64. *Ibid.*, 87.
65. *Ibid.*, 88.
66. *Ibid.*, 137.
67. *Ibid.*, 139.
68. *Ibid.*, 142.
69. *Ibid.*, 140.
70. *Ibid.*, 148.
71. M. Foucault, *Naissance de la Clinique: Une Archéologie du Regard Médical* (Paris: Presses Universitaires de France, 1963), trans. by A. M. Sheridan Smith as *The Birth of the Clinic* (London: Tavistock, 1973).
72. A parallel would be Ticehurst House. See Charlotte Mackenzie, 'A Family Asylum: A History of the Private Madhouse at Ticehurst in Sussex, 1792–1917' (Ph.D. Dissertation, University of London, 1987).
73. Ian Dowbiggin, 'Degeneration and Hereditarianism in French Mental Medicine 1840–1890: Psychiatric Theory as Ideological Adaptation', in W. F. Bynum, Roy Porter and Michael Shepherd (eds), *The Anatomy of Madness*, Vol. 1 (London: Tavistock, 1985), 188–232; *idem*, 'French Psychiatry, Hereditarianism, and Professional Legitimacy, 1840–1900', in Andrew Scull and Steven Spitzer (eds), *Research in Law. Deviance, and Social Control*, Vol. 7 (Greenwich, Conn.: JAI Press, 1985), 135–65; Daniel Pick, *Faces of Degeneration: Aspects of a European Disorder c. 1848–1918* (Cambridge: Cambridge University Press, 1989). Valuable general remarks about the relations between architectural space, cognition and psychiatry are to be found in T. A. Markus (ed.), *Order in Space and Society* (Edinburgh: Mainstream Publishing Co., 1982).

11

Vitalism, Disease and Society

Roselyne Rey

The title of this paper, 'Vitalism, disease and society' requires some explanations and raises three difficulties I would like to analyse before going into any detail. First of all, in classical histories of the medical enlightenment[1] vitalism has been defined more from a physiological than from a pathological point of view. Too much attention has probably been payed to the vital principle, in spite of the hesitations of vitalists themselves as to what it is and if it is something more than a word, a mathematical variable, X, Y, or Z, as Barthez himself claims in his *Nouveaux eléments de la science de l'homme.*[2] To clarify the following discussion, I just want to record some features the vitalists share: a) this medical philosophy, criticising the mechanistic, reductionist view of man, as well as the animist one,[3] stresses the specificity of life, not as a result of organization, but as the expression of vital forces or properties of living matter; among these properties, the most important is sensibility, which contains all the others,[4] b) the existence of vital forces or sensibility does not completely exclude mechanical or chemical explanation, but it subordinate them to a more powerful order, the order of life and teleology; c) the third feature frequently invoked is the idea of mutual dependance and solidarity between all the organs of the body, according to the famous comparison of the living body as a swarm of bees,[5] which leads to the concept of organism; d) the last characteristic is the interaction between mind and body, not only in the sense that organic disorders are able to disturb intellectual functions, but in a more general sense, since the passions of the soul are in turn responsible for organic disorders like ulcers and for delay in the recovery from disease or in the cicatrization of wounds.[6] It is only through this last feature that a link has usually been established between vitalism and pathology, especially mental diseases. The problem of knowing whether there is a vitalistic conception of disease or not, remained unsolved. One of my concerns is precisely to try and answer this question.

The second difficulty arises from the analogy between vitalist claims and other traditions: the question is whether there is something particular in their views of disease, or whether there is nothing else, nothing more than an Hippocratic tradition, revised by Stahl. As far as the Hippocratic tradition is concerned, there is no need to emphasize the importance of the work on *Airs, Waters and Places*, and what must be the attitude of a physician when he arrives for the first time in a town: he has to investigate not only the climate, the winds, the nature and quality of water, but also the way of life of the inhabitants, and the political system that rules them[7]. The British physician John Arbuthnot, in his work *An Essay Concerning the Effects of Air in Human Bodies*, first published in 1733 and translated into French in 1742,[8] was rightly considered by Montesquieu as a valuable source for neo-Hippocratic ideas,[9] which integrate social and political conditions, as well as natural environment into the field of pathology. The popularity of medico-topographical monographs in the second half of the century in France,[10] the attempts to look for the causes of epidemics in both natural and social circumstances are well known. The importance of the Hippocratic tradition among vitalist physicians, especially in the Montpellier school, probably explains why they are so involved in the general framework of the struggle for hygiene and medical policy; but of course, we have to recognize that this is not a specific attitude towards disease. We could sum up this point by the following formula: all vitalist physicians are in favour of Hippocratic ideas, but not all Hippocratic physicians are vitalist.

On the other face of the tradition, that of Stahl's animism, vitalists are said to have accepted the idea of Nature as a powerful healthy force, so that the physician has only to follow and help Nature to carry out its healthy crisis.[11] In this view, there is a permanent conflict between life and inanimate bodies. But we will see, through Théophile Bordeu's works, for instance, that things are not so simple and that 'expectant medicine' versus 'active medicine' is not appropriate to characterize vitalist medical practice. Any way, this kind of approach does not enable us to discover the exact relations between vitalism, disease and society. So we have to explore another way to define a strong relation between them. I hope to show that to link these three words was not a mistake or an artificial construction, but something which has a more solid foundation.

We come now to my third preliminary remark, namely the

relationship between disease and society. The most obvious approach would be to study the social and political background of the vitalistic conception of disease in the second half of the 18th century:[12] this will not be my approach. We can stress, as a matter of fact, that very similar conceptions of disease are found in Great Britain, with John Hunter, and in France, in quite different contexts. Is there then a possibility of binding more closely disease and society? By this, I do not exactly mean that disease is a social and cultural construction as well as a biological data: of course, it is, but this idea seems to be too general. I wish to point out that since disease is rather a process than a state, and since there is an identity of physiological and pathological processes, then, the physician has not to look for morbid entities, but for how society is involved in pathological process. Bordeu, in his *Recherches Anatomiques sur la position des glandes et leur action*, published in 1751, compares the pathological process of inflammation with the normal one of a gland secretion, consisting of three phases, stimulation, work and excretion,[13] and in his *Recherches sur les maladies chroniques* (1775), he compares the whole life with a disease divided into its periods of preparation, coction and crisis.[14] Society is related to disease not only in the way it appreciates, learns, cures or controls disease, but mainly in the way it participates in the production of disease. To remove all possible ambiguities in this interpretation, it may be useful to state that society is responsible for disease exactly in the same way that sensations, passions and social relations, are necessary to maintain and stimulate life itself. To some extent, the links between vitalism, disease and society, have to be sought in the vitalist conception of 'animal oeconomy', as well as in the similarity between normal and pathological processes, so that social data such as diet, social position, kind of job and so on, are not added circumstances in a causal process, but are at the heart of life and disease. In other words, society is a masterpiece in the dialectic between the organism and the environment,[15] between inside and outside: it is both a source of trouble and a source of self-regulation. I will concentrate on the Paris physician La Caze, who is the common source of the Montpellier school,[16] and on its main representatives, Bordeu, Ménuret de Chambaud, Barthez, and also on the German physician C. W. Hufeland.

La Caze's Theory of Centre of Action and Reaction

A few words on Louis La Caze (1703–1765) may be useful. We know little about him: he was born in Lambeye in the Bearn, was received as a doctor in Montpellier in 1724 and then went to Paris where he obtained the position of ordinary physician to the Regent. He was also the uncle of Bordeu whom he lodged in Paris for some years. Bordeu tried to give credit to the idea that he worked for La Caze who took from him his main ideas.[17] In fact, Bordeu was not yet in Paris when La Caze published his first book in 1749, *Specimen Novi Medicinae Conspectus,* whose second edition appeared in 1751.[18] The most well-known of his works is *Idée de l'Homme Physique et Moral,* on sale in 1755, a book which obtained an enormous success, since Buffon in his *Histoire des animaux carnassiers* (1758) adopted his main ideas,[19] and many articles of Diderot's *Encyclopédie* are devoted to presenting La Caze's views. In articles such as 'Animal Oeconomy', 'Inflammation', 'Spasm', 'Sensibility' (all by Ménuret, except the last one), La Caze is presented as a man of genius, who completely changed the face of medicine, a man who wrote both 'a treatise of morality and happiness'.[20] Bordeu, Barthez, Cabanis and many other took up his theory of the living body.

La Caze's views on 'animal oeconomy' are based on the existence of a permanent action and reaction in the body: but, instead of imagining this movement as the mechanistic process of a spring, he argues that life depends upon the relations between three centres of action and reaction, which will become in Cabanis' thought three focuses of sensibility:[21] two of them are traditional, they are the brain and the epigastric region, but the third one is much more original in so far as it is what he called 'the general external organ', something that involves skin as a whole envelope which wraps all the body, the integuments and the cellular tissue under the skin.[22] This organ is quite concerned with all the outside stimulations and need them to react and transmit its impressions to another centre in the body. Life is a complex process of action and reaction from the periphery to the centre (which is the region of phrenic forces) and vice versa, from outside to the depths of organism. Thanks to what he called the tripod or triumvirate of life, he sees animal oeconomy as a field of forces which circulate from one point to another, from skin to brain, and from brain to epigastric region, breaking up the regularity and monotony of a binary system. These ideas can also be found with many details in the article 'Oeconomie Animale' of Diderot's *Encyclopédie.*[23] In his *Researches sur les maladies chroniques* Bordeu completely agrees with this view of the organism as a triumvirate, except that he is reluctant to choose the brain or the heart as one of the centres. Nevertheless, he states that sensibility, as a general property, quite different from those which dominate in inanimate bodies, is constantly awakened by many sensations and actions, some of them physical, such as changing atmosphere, climate, food, some others moral: unceasingly, the living body is trembling, quivering, restless and moving about in the deepest and the smallest part of its fibres, with vibrations and oscillations which spread to the cellular tissue. The general external organ is like a gate wide open to all the external impressions.

It is easy to recall Van Helmont's duumvirate[24] but the attention paid to the skin, a boundary between inside and outside, and the organ which is most in contact with all the external influences is something quite new, a discovery, Ménuret claimed.[24] This organ reacts immediately with the centre of phrenic forces, especially with the diaphragm, first set in motion by breathing at the birth of the individual, which is like a trigger of all the vital processes. But it needs immediately a counterpoint, an antagonistic force opposed to itself. Every sensation, every action is a beneficial opportunity to sustain the life of the brain and, above all, of the phrenic centre formed by the connections of nerves from the diaphragm, like a spider in the centre of its web.[25] It is easy to understand that in such a view of the 'animal oeconomy', the lack of sensation, as well as the excess of actions in one of the centre can bring several diseases. Of course, here, we are not far from a methodist theory of spasm and atony, like the one found in Hoffmann's *Medicina Rationalis* [26] but Hoffmann does not provide such a great integration between life and sensation, and does not see spasm and atony at the level of functional centres but only at the level of a single fibre. In addition, no other model of the living body contains such an interaction between moral and medicine. As Ménuret claims, 'to be a good moralist, it is necessary to be previously an excellent physician'.[27]

Vitalists such as Bordeu and Ménuret were soon to transpose these three organic centres into centres of sensibility, as a general and common property. Each of these centres has its own department of action and the living body then becomes like a dynamic space criss-crossed by roads and paths of sensibility, intersecting each other, according to axes of circulation which separate the body into two symmetric parts, and into an upper and lower level whose limit is the diaphragm. The nervous connections between each centre form the basis for an extensive application of the doctrine of sympathies, as Barthez for example points out,[28] and no kind of living tissue or fibre is free from nerves and sensibility.[29]

The Need for Sensations, or How to Reconcile Nature and Society

In this general view of the organism, every being has to seek a continuous stimulation of its sensibility, in a way very similar to what John Brown was to defend thirty years later.[30] Each sense, touch, sight, hearing, is said to be the source of useful solicitations, and at the same time, it is a medical and moral duty to excite and use one's senses. Needs, wishes, desire, anxiety, far from being the sorrowful condition of mankind are powerful ferments of life and happiness. Nevertheless, these ideas do not lead to a simple formula such as 'the more everyone exercises his own senses, the more he is healthy and happy'. These maxims, which imply an apology for passions, are not quite appropriate to describe exactly the vitalistic medical thought, for two reasons. The first one is that La Caze, like Ménuret, Bordeu, or Fouquet,[31] is perfectly aware of the morbid consequences of exercising one's senses without measure or control, aware of the danger of giving into all one's desires. It is a topic in medicine that to give oneself over to the passions brings many diseases which are, by themselves, a medical sanction for misdeeds. The second reason is that society prevents individuals from trying to fulfil their duty of pleasure and happiness. Frequently, vitalists deplore the limits and the social laws which hinder the freedom of sensibility. Society puts obstacles in the way of passions and vitalists agreed that convent closures or the bad education of women are the causes of a lot of diseases, not only mental diseases like melancholia, hysteria, vapours, but also organic disorders, like dyspepsia, amenorrhea, and so on.[32] Their position cannot be reduced to a permissiveness that gives in to all the passions; it is rather a call for reforms and changes in the organization of social rules. For La Caze especially, the choice is not between nature and society, or between individual claims and social organization; he argues that the various, diverse passions are by themselves a means of regulation or control, able to prevent disease. One passion alone is dangerous, but several are not. Diversity is the best way to moderate and compensate their energy. In this general context, every man has to cultivate his different passions. The change from normality to disease proceeds from a difference in degree, intensity or length of sensibility, not from a difference in nature. Society also provides a lot of opportunities to arouse needs and passions, and the result of this is to allow man to live within social constraints. Instead of a strong opposition between nature and society, La Caze points out the human need for social relations, emulation, culture and science, work, desire for knowledge, duties and rights of the citizen; all that provides a wide range of necessary stimulations. Individual nature is also a social construction and there is not a primitive state of human nature opposed to a social state. La Caze wrote: 'We need sensations as essentially as we need food, and the air we breath is no more necessary for us than sensation'.[33] And he adds: if man was bounded in his search for the satisfaction of his elementary needs, he would be in a state very near to sleep or even death.[34] The more activities we indulge in, the more diverse stimulations we have, and the more fully we feel the internal sensation of our life. La Caze draws a picture of human life which is an inversion of Rousseau's. The feeling of one's own existence is the starting point of happiness, but this feeling is not a movement of withdrawal into oneself, but an organic situation of disponibility, of looking forward to all impressions and stimulations. The comparison between civilized man and savage man gives the advantage to the former.

Conception of Disease: a Bad Management of Life

Hence, it is possible to understand better what disease is: it is not merely an attack from outside against the vital forces, and there is a slight difference between the Stahlian and the vitalist definitions of disease.[35] Disease is not only an internal disturbance, but an error in the distribution of sensibility, a mistake in the proportion, balance, equilibrium, in a more complicated system of communication between the three poles we have described, one of which, the general external organ, is especially in relation with the outside world. Stimulation becomes morbid irritation, not by itself when its intensity is increasing, but when one of the centres of sensibility becomes dominant at the expense of the others.[36] More often than not, says La Caze, the starting point of the disturbance is no more than a lack of appropriate reaction from the centre of the phrenic forces which is continually being pulled about by the actions it had to counterbalance. It leads the two other centres to more general disorders.

Each man is responsible for the good regulation of stimulation in the three centres because habits of action as well as excess or lack of passions engender diseases. But disease is not only a problem of excess or shortage, and it is not a conflict between the physical and moral; it is a problem of management of life. La Caze concludes his work with what we could probably call a utopia, a utopia of health which is confused with happiness, exactly as physiology and medicine can be a substitute for morality: 'the best plan of life is the one that ties us to the general interest and to our specific society, so that people wish to keep relations with us and vice versa.[37] Disease then is not, as in a mechanistic view, an interruption in the circulation of fluids, provoking obstructions; it is not a break in the equilibrium between fluids and solids; and it is not merely a vital reaction, sometimes excessive in comparison with the cause which produces it; it does not appear only when an organ or a centre captures all the activity and energy of the body. It can be deduced from an unequal distribution of vitality, a discrepancy in the sharing out of sensibility. Briefly speaking, disease is a problem of management of resources, a problem of self-government, a political and economic problem. Every man has the possibility and even the duty to act on his own centres of sensibility. Of course, every body is not able to prevent disease, and the physician has to interfere in the course of disease. The strategy used by vitalistic physicians corresponds to a double purpose: first, as it is well known, to shake, excite and awaken sensibility, deficient in one part because it is intemperate in another one; second, to change the direction of energy and its distribution in the body. To make it possible, it is necessary to provoke a general revolution in all the 'living machine', especially in order to convert a chronic disease into an acute one. The good effect of mineral waters, for example, is not produced by the quality of water, but, among all the aids provided by medicine, it is, Bordeu says in his *Recherches sur les maladies chroniques*, 'the most able to carry out, both for the physical and for the moral sphere, all the necessary and possible revolutions in chronic diseases: all the objects contribute to this aim: travelling, expectations of success, the diversity of food, changing air, amazing and wonderful new places, shift in usual sensations, minor passions that begin in these occasions, agreeable freedom; all these changes distress and distry the habits of uneasiness and disease of the town inhabitants'.[38] This is not only a common therapy of diversion and entertainment, frequently used for nervous disorders and taken from Hippocratic ideas; it is supposed to be really useful for any kind of diseases. Barthez, another vitalist physician, was to call it a therapy of 'perturbation'.[39]

Some of these ideas are still more obvious in the work of the German physician C.W. Hufeland, who published in 1796 his *Macrobiotics*, a book about hygiene, intended both for physicians and for the ordinary reader, which was soon to be translated into French as *L'art de prolonger la vie humaine.* He was professor of 'popular medicine' at Jena University, a chair without any equivalent in France, and he tried to lay down the difference between medicine as a selective, limited intervention, and the art which consists in examining the conditions of life, defined as a 'physico-animal operation'. He was vitalist in the special meaning of the word in German speaking countries, that is to say that he conceived the vital principle as a property of living matter, subordinate to particular chemical processes. Like La Caze, Hufeland wanted to integrate individual experience into general rules for a long life: 'If we lay down certain recognized principles concerning its nature and its needs, in the light of experience, we can determine which conditions speed it up and which conditions delay it and hence prolong it. We can deduce the rules to be observed in the natural and medical regimen of life, which can prolong it. The result is a particular science, macrobiotics or the art of prolonging life. This science is the subject of this work'.[40]

Dismissing all the elixirs of life and waters of youth, Hufeland defined life as a fixed quantity of energy, given to each individual: this notion did not have a very clear scientific meaning, and combined traditional metaphors of the vital flame or innate heat, with conceptions taken from electricity and magnetism, in the melting-pot of an all-embracing philosophy of Nature. Though the quantity of life is determined once and for all, it is possible to extend it or to shorten it according to the the way we use it. Necessity and freedom could be reconciled if each individual endeavoured to know himself and to 'manage' the quantity of life he had at his disposal. Vital energy is consumed in proportion to the intensity with which it is expended, i.e., according to the stimuli it receives: 'the principle of life can exist both in a state of development and of non-development, and thus, it looks like fire or electrical principle'.[41] It may remain hidden for a long time without revealing itself, simply preventing the body from corruption. The originality of Hufeland's ideas compared to those of romanticism in medicine, of stimulation and counterstimulation, which were popularised in conjunction with brunonianism, consists in the fact that he did not systematically advise awakening and stimulating the vital principle. In Nature, some elements such as light, heat, oxygen, water favour the good working of life and every body must do his best to 'manage' his quantity of life, while being aware of the dangers: any increase in the vital forces or in their intensity tends to reduce the length of life. Excessively prolonged activity leads to exhaustion and a frantic rhythm in the consumption of the vital principle leads to disastrous consequences. 'He who consumes in one day twice as much vital principle as another man will also exhaust twice as quickly his total sum of vital principle [...]. Thus vital energy is in adverse proportion to its length; the more intensively one lives, the shorter is one's life. The expression "to live fast", which, like the thing has become so fashionable, is perfectly correct. It is perfectly possible to accelerate or slow down the consumption of life, whether it is in action or enjoyment. Thus, one can live fast or slowly'.[42] Macrobiotics put in the hands of the individual, whether physician or not, the keys to his own fate.

Starting with a fund of vital energy that did not depend on himself, each person could increase or dilapidate it according to his choices, which compensates the unequal distribution of energy among individuals. Thus macrobiotics, which is both an economic and political science, instead of laying down hygienic precepts and injunctions, rather defines the laws of rationality which should govern individual behaviour: he should increase his vital faculties, strengthen his organs, reduce the consumption and facilitate or perfect the restoration of his forces. Self control, combining the physical and the moral as the notion of energy concerns them both, implies patient listening to oneself, the slow appropriation of the resources of one's own body. In the unceasing conflict between vital and destructive forces, there exists an art of management which is nevertheless not the same thing as the parcimonious exercise of life. To be a man, according to Hufeland, one 'must act, influence, enjoy'.[43] This conception of hygiene implies a transferral of responsibility from the physician to the layman, from nature to a social being, from general social factors to individual behaviour in the city. At the same time, this conception of hygiene gives an explanation of the production and the nature of disease and explains why medicine is 'a science of man'.

I would like to submit some conclusions: there is indeed a vitalistic conception of disease, which is taking shape and form in France around the second half of the eighteenth century, with the works of La Caze and which grow up along with the the works of the Montpellier School. As we have seen with Hufeland's example, it is a European movement.

The specificity of disease for vitalists should not be looked for in the traditional definition of a morbid state opposed to nature, which is able by its healing forces to win, but rather in the idea of a natural process (there is a physiology of disease) which society is completely involved in. In so far as the individual is a social being who needs society and social emulation for his health and happiness, his relations with society are the touchstone of medicine, not only for moral diseases, but for any kind of disease. Thus, we could speak of a double shift: from the body as a machine towards an organism where all the parts are sensible and in mutual dependance; from a problematic of mere struggle between two opposing categories – living body versus environment – towards a problematic of management of relations which may include both exchanges and conflicts. This view leads to a dialectic of inside and outside. Medicine, then, is a political problem, a problem of self government by a person who is able to choose his way of life and, to some extent, his kind of disease. By this, I do not mean this transferral of responsibility is no more than the old religious idea that disease is a punishment for some sin, but on the contrary, that each individual, responsible for his life, may have the diseases that he, or the society he lives in, deserves.

Notes

1. See for instance, J. Roger, *Les sciences de la vie dans la pensée française du XVIIIeme siècle* (Paris: Armand Colin, 1971); F. Duchesneau, *La physiologie des Lumières, Empirisme, modéles et théories* (La Haye: Nijhoff, 1982); E. Haigh, 'Xavier Bichat and the Medical Theory of the Eighteenth Century', *Medical History*, Supplement, 4, (1984), 146 p.; R. Rey, *Naissance et développement du vitalisme en France, de la seconde moitié du dix-huitiéme siècle à la fin du Premier Empire*, Thèse d'état, Université de Paris 1, 3 vols (forthcoming in *Studies on Voltaire and the eighteenth century*).
2. P. J. Barthez, *Nouveaux Eléments de la science de l'homme* (Paris: Goujon et Brunot, 1806), 2 vols; this comparison is in Vol. 1, Notes, p.16.
3. Critical claims against the animistic assumption of soul as involved in organic functions can be found in Menuret de Chambaud's many articles in Diderot's *Encyclopédie*; see *Encyclopédie ou Dictionnaire raisonné des sciences, des arts et des métiers*, par une Sociéte de gens lettres, mis en ordre par M. Diderot, et quant à la partie mathématique par M. D'Alembert, (Paris: Briasson, David, le Breton, Durand; puis Neufchátel: S. Faulche. 1751–65), 17 vols in folio (hereafter *Enc.*), especially 'Inflammation', Vol. 8, 712b and 'Tenesme', Vol. 16, 13a.
4. Vitalists disagree with Haller's distinction between muscular irritability and nervous sensibility, because they consider both as distinct fibres reactions of one and the same property, which is sensibility a property which may be conscious or not.
5. The metaphor of the swarm of bees, which means that every fibre is sensible and every part is dependant on each other, can be found in Ménuret's articles 'Observation', *Enc.*, Vol. XI, 318b and in Bordeu's *Recherches Anatomiques sur la position des glandes et leur action*, in *Oeuvres Complètes* (hereafter *O.C.*), précédées d'une notice sur sa vie et sur ses ouvrages par M. Le chevalier Richerand (Paris: Caille et Ravier, 1806, 2 vols) (first edn 1751), Vol.1, 187; for more details, see R. Rey, *op. cit.* (note 1), vol.1, 315–21.
6. See *Enc.*, Vol. 8, article 'Inflammation', and the same idea in John Hunter's work, *A Treatise on the Blood, Inflammation, and Gun-shot Wounds* (1793), in *The Works of John Hunter*, J. F. Palmer (ed.),

London: Longman, 1837), Vol.III; French translation by G. Richelot (Paris: Béchard jeune, 1839–40); on Hunter, see S. J. Cross, 'John Hunter, The Animal Oeconomy and Late Eighteenth Century Physiological Discourse', *Studies in the History of Biology*, V (1981), 1–110, and F. Duchesneau, 'Vitalism in Late Eighteenth Century Physiology: the Cases of Barthez, Blumenbach and John Hunter', *William Hunter and the Eighteenth Century Medical World*, W. F. Bynum and Roy Porter (eds), (Cambridge: Cambridge University Press, 1985), especially 279–95.

7. *Traité Des Airs, des Eaux et Lieux*, in *Oeuvres Complètes d'Hippocrate*, trad. E. Littré (Paris: J. B. Baillière, 1839–61), 10 vols.
8. John Arbuthnot, *An Essay Concerning the Effects of Air in Human Bodies* (London: J. & R. Tonson & S. Draper, 1733), XI–224; French translation by Boyer de Pébrardié, *Essai sur les effets de l'air sur le corps humain* (Paris: J. Barrois le fils, 1742).
9. Montesquieu quotes J. Arbuthnot twice, in his *Spicilège* and in *L'Esprit des Lois* (1748), *Oeuvres complètes* (Paris: Seuil, 1964), 424 and 626. He refers to Hippocrates in his climate theory.
10. See R. Favre, 'Du Medico-topographicque à Lyon en 1783', *Dix-Huitième Siècle, La Sain et le Malsain*, 9 (1977), 151–9; Ménuret de Chambaud wrote a medico-topographical report about Montelimar and about Paris, and Fouquet about Montpellier.
11. G. E. Stahl, *Theoria medica vera* (Halae: Literis Orphanotrophei, 1708), 7 parts in 2 vols; the idea of natura medicatrix is scattered in many works, for example in 'Du mixte et du vivant', *Oeuvres Médico-philosophiques et pratiques, traduites et commentés par T. Blondin* (Paris: J. B. Baillière, 1859–64), II–VI vols (first volume never appeared), II, 454.
12. The political background of vitalist conception of disease seems to give little illumination, at least for the second half of the eighteenth century; we can find more or less the same ideas in all European countries, in spite of strong differences between the political systems; the philosophical background is more significant.
13. T. Bordeu, *Recherches Anatomiques sur la position des glandes et leur action, O.C.*, I, 144 sqq.
14. T. Bordeu, *Recherches sur les maladies chroniques* (first edn 1775), *O.C.*, II, 845; see R. Rey, 'La théorie de la sécrétion chez Bordeu, modèle de la physiologie et de la pathologie vitalistes', *Dix-Huitième Siècle, Physiologie et Médecine des Lumières*, 23 (1991), 45–58.
15. L. Jordanova stresses the importance of the idea of environment for instance in her work, *Lamarck* (Oxford: Oxford University Press, 1984), ch. 6, 58–70; in 'Policing Public Health in France 1780–1815', *Public Health*, Proceedings of the 5th International Symposium on the Comparative History of Medicine East and West, Teizo Ogawa (ed.), (Tokyo: Saikon Pub. Comp., 1981), 12–32.
16. L. La Caze, *Idée de l'homme Physique et moral* (Paris: H. L. Guérin,

1755); he is not completely devoid of ambiguities in his definition of life; but he provided decisive tools against mechanistic views.

17. T. Bordeu, *Correspondance,* édition critique présentée etannotée par M. Fletcher, avec la collaboration de Nadine Labé et d'Aloys de Laforcade (Montpellier: CNRS–Université Paul Valéry, 1980), 4 vols, especially Vol. 2.
18. For a detailed account of La Caze's views in his Latin work, *Specimen Novi Medicinae Conspectus* (s.1, 1749; 2nd edn, Paris: H. L. Guérin), see Rey, *op. cit.* (note 1), Vol.1, 355–68.
19. On this aspect, see R. Rey, 'Buffon et le vitalisme', *Buffon* 88, Actes du Colloque International Paris-Montbard-Dijon, Préface d'E. Mayr, Postface de G. Canguilhem, sous la direction de J. Gayon (Paris: Vrin, 1992), 399–413.
20. 'Un des principaux avantages de ce nouveau plan de médecine, et en quoi il est éminemment préférable et véritablement unique, c'est le grand jour qu'il répand sur l'hygiène ou la science du régime, cette branche de la médecine si précieuse et si négligée et d'embrasser le régime des sensations et des passions d'une manière si positive et si claire qu'il en résulte un traité médical de morale et de bonheur', claims Ménuret, *Enc.,* Vol. XI, article 'Oeconomie Animale', 366b.
21. P. J. G. Cabanis, *Rapports du physique et du moral de l'homme* (Paris: Caille et Ravier, an X), Septième Mémoire, 'De l'influence des maladies sur la formation des idées et des affections morales'; I refer to Dr Cerise's edition (Paris: Fortin, Masson & Cie, 1843), 270. For a more general account on Cabanis, see M. S. Staum, *Cabanis, Enlightenment and Medical Philosophy in the French Revolution* (Princeton: Princeton University Press, 1980); for 'action and reaction', see J. Starobinski, 'Le mot "réaction" de la physique à la psychiatrie', *Diogène,* 93 (1976), 3–30.
22. La Caze, *op. cit.* (note 16), 428; we find the same idea in *Enc.,* Vol. XI, article 'Peau (médecine sémiotique)', 366 b.
23. *Enc.,* Vol. XI, article 'Oeconomie Animale', 366 b.
24. J. B. Van Helmont, *Ortus Medicinae, id est initia physica inaudita, progressus medicinae novus, in morborum ultionem ad vitem longam* (Amstelodami, apud L. Elzevirium, 1648), Tractatus De Anima, 349–52.
25. This image of the spider in the centre of its web can be found in La Mettrie's *L'homme machine,* Bordeu's *Recherches sur les maladies chroniques,* 923–27 and in Diderot's *Rêve de D'Alembert, Oeuvres Complètes,* Lewinter (ed.), (Paris: Club français du livre, 1971), VIII, 99.
26. F. Hoffmann, *La Médecine Raisonnée,* translated by J. Bruhier (Paris: Briasson, 1739–43), 9 vols, Vol 1, 70–1.
27. *Enc.* t. XI, 'Observation' (signed 'm', i.e. J. J. Ménuret de Chambaud): 'peut-étre est-il vrai que, pour un bon moraliste, il faut être un excellent médecin', 319 b.
28. Barthez studies the different kinds of sympathy, not only between

organs directly connected together by the nervous system, but also between organs located in two symmetrical parts in the body, or even between organs separated by cellular tissue. On sympathy, see *op. cit.* (note 2), Vol. 2 especially 5–99, and also in the first edition of his work (Montpellier: J. Martel aîné, 1778), 142–62.

29. See Fouquet's article 'Sensibilité', *Enc.*, Vol. XV; Ménuret's articles 'Pouls', *Enc.*, XII, and 'Oeconomie Animale', *Enc.*, XI; Bordeu *op. cit.* (note 14), Théorème CXXXIV: 'Quoi qu'il en soit, il n'y a aucun sujet de douter que les parties du corps vivant ne soient toutes douées de la faculté sensible', 925.
30. John Brown's *Elements of medicine* were translated in France (*Eléments de Médecine,* traduits de l'original latin avec des additions et des notes de l'auteur, par Fouquier (Paris: Demonville et Gabon, an XIII; there is another translation by R. J. Bertin, Paris: J. Barrois le Père, an XIV) but never received great approval, except among surgeons, may be because vitalism had already won in medical circles in Paris as well as in Montpellier; however, there are some discrepancies between vitalism and brunonianism: for one, specific vital properties belong to all living beings, had they stimulation or not, and the power of life may remain latent and its energy asleep; for brunonianism, without stimulation, there is no life at all. For a more general account, see G. Canguilhem, 'Une idéologie médicale exemplaire', *Idéologie et Rationalité dans l'histoire des sciences le la vie* (Paris: Vrin, 1977), 47–54, and *Brunonianism in Britain and Europe,* W. F, Bynum and Roy Porter (eds), *Medical History,* Supplement (1988), 104.
31. Henri Fouquet, author of some entries in Diderot's *Encyclopédie,* such as 'Sensibilité', 'Sécrétion', 'Vésicatoire', is a vitalist physician from Montpellier.
32 These ideas are expressed in many *Encyclopédie' s* articles, such as 'Manustupration', 'Mariage', 'Mélancolie', 'Pouls', as well as Bordeu's *Recherches sur les maladies chroniques* and Barthez's *Consultations de Médecine* (with Bouvart, Fouquet, Lorry and Lamure) (Paris: L. Collin, 1807), 2 vols.
33. (My translation), La Caze, *op. cit.* (note 16), 414: 'Nous avons besoin de sensations aussi essentiellement que de nourriture, et l'air qui nous fait respirer ne nous est pas plus nécessaire pour le soutien de la vie que les sensations'.
34. *Ibid.*, 391–2.
35. Stahl's definition of disease combines two levels of analysis: The soul (*logos,* not *logismos*) is responsible for disease exactly in the same manner as it is responsible for all the organic motions; thus, disease is nothing else than a vital reaction against the natural tendency of the body towards corruption, within a framework of struggle between the living body and the physical laws; but at the second level, Stahl needs mechanical explanations for disease, i.e., plethora, thickening of blood

or stasis, unusual motions; see 'Pathologie très spéciale', *op. cit.* (note 11), Vol.V.

36. See for example La Caze, *op. cit.* (note 18), 49–51, and Ménuret's comment in 'Spasme', *Enc.*, XV, 435 b.
37. 'Le meilleur plan de vie est donc celui qui nous lie assez à l'intérêt général et à notre société particulière pour qu'on désire conserver des rapports avec nous comme l'inverse', La Caze, *op. cit.* (note 11 or 16), 435.
38. Théophile Bordeu, *Recherches sur les maladies chroniques, O.C.*, II,. 806.
39. See Barthez, *op. cit.* (note 2), II, 178 and also in his *Traité des Maladies Goutteuses* (Paris: Déterville, 1802), 2 vols.
40. (my translation); 'En posant des principes avérés sur sa nature et ses besoins, et à l'aide de l'expérience, on peut déterminer les conditions qui la précipitent ou la retardent et par conséquent la prolongent. On en tire des règles à observer dans le régime naturel et médicinal de la vie, qui peuvent en procurer la prolongation: et il en résulte une science particulière, la macrobiotique, ou l'art de prolonger la vie; et c'est cette science qui fait le sujet de cet ouvrage', C. W. Ihufeland, *L'art de prolonger la vie humaine* (Lausanne, Hignou & Cie, et Lyon, Savy) p.VIII (1st edn 1796).
41. 'Le principe de vie peut également exister dans un état de développement et de non-développement, et il a, en cela, beaucoup de rapport avec le feu et le principe électrique, de même que ceux-ci peuvent exister dans un corps sans se montrer d'aucune manière jusqu' à ce qu'un stimulant proportionné à sa force le mette en mouvement, ainsi le principe de vie peut être dans un corps organisé dans un état de développement et de non-développement pendant très longtemps, sans s'annoncer autrement qu'en conservant ce corps et en l'empêchant de se dissoudre', *ibid.*, 25.
42. 'Celui qui en un jour consume deux fois autant de principes vitaux qu'un autre épuisera aussi deux fois plus vite la somme des principes vitaux qu'il renferme [...]. Ainsi l'énergie de la vie est en rapport opposé avec sa durée; plus un être vit intensivement, moins sa vie est-elle extensive. L'expression "vivree vite", qui, ainsi que la chose, est devenue si à la mode, est parfaitement juste. Il est parfaitement possible d'accélérer ou de ralentir la consomption de la vie, soit qu'elle existe en action, ou en jouissances; ainsi, l'on peut vivre vite ou lentement' *ibid.*, 40).
43. *Ibid.*, 140.

12

The Weight of Evidence and the Burden of Authority: Case Histories, Medical Statistics and Smallpox Inoculation

Andrea A. Rusnock

Statistical evaluation of medical practice is regarded as one of the pillars of modern scientific medicine. Whether through the agency of government commissions, universities or modern hospitals, statistics are generally the product of bureaucracies, which both legitimate and obscure the difficulties in collecting and evaluating the numerical data produced within them. In light of this, it is instructive to examine in detail an example of the collection of statistics, or more precisely, numerical figures, in a pre-institutional setting.[1] Without the structural support of bureaucracies, the fissures, flaws, strains and tensions of reducing individual case histories to numerical data become readily visible.

The introduction of statistics into medicine, usually located in early nineteenth-century Paris hospital medicine, has significant roots in eighteenth-century Britain, as Ulrich Troehler and others have shown.[2] In this essay I will concentrate on arguably the first use of numerical evidence to evaluate a medical practice, namely the introduction of smallpox inoculation in early eighteenth-century Britain. Numerical arguments formed an important part of the debates over inoculation, and their use in these debates established a novel approach to evaluating medical practice that would be employed by later writers.

The chief architect of this numerical approach was the physician James Jurin (1684–1750), who served as secretary to the Royal Society for the years 1721 to 1727. Educated at Trinity College Cambridge (BA 1705, MA 1709), he briefly studied in Leiden and received his MD from Cambridge in 1716. He moved to London and wasted little time in advancing his position both as a physician and a natural philosopher. In 1718 he became a Fellow of the Royal Society, and in 1719, a Fellow of the Royal College of Physicians. Perhaps best known for his contributions to the Analyst controversy over the epistemological status of the calculus, Jurin's scholarship extended into many fields including iatromechanics, mechanics, optics, cures for the stone and, most importantly smallpox inoculation.[3]

In a series of pamphlets published between 1723 and 1727, Jurin argued the case for inoculation using a novel method of quantification. Presenting comparative mortality figures for natural and inoculated smallpox, he showed that the hazard of dying from inoculated smallpox was much less than that of dying from natural smallpox.[4] His figures were widely cited in England and on the Continent and very few attempted to duplicate his numerical ratios until the end of the eighteenth century. Despite this widespread acceptance, many difficulties beset Jurin's numerical investigations in medicine. To construct mortality ratios, he had first to collect and collate case histories, which required extensive correspondence with a group of geographically widespread practitioners. Building such a network took considerable effort and maintaining the goodwill of voluntary correspondents demanded diplomatic skill. The creation of standard narratives from the numerous individual case histories involved the extraction of consistent, quantifiable information, which then could be tallied and tabulated in established categories.[5] Jurin's indisputable ratios of the number of inoculated and natural smallpox cases were thus the result of an arduous and at times controversial process of soliciting, selecting and sorting varied case histories.

In many ways, Jurin's methods followed the precepts of the Royal Society at the time: a combination of Baconian induction and Newtonian natural philosophy. In accumulating numerous instances of inoculation Jurin sought to demonstrate mathematically that it was an effective medical practice. But this method raised the problem of what to do with unsuccessful cases, in which inoculation caused death or failed to have any effect whatsoever. Negative case histories were matters of constant debate in the inoculation literature and they posed an acute problem to Jurin. His numerical ratios rested on the accuracy and trustworthiness of the testimony given in the case histories. The question of authority in the late seventeenth and eighteenth centuries was particularly charged in large part because the more traditional forms of authority were increasingly untenable in the rapidly changing world of commercialization, social mobility and political unrest.[6] Steven Shapin has described some of the mechanisms used in experimental practice in late seventeenth-century England in which authority was established by controlling space (such as in the public rooms of Robert Boyle's house or in Royal

Society meetings); however, these stratagems do not apply to written forms of evidence. Correspondence demanded different means to ensure trustworthy testimony.[7]

Jurin's method of analysing smallpox inoculation constituted a new approach to gathering information and evaluating its sources. In the first section of this essay, I examine the methods Jurin used to establish and maintain a correspondence network. Jurin's calculations of the risks of inoculation are the subject of the second section, and his attempts to resolve negative case histories form the subject of the third. In the final section, I analyse the public reception of Jurin's approach to medical evidence.

Establishing a Correspondence Network

Prior to its introduction into Europe in the early eighteenth century, inoculation was a widespread folk practice found in Turkey, China and parts of Africa. The actual procedure consisted of making a scratch or small incision, typically on two limbs (some combination of arms and legs), and placing a thread covered with the pus from a virulent pock on that incision. The scratch was covered with bandages for a day or so to ensure that the graft would take. The incisions would become inflamed approximately four days after they were made. The inoculee would then develop a fever on the seventh or eighth day, and a few pocks on the tenth or eleventh day. The individual normally recovered by the 15th or 16th day.

Members of the Royal Society became informed of inoculation at an early date. In 1713 and 1714, accounts were read before the Society and later published in the *Philosophical Transactions*.[8] The historian Genevieve Miller has stressed the roles played by Sir Hans Sloane, president of the Royal College of Physicians and later president of the Royal Society, and leading members of the royal family and aristocracy in publicizing and promoting inoculation in England.[9] An extensive pamphlet war took place during the early 1720s involving the religious, medical and nationalist objections to the practice. Religious men argued that inoculation interfered with divine providence, while medical opponents focused on the ethics of such a practice. Inoculation could not properly be classified as a therapy: who would give an illness to prevent an illness? Surely, this was beyond the proper bounds of medicine and violated all maxims of ethical practice. Because of its non-European origins, much of the anti-inoculation literature disparaged the practice as something performed 'by a few *ignorant women*, amongst an illiterate and unthinking People.'[10] And finally, English nationalists raised Hippocratic objections to a practice developed in a foreign land (Turkey) for a foreign people: it could not possibly suit the needs of Christian, meat-eating, English.[11]

Jurin entered the fray with the stated goal of avoiding entanglement in the heated, ongoing disputes and providing instead only 'matters of fact'. In his first publication on inoculation in 1723, he announced:

> I have no Inclination to enter into this Controversy; it is in better and abler Hands: but, as the Point in Dispute is of the utmost Importance to Mankind, I heartily wish, that, without Passion, Prejudice, or private Views, it may be fairly and maturely examin'd. In order to which, if the following Extracts and Computations, concerning the comparative Danger of the Inoculated and Natural Small Pox, may be of any Use to your self, or to other impartial and disinterested Judges, I shall think my Labour well bestowed.[12]

These statements fit nicely with the aims of the Royal Society, and as many historians have shown, members of the Royal Society in the late seventeenth century sought to avoid political and religious controversy by relying on an experimental approach to knowledge.[13]

Jurin's method of providing matters of fact was to compare the mortality rates of inoculated and natural smallpox, as suggested to him by one of his correspondents, Dr Thomas Nettleton of Halifax.[14] Nettleton seemed to have been genuinely driven by the shortcomings of contemporary medicine in easing the pain of those suffering from smallpox, and he began practising inoculation having learned of it solely from the *Philosophical Transactions*.[15] In a letter to Jurin, he wrote that the only way to prove that the inoculated smallpox was less dangerous than the natural smallpox was 'by making a Comparison so far as our Experience will extend'. To that end, he collected smallpox mortality figures for Halifax and surrounding towns.[16] In his reply, Jurin praised Nettleton's efforts and informed him that he was 'collecting all the accounts I can procure concerning the number of Persons, that have been inoculated here in England, & the mortality of the Natural Small Pox'.[17]

Jurin gathered these accounts through a network of correspondence dating from 1723 until 1727, when he stepped down from his position as secretary to the Royal Society. This correspondence network was created in large part by well-placed publicity. In 1723 Jurin issued an advertisement, initially published in the *Philosophical Transactions* and in his pamphlet, *A Letter to the Learned Caleb Cotesworth*, and reissued in each yearly pamphlet entitled *An Account of the Success of Inoculating the Small Pox for the Year....*[18] The advertisement read as follows:

> All Persons concern'd in the Practice of inoculating the Small Pox, are desir'd to keep a Register of the Names and Ages of every Person inoculated, the place where it is done, the Manner of the Operation, the Days of sickening and of the Eruption, the Sort of small Pox that is produc'd, and the Event.
>
> They are intreated to send these Accounts, or an Extract from them, comprehending all Persons inoculated from the Beginning, to the end of the present Year, to Dr *Jurin*, Secretary to the Royal Society, some time in *January*, or at farthest *February* next, that so the Result of them may be publish'd early in the spring.[19]

Numerous individuals throughout the British Isles responded to Jurin's request and their letters provide rich details about the actual practice of inoculation and the reception of Jurin's project.[20]

Complete, faithful and accurate case histories were central to Jurin's project, especially in the first year or so when inoculation was an unfamiliar procedure to most people in Britain. In his first published *Account of the Success of Inoculating the Small Pox* (1724), Jurin gave a composite account of the procedure and the typical course of illness in an inoculated patient. 'I shall here give some Account of what is to be done, and what is usually observ'd in Inoculation,' Jurin instructed, 'as I have extracted it from a careful Examination and Comparison of the several Relations transmitted to me.'[21] This section was excluded in his subsequent pamphlets, presumably because the actual procedure of inoculation had become fairly well known.

Respondents to Jurin's advertisement ranged socially and geographically. Medical men – apothecaries, surgeons, and physicians – were by far the majority of contributors, but there were also letters from the gentry (for example, Sir Thomas Lyttelton and Lady Catherine Percivall provided detailed accounts of their children's inoculation), from local ministers who vouched for the legitimacy of certain reports, and from a weaver turned medical practitioner who became embroiled in a particularly disputed case, which I will discuss below.

Certainly part of Jurin's success in collecting inoculation accounts must be attributed to his position as Secretary to the Royal Society. The Royal Society provided crucial institutional support ranging from such mundane, but necessary, matters as covering postage costs to the less tangible factors of legitimation.[22] Jurin's ability to utilize the prestige and patronage of the leading scientific society of England at that time – whose president was the formidable Sir Isaac Newton –

gave credence and authority to a practice which initially occasioned much hostility and doubt. Even in this world of pre-state bureaucratic statistics, some sort of institutional affiliation served to guarantee the accuracy and truthfulness of the numbers produced.

Correspondents, too, profited from participating in Jurin's correspondence network, primarily through connection with the Royal Society. Thomas Nettleton, for example, wrote that it was 'the greatest of my ambition that my Letter may be inserted' in the *Philosophical Transactions.*[23] And in a subsequent letter, he confessed: 'The Approbation of that Illustrious Body [the Royal Society] will far overballance all the hard censures, and injurious reflections, which every man must expect to meet with, who endeavours to promote a thing so uncommon, and so disagreable to the general Humour of the People, as this has hitherto been.'[24]

From the numerous letters he received, it is evident that Jurin had a wealth of information at hand. Some of his respondents delighted in detail: Dr Henry Jones of King's College, Cambridge penned a four-page report of four sisters who had been inoculated, which in his words, was 'a *Minute* and *Impartial* Account of all the Particulars that occurr'd during the Time of the Distemper....'[25] Similarly, Dr William Oliver contributed a four-page description of the inoculation of two children in Plymouth.[26] Reports of this length took the form of medical case histories. Details concerning the health of each inoculated individual were recorded from the initial incision until the last pock dried and flaked off the skin. Each day symptoms were noted including changes in urine, stools and temperature. The incisions were watched closely and often kept open in order to ascertain if the small pox graft had taken, and the process was generally conceived in humoral terms: '... the running of the Incisions may probably be of great Service, the matter issuing from them being of the same nature with what fills the Pocks....'[27] The outbreak of pocks on the seventh or eighth day was agreed to be the true sign of whether the inoculation had been successful. The number of pocks was frequently recorded, and it was widely believed that those who had smallpox through inoculation suffered fewer pox, leading Jurin to conclude: 'The Small Pox given by Inoculation are generally fewer in Number, and all the Symptoms more favourable, than in the natural way.'[28]

Many of Jurin's correspondents, however, were not as diligent in reporting case histories as Dr Jones and Dr Oliver, and Jurin frequently requested additional information. In a letter to the surgeon Mr. Hepburn of Stamford in Lincolnshire, Jurin appealed to the public good as a means to soften his further demands. 'I am favour'd with yours of Jan. 21st in which you are pleas'd to give me an account of your success in inoculating the Small Pox upon the two Sons of Mr Richards. The same publick Spirit, which has moved you to send me that relation, will I hope induce you to satisfie me in the following particulars, which are not so expressly set down in your Letter, as I could wish.'[29] Correspondents replied promptly to Jurin's additional queries, and one writer even apologized for his negligence: 'I shall be more carefull for the future to transmit Names or any other particulars, that you may not have so troublesome a Correspondent....'[30]

Details about names, ages and place where the inoculation was performed were the most frequent of Jurin's requests.[31] A complete case history needed as its bare essentials precisely these elements along with outcome, and increasingly only these elements as the typical course of inoculated smallpox became more widely. known and agreed upon, and hence standardized. Name and place provided Jurin with the means of securing further information should any questions arise about a specific case. 'I am obliged to you for the Favour of yours of March 18, ' Jurin wrote to Nehemiah Towgood of Somerset, 'but am under a necessity of giving you this trouble to desire the names of your two Patients. My intention is not to print those names, but only to keep them by me, as I do all the rest, in order to be provided for any dispute that may happen afterwards.'[32] In this way, Jurin's register of the names of inoculated individuals served to guarantee the accuracy of reported inoculations.

Tallying the Typical

The next step in Jurin's project was to assemble the case histories and create a numerical account of the state of inoculation within a given year. By reporting the numbers of persons successfully inoculated, Jurin skirted the issue of impropriety as suggested in the letter to Towgood. Many of Jurin's correspondents in fact requested that the names of their patients not be published. 'You are desired by the parents to conceal their Names', wrote the surgeon Hepburn; 'the Father desires the Child may not be mentioned in print', reported the apothecary Brady; and again, James Burges stated 'As you see by Mr Grenvill's Letter, Names are not to be printed....'[33] In at least one instance, the propriety of printing women's ages was challenged by the Royal Surgeon Claude Amyand whose patients were primarily members of the gentry: 'T'were to wish the fair sexes Ages did not Stand upon Records.'[34] The desire for privacy, particularly among the upper classes, made Jurin's strategy of reporting only the number of people inoculated all the more appealing.[35] Numbers provided anonymity.

Essential to quantification – broadly conceived as the process of assigning numbers to represent things – was categorization. In order for Jurin to quantify the success of inoculation, he had to develop categories to enumerate. In his pamphlets, he addressed two questions which he regarded as central to evaluating the efficacy of inoculation: first, whether inoculation provided 'effectual Security' against natural smallpox; and second, 'Whether the Hazard of Inoculation be considerably less than that of the natural Small Pox?'[36] By framing the questions in this way, Jurin negotiated a complex issue by reducing the number of potential objections to inoculation. Throughout his inoculation correspondence, one can find evidence of Jurin's efforts to restrict the inquiry to these two questions.

To answer the first question, he had to rely upon the experience of inoculated individuals – or as Jurin put it:

> For tho' many Trials have been purposely made by Physicians and others, both upon Children and grown Persons, who have had the Small Pox by Inoculation, causing them not only to converse with, but to handle, to nurse, and to lie in the same Bed with others Sick of the natural Small Pox; yet there is no Instance as far as I have been able to learn, of any one Person, either in Turkey, New England, or here at Home, who has received the Small Pox by Inoculation, that has afterwards had it in the natural Way.[37]

The issue of permanent immunity was a difficult point to prove: collecting reports of negative results of a form of human experimentation in order to convince others that inoculation prevented subsequent natural smallpox infection was not an easy task. Although Jurin never explicitly requested information on this score, some individuals did perform and report human experiments. As late as 1730 Jurin received a letter from Dr William Oliver relating the case of two boys who had been inoculated six years earlier and who had just been exposed to a virulent form of smallpox with no ill effects. Oliver concluded his letter with the following plea: 'I find it urg'd as a Strenuous Argument against Inoculation that the Inoculated are liable to have the Small Pox again by Infection in the Natural Way. Some more Trials of this kind wou'd finally determine that Part of the Dispute.'[38] Strikingly, Jurin did not solicit instances of such trials, perhaps because of the questionable ethics of exposing inoculated patients to infected individuals.

To answer his second question about the hazard of inoculation, Jurin turned to a numerical approach. Here his task was simpler: he sought to enumerate the number of people who were inoculated, and of those how many survived and how many died, for in fact some did die from inoculation. A quick look at his categories, however, suggests that this process was not quite so straightforward. In his account for the year 1723, for example, Jurin listed 34 inoculators (17 surgeons, 7 apothecaries, 6 physicians, 2 ministers and 2 women) who inoculated 483 persons. Of those 483:

> 440 had the small pox by inoculation,
> 5 had an 'imperfect small pox by inoculation',
> for 29 individuals the procedure had no effect,
> and 9 persons were 'suspected to have died of inoculation'l.[39]

After exhibiting this tally, he subtracted the number of individuals on whom the operation had no effect, leaving the hazard of dying of inoculated smallpox to be 9 in 445, or roughly 1 in 49 or 50.

The category 'imperfect small pox by inoculation' immediately leaps out from the above list, raising myriad questions about how individuals identified smallpox, how they distinguished an 'imperfect' sort and so on. A difficulty encountered by all concerned in inoculation stemmed from the vagaries of diagnosis. How did individuals determine whether they had contracted smallpox from inoculation? Were the symptoms of inoculated smallpox similar enough to natural smallpox to facilitate diagnosis? From the various reports it is clear that individuals reacted to inoculation in a variety of ways, and that although a generalized case history could be abstracted (as Jurin and others did), many inoculated persons did not suffer from the typical symptoms. To illustrate these difficulties encountered in diagnosing one of the most externally visible diseases, I will discuss one hotly disputed case.

George Percivall, age three, according to his mother Lady Catherine Percivall, was inoculated by the royal surgeon Claude Amyand on 5 May, 1725.[40] Eight days following the operation, several smallpox began to appear on his face and the boy had a slight fever and quicker pulse. Over the next few days, approximately 120 pocks appeared on his body, but his mother wrote, 'they never were so bad but that he cou'd whip a Top and beat a drum'. Eleven days after the first pocks appeared, all the pocks had dried and flaked off, and after a few purges, Lady Percivall wrote 'I thank God he is as well as ever he was in his life.'[41] Three weeks later, however, George became ill, and he was attended by several physicians who offered their opinions on the case in letters to Jurin. Most of those who testified in this case agreed that George had 300 or 400 pustules that stayed from two to three days, and five or six larger pustules, which stayed much longer. Beyond this no one agreed. Dr

Monro, in a letter dated 14 April, 1726, indicated that he met Amyand at the boy's house: 'It was his [Amyand's] opinion it was the chicken pox in which the thickness of the Skin had pent the matter longer than usuall, to which I answered poynting to that on his right hand, that I beleived we might from that pimple inoculate the small pox.'[42] Later in this letter, he stated that he told Lady Percivall that the larger pustules 'were in all their circumstances so like the small pox, that I cou'd not tell what else to call them, that the rest might be the chicken pox.'[43]

In August of the same year, the surgeon Amyand wrote to Jurin that because 'the Case of the honourable Master George Percivall having been differently reported; the Right Honourable the Lady Percivall his Mother has given me leave to take a Copy of her Journal of that Case, which for the publicks Satisfaction she is pleased to allow to be printed, as well as the Enclosed Letter....' Amyand concluded his letter by asserting that George's second eruption 'was Nothing more than the Chicken Pox'.[44] Jurin published selections from the letters written by Monro, Amyand, and Lady Percivall in his *Account* for the year 1725, and concluded: 'From these Accounts it plainly appears, that this young Gentlemen had the Small-Pox by Inoculation; and whether the second Eruption deserves to be call'd the true Small-Pox, is left to the Reader's Judgment.'[45]

Throughout his published writings and in his correspondence, Jurin sought to downplay these difficulties in diagnosis and classification by rigidly reducing the variety of inoculation experiences to a limited number of categories. For perhaps polemical reasons or simply exigency, Jurin selected the binary categories of life and death. 'I need not give you the trouble of drawing up an account of the accidents happening to any of your inoculated Patients,' Jurin wrote to Dr Nettleton. 'I think a Comparison between the natural and inoculated Small Pox, in point of Life or Death will be sufficient....'[46] In Nettleton's case, a young girl had been left deaf and mute after inoculation, but regardless of these afflictions which might or might not have been the result of inoculation, Jurin counted the girl's inoculation experience as a success because it had not resulted in death.[47] Any disability that might have resulted from inoculation was thus pushed to the margins. In Jurin's scheme inoculation failed in only two instances: 1) by causing death; or 2) by failing to protect the inoculated individual from a subsequent attack of smallpox. To be sure, Jurin offered some justification for this position. In his account for 1723, he argued that if accidents other than death resulting from inoculation were to be reported, so too would conditions emanating from natural smallpox.[48]

After categorization and enumeration, Jurin completed his numerical argument by comparing the odds of dying from inoculated smallpox with those of dying from natural smallpox, which he initially calculated from the London bills of mortality. In his first publication on inoculation, 'A Letter to the Learned Dr Caleb Cotesworth ... containing a Comparison between the Danger of the Natural Small Pox and of that given by Inoculation,' he included two tables drawn from the London bills of mortality which show his calculations.[49] [See Figures 1 and 2.] The first table indicated mortality figures for the years 1667–86, and the second for 1701–22. Jurin omitted the intervening years (1687–1700), because deaths due to smallpox and measles were counted together.[50] From these tables he initially calculated the odds of dying from natural smallpox as 1 in 14, but he went on to adjust these odds.

Jurin was careful to distinguish morbidity and mortality rates, indicating the sophistication of his argument. His reasoning hinged on the recognition of a high infant mortality rate – something that John Graunt had pointed out in his pioneering work published in 1662 which also relied on the bills of mortality.[51] Jurin argued:

> For since one fourteenth part of Mankind die of the Small Pox, and the other thirteen parts die of other Diseases; if these thirteen have all had the Small Pox, and recover'd from it, before they fell ill of those other Diseases of which they died, then just thirteen will have recover'd from the Small Pox, for one that dies of that Distemper: but, as it is notorious, that great Numbers, especially of young Children, die of other Diseases, without ever having the Small Pox, it is plain, that fewer than thirteen must recover from this Distemper, for one that dies of it.[52]

Again following Graunt, Jurin subtracted the number of deaths due to certain diseases associated with infants, for example, 'Overlaid, Chrysoms and Infants, Convulsions, Horseshoehead, Headmoldshot, Teeth,' which together amounted to 386 deaths per 1,000 over the 22 year period. Thus deaths due to smallpox must now be reckoned as a fraction of the remaining 614 deaths per 1,000. Jurin made the further assumption that everyone after 2 years of age contracted smallpox at some point in their life.[53] He concluded his argument as follows:

> Allowing therefore, that out of every 1000 Children that are born, 386 die under one or two Years of Age, without having the Small Pox, and 72 do some time or other die of that Distemper; it follows, that the Hazard of dying of it, to the remainder of Mankind, above one or two Years of Age, who are all supposed to undergo that Disease sooner or later, is that of 72 out of 614, or

> nearly 2 out of 17: so that *no more, than between 7 and 8, can recover from that Distemper, for one that dies of it.*[54]

He supported these adjusted figures with local parish surveys undertaken by some of his correspondents, who assured Jurin of the accuracy of their figures. For example, Dr Thomas Dixon of Bolton Le Moors wrote: 'The Account I here send You, will I hope be acceptable, being carefully and faithfully taken from House to House thro' this Town. The Small Pox visited this place in May 1725, and did not leave us 'till Christmas. The Number that have, in the time mention'd, been seized with the Small Pox is 341. The Number that died of the Small Pox is 64.'[55] Indeed a house-to-house survey was the only way to arrive at a precise figure. 'This is a faithfull account,' testified Dr George Lynch of Canterbury, 'and I believe may be depended upon, being taken by a proper Person going about from House to House.'[56] But as with more general censuses, such enquiries provoked suspicion. Dr Beard, after reporting smallpox mortality figures for Romsey, added: 'I shall do the same for Worcester as soon as I can break thro that formidable Objection of our Solemn Clarks, viz numbering the people.'[57] Smallpox was viewed as a negative mark on a community, and hence some towns did not want mortality figures made public.[58]

When Jurin published this numerical information, he assured his readers that it was 'communicated to me by Persons of Credit,' highlighting his concern for authority and legitimacy.[59] In the conclusions to his pamphlets, Jurin simply reiterated the hazards of dying from inoculated and natural smallpox, thus reinforcing his claim to present only matters of fact.

Challenging the Atypical

In a letter to Dr Richard Beard, Jurin made explicit his decision to suppress 'typical' case histories: 'I have made it a rule to my self to publish no particular cases out of the great number that are sent me, except upon the death of the Party, or any dispute about his having the distemper a second time.'[60] After his initial publication, the unique and atypical case history became the subject of concern and publication, reflecting the overwhelming power of one case to dissuade individuals from inoculation. '...[I]f any thing goes amiss, or seems to do so, the world presently rings of it with all the aggravations imaginable, but on the other hand many successful Experiments are, I believe, buryed in silence,' wrote Edward Edlin to Jurin in 1726.[61] Dr Bayly writing from Havant conveyed similar sentiments, referring to a patient who did not contract smallpox from inoculation: 'In 2 or 3 Days afterwards the Incisions were quite healed up and the Patient perfectly well in Body but greatly mortify'd at this Disappointment which also discourag'd some others who were resolved to have been Inoculated if this Case had Succeeded as well as the former. Thus a Stop was put to the Practice of Inoculation in this Place.'[62]

Jurin himself, painfully aware of this situation, acknowledged the limitations of his quantitative approach in his *Account* for the year 1725: 'But though the affirmative Side of this Question cannot be fully establish'd under a considerable Length of Time, and a great Number of Experiments; the Negative may indeed admit of an easier Proof: For a small Number of Instances of Persons receiving the Small-Pox by Inoculation, and having them afterwards in the natural Way, will be sufficient to convince the Publick, that Inoculation is no Security from the naturall Small-Pox.'[63] Reflecting these concerns for negative reports of inoculation, the atypical case became the subject of case histories in Jurin's later pamphlets, while those individuals who suffered no unusual complaints or symptoms in their course of inoculated smallpox were simply added to his list of successful cases. In his 1725 account, for example, Jurin devoted only ten pages to a general discussion of inoculation and 43 pages to three particularly disputed cases.[64] Underlining this change in focus was the addition of two paragraphs to Jurin's advertisement asking for detailed reports of any inoculation cases which either produced no illness or resulted in death.[65] He devoted considerable energy to investigating cases which called inoculation into doubt and the majority of his later pamphlets were devoted to eyewitness accounts of these contested cases, underscoring once again the evidential power of negative evidence. I will concentrate on one colourful example which appeared in the account for the year 1725.

The disputed case concerned a child who was supposedly inoculated in the town of Oswestry in 1725 by a surgeon named Mr Jones. In the appendix to a pamphlet published in 1725, Dr William Clinch cited this case as an instance when an inoculated individual later succumbed to natural smallpox.[66] In response to this pamphlet, Jurin sent letters to a local minister, Mr Parry, and to Jones, both dated 22 February, 1726, in an attempt to assess the veracity of Dr Clinch's claims. In his letter to Jones, Jurin wrote: 'this matter has occasion'd a great deal of talk here in Town, and some Persons have made it a Question, whether the Child was really inoculated, or no. I am sensible, Sir, how dear every honest Man must hold his Reputation, and therefore am concern'd to tell you how far yours is affected by these disputes: but the Remedy lies in your own hands, by clearing up the Truth in such a manner as may be satisfactory to the World.'[67]

Jurin received a prompt response from the minister Parry, in a letter dated 1 March, 1726, who doubted Jones' claims to have performed the inoculation because he would neither show the incision marks on the child nor identify the person from whom he had taken the infectious matter. Parry cast further doubt on Jones' character in a postscript by suggesting that he had been inspired by greed: 'What he says in answer to your's is, that if you will give him an handsome reward, he will come up to London, and declare to you the whole State of the Case, and will bring witnesses along with him to prove it upon oath.'[68] Jurin wrote Parry on 5 March, thanking him for his letter, agreeing that the credibility of Jones was severely undermined, but none the less asked for further inquiries. In a rather self-righteous tone, Jurin charged that he did not understand 'why he [Jones] should expect what he calls a handsome reward from me, who neither have, nor desire any other recompence for the pains I have taken in my Enquiries about Inoculation, than the satisfaction of doing some Service to my Country....'[69]

Almost two weeks later Jones himself wrote to Jurin and confessed 'I cannot say that I have Inoculat[*sic*] my own Child nor any body els[*sic*] because I do not know what Reall Inoculation is.'[70] And Parry added his own postscript to the affair: 'What Mr Jones has said concerning Inoculation is all rodomontade...'[71] In a final letter concerning this matter, Mr. Tomkies, a surgeon in Oswestry, stated that Jones 'is a fellow of no consideration nor ought to be allow'd of the profession. He was brought up a weaver and follow'd that occupation till I know not by what inspiration he undertook the healing faculty of physick and surgery without being able to read english....'[72] Jones' report became thoroughly discredited in part because of his own confession of ignorance regarding inoculation, but also in part through the knowledge of his social origins. In this instance and others, Jurin relied upon social status as a way to guarantee the accuracy of the accounts sent in by unknown correspondents.

From this detailed discussion of a case history, one may conclude that individual case histories continued to be very powerful tools for convincing others. The fact that Jurin devoted considerable effort to challenging those case histories which undermined inoculation, along with the fact that he published the correspondence relating to disputed cases in his annual account, indicates that he was fully aware of the limitations of his numerical approach. Yet at the same time it is important to stress the vulnerability of case histories as the above instance demonstrates. By their very nature, case histories give rise to questions of authority and testimony. Whose case histories in correspondence are to be regarded as accurate and admitted as evidence? Since Jurin did not know the majority of his correspondents, whose testimony was he to believe and on whose authority? Part of his campaign was precisely to undermine the testimony of those who presented case histories which purportedly demonstrated the ineffectiveness or danger of inoculation.

The published inoculation literature addressed these same concerns. For example, in 1722 Daniel Neal suggested that stories from African blacks concerning inoculation practices should not be accorded full credibility. Referring to an account of inoculation that originated in New England, Neal wrote 'but the Truth of this Relation depending chiefly upon the Testimony of *Negroes*, I should think it worth while to consult some of our English Traders to those Parts, before we give entire Credit to it'.[73] On the other extreme, one pamphleteer stated that the testimony 'given by *Gentlemen* of *Learning* to such a Body as that of the *Royal Society*' concerning inoculation left him no choice but to '... give Credit to their *Testimony*, in a Matter of Fact whereof they were Eye-Witnesses.'[74] In between Africans and members of the Royal Society were the testimonies of among others, doctors, surgeons and apothecaries. Jurin's correspondence reveals these processes of weighting, judging and legitimating testimony in the form of case histories.

Persuasiveness of Jurin's Approach

Jurin received many testimonials to his approach of comparing the mortality of inoculated and natural smallpox. For example, Dr John Woodhouse of Nottingham wrote to him in February of 1726 returning 'Hearty thanks for your good Intentions to the Publick by continuing This Annuall Account which will I doubt not soon Convince all Enemys to this Practice and Establish it for the Great Benefit of Mankind.'[75] Others, such as Dr Dixon, focused on the advantages of Jurin's numerical method: 'I think the Method you pursue of convincing the World by matter of Fact is fair and Just, and Prejudices, in reference to Inoculation, can, I think, be remov'd by no other Means.'[76] Dr Perrott Williams writing from Haverfordwest in Wales praised Jurin's method, stating 'yet I doubt not, but Posterity will hold 'emselves obliged to you for the pains you have taken in drawing up your accurate Calculations, together with the undeniable Conclusions, necessarily flowing from 'em.'[77] And Nettleton wrote in May 1725 about Jurin's annual account for 1724: 'Your Pieces have been every where well received so far as I can learn, and the more because of the strict Neutrality you observe between the contending Partys. The less you appear to favour the side of Inoculation and the more weight your impartial Representation of it will have with the generality of Mankind who are very much prejudiced against it.'[78] And most telling of all, at least one individual declared that Jurin's numerical arguments had persuaded him to inoculate his only daughter. Mr Edlin writing from Holborn in London stated that 'the Disproportion between the Chance of death in the small Pox by natural infection and by Inoculation as it appears in your Books, be such as makes me entertain thoughts of Inoculating the only Child I have as soon as she is able to give so distinct an account of what she ails to enable us to apply proper remedyes....'[79] Among those who objected to Jurin's approach, very few questioned the relevancy of calculations to medicine. Jurin's most prominent opponent, Dr William Wagstaffe, who pointed out that inoculation could not be explained theoretically, summarily dismissed Jurin's figures, describing them as 'some obscure and improper Calculations, scarcely intelligible to any body, or if intelligible, altogether foreign to the Purpose'.[80] But his voice of rejection was a lone one. More typical criticisms addressed the adequacy of Jurin's calculations and figures.

Two apothecaries, Francis Howgrave and Isaac Massey, for example, criticized Jurin by addressing what they saw as fundamental differences between the two groups of people, those with natural smallpox and those with inoculated smallpox, that were implicitly compared. Howgrave's argument focused on the fact that inoculators recommended that only the strong get inoculated.[81] Massey's critique was even more sophisticated, incorporating both economic and health considerations. He disputed Jurin's use of the bills of mortality, 'wherein no Account is made or supposed of those who die of that Distemper for want of proper Necessaries, and by the ignorance of practising Nurses....'[82] He continued:

> The Use I would make of this Observation, is, to shew how insufficient and improper any comparison must needs be between such indigent sick, and the *Inoculated*, who have all imaginable Care and Help afforded them, and for any Person to estimate and compare the success between Patients, *under such unequal Circumstances*, is what, I believe, you did *not well attend to*, or will hereafter *think pertinent to the case in Hand*.[83]

Only the healthy and wealthy were inoculated, while the deaths attributed to smallpox recorded in the bills of mortality generally referred to the poor. Massey put his point succinctly: '... to form a just comparison, and calculate right in this case, the Circumstances of the Patients, must and ought to be as near as may be on a Par'.[84] Arguments such as these focused not on the relevancy of numerical arguments in medicine but on the representativeness and accuracy of calculations.

Conclusions

This essay illustrates the obstacles faced by proponents of a numerical approach to evaluating medical procedures. Jurin's motivations for turning to a numerical approach – that is, to quantify mortality – stemmed from scientific and cultural reasons. Regarding the first, he applied Baconian methods to a new area of knowledge, namely medical practice, which enabled him to pursue a medical topic in the Royal Society.[85] His advertisements requesting case histories allowed him to collect information in a good Baconian fashion and his use of numerical arguments was an explicit appeal to a Newtonian world view and to the methodological precepts of the Royal Society.

Medical practice and therapy raised dilemmas in ways that natural philosophy did not, and the use of numerical arguments provided a means to avoid them. First, by presenting only the number of those inoculated, Jurin avoided the impropriety of printing the names and ages of individuals who preferred to remain anonymous. Second, by focusing on the success rate of inoculation Jurin sidestepped the religious, medical and ethical debates surrounding inoculation. Third, numerical arguments avoided the charges of empiricism – a charge that could damage Jurin's career as a London physician. Typically, only quacks and empirics justified their remedies solely on the basis of success. Jurin's use of a quantitative method was an attempt to make the practice of inoculation appear more philosophical and hence, legitimate. His success was predicated on the reliability of his lists and tables of numbers published in his pamphlets, which, in turn, were dependent on accurate case histories, communicated to him by reliable reporters and correspondents. With the absence of state-sanctioned statistical bureaus, Jurin himself became the guarantee of accuracy. The importance of his position as Secretary to the Royal Society is clear in this context.

These considerations raise an important theme: whether statistics have been deployed in medicine when contemporary medical theory has been incapable of providing a satisfactory theoretical account for why a particular practice might or might not work. The correspondence and publications addressing inoculation in eighteenth-century Britain indicate that numerical and probabilistic arguments were enthusiastically embraced, at least by some members of the public, thus confirming observations made by historians such as Patricia Cline Cohen, James Cassedy and John Money, that numeracy in all its many facets was on the rise in the eighteenth century.[86] Indeed the story of the role of numerical arguments in the inoculation controversy is in part a social history of the reception and acceptance of probabilistic and quantitative reasoning and complements the recent histories of probabilistic ideas by Lorraine Daston, Ian Hacking, and others.[87]

It is, however, a story about medical practice, not natural knowledge, and this is an important difference. This story shows the important role of individual case histories, particularly in disputed cases, and raises the question of what is the persuasive power of a case history. Perhaps case histories are powerful because they are narratives about individuals, invoking a range of human sentiments that numerical odds simply do not. Numbers are inherently *impersonal*, and perhaps for this reason they are less persuasive to individuals, especially patients and healers, who generally perceive and present their lives and illnesses in narrative fashion.

Acknowledgement

I would like to thank the Wellcome Trust for a grant which has given me the opportunity to edit the James Jurin correspondence with Professors W. F. Bynum and Roy Porter at the Wellcome Institute for the History of Medicine. I presented an earlier version of this paper to the workshop 'Questions of Evidence, Medicine in the 18th and 19th Centuries', at the University of Essex, 5 June, 1993, and I would like to thank the participants for their questions and comments. In addition, this essay has been improved immeasurably by the critical readings of Ken Arnold, John Carson, Paul Lucier, Roy Porter, Molly Sutphen and Andrew Wear.

Figure 1

TABLE I.

Years	Total N° of Burials	Died of the Small Pox. In all.	In 1000	In Proportion.
1667	15842	1196	75	$\frac{1}{13}$
1668	17278	1987	115	$\frac{1}{9}$
1669	19432	951	49	$\frac{1}{20}$
1670	20198	1465	73	$\frac{1}{14}$
1671	15729	696	44	$\frac{1}{23}$
1672	18230	1116	61	$\frac{1}{16}$
1673	17504	853	49	$\frac{1}{21}$
1674	21201	2507	118	$\frac{1}{8}$
1675	17244	997	58	$\frac{1}{17}$
1676	18732	359	19	$\frac{1}{52}$
1677	19067	1678	88	$\frac{1}{11}$
1678	20678	1798	87	$\frac{1}{12}$
1679	21730	1967	91	$\frac{1}{11}$
1680	21053	689	33	$\frac{1}{31}$
1681	23971	2982	125	$\frac{1}{8}$
1682	20691	1408	68	$\frac{1}{15}$
1683	20587	2096	102	$\frac{1}{10}$
1684	23202	156	7	$\frac{1}{149}$
1685	23222	2496	107	$\frac{1}{9}$
1686	22609	1062	47	$\frac{1}{21}$
20 Years	398200	28459	$71\frac{1}{2}$	$\frac{1}{14}$
Each Year at a *Medium*	19910	1423	$71\frac{1}{2}$	$\frac{1}{14}$

James Jurin, 'A Letter to the Learned Dr Caleb Cotesworth',
Philosophical Transactions xxxii (1723), 217.

Figure 2

TABLE II.

Years	Total N° of Burials	Died of the Small Pox.		
		In all.	In 1000	In Proportion.
1701	20471	1095	53	1/19
1702	19481	311	16	1/63
1703	20720	898	43	1/23
1704	22684	1501	66	1/15
1705	22097	1095	50	1/20
1706	19847	721	36	1/28
1707	21600	1078	50	1/20
1708	21291	1687	79	1/13
1709	21800	1024	47	1/21
1710	24620	3138	127	1/8
1711	19833	915	46	1/22
1712	21198	1943	92	1/11
1713	21057	1614	77	1/13
1714	26569	2810	106	1/9
1715	22232	1057	48	1/21
1716	24436	2427	99	1/10
1717	23446	2211	94	1/11
1718	26523	1884	71	1/14
1719	28347	3229	114	1/9
1720	25454	1440	57	1/18
1721	26142	2375	91	1/11
1722	25750	2167	84	1/12
22 Years	505598	36620	72	1/14
Each Year at a *Medium*.	22982	1665	72	1/14
42 Years	903798	65079	72	1/14
Each Year in 42 at a *Medium*.	21519	1550	72	1/14

James Jurin, 'A Letter to the Learned Dr Caleb Cotesworth'. *Philosophical Transactions* xxxii (1723), 218.

Notes

1. As Theodore Porter has pointed out, the word statistics originated in Germany (*Statistik*), and referred to a thorough, but not necessarily quantitative description of the state. It was first used in Britain by John Sinclair at the end of the eighteenth century, and did not become

primarily associated with numbers until the 1820s. For these reasons, I have chosen to use phrases such as 'numerical evidence' and 'numerical arguments' to refer to eighteenth-century activities. See Theodore M. Porter, *The Rise of Statistical Thinking 1820–1900* (Princeton: Princeton University Press, 1986).

2. Erwin Ackerknecht, *Medicine at the Paris Hospital 1794–1848* (Baltimore: Johns Hopkins Press, 1967); Ulrich Troehler, 'Quantification in British Medicine and Surgery 1750–1830, with Special Reference to its Introduction into Therapeutics', Ph.D. Dissertation, University of London, 1978; *idem*, '"To Improve the Evidence of Medicine": Arithmetic Observation in Clinical Medicine in the 18th and Early 19th Centuries', *History and Philosophy of the Life Sciences Supplement* x (1988), 31–40; Andrea A. Rusnock, 'The Quantification of Things Human: Medicine and Political Arithmetic in Enlightenment England and France', Ph.D. Dissertation, Princeton University, 1990.
3. During the Analyst controversy, Jurin published under the pseudonym Philalethes Cantabrigiensis. See *Geometry no Friend to Infidelity; or a Defense of Sir Isaac Newton & the British Mathematicians* (London: 1734); and *The Minute Mathematician; or the Freethinker no Just Thinker* (London: 1735). For examples of Jurin's other works, see: *Dissertationes Physico-mathematicae* (London: 1732); *On Distinct and Indistinct Vision*, appended to Robert Smith's *Optics* (London: 1738); *An Account of the Effects of Soap-Lye taken Internally for the Stone* (London: 1742); and *Lettre à M. de Buffon...En réponse à quelques Censures contenuès dans le traité du Coeur de M Senac* (Paris: 1749).
4. See James Jurin: 'A Letter to the Learned Caleb Cotesworth, MD, FRS, of the College of Physicians, and Physician to St. Thomas's Hospital, Containing A Comparison between the Mortality of the Natural Small Pox, and That Given by Inoculation,' *Philosophical Transactions*, xxxii (1723), 213–24, and published separately as a pamphlet with additions, *A Letter to the Learned Caleb Cotesworth ... To Which is Subjoined an Account of the Success of Inoculation in New-England; As Likewise an Extract from Several Letters concerning a Like Method of Communicating the Small-Pox, That Has Been Used Time Out of Mind in South Wales* (London: 1723); *An Account of the Success of Inoculating the Small Pox in Great Britain with a Comparison Between the Miscarriages in that Practice, and the Mortality of the Natural Small Pox* (London: 1724); *An Account of the Success of Inoculating the Small Pox in Great Britain, for the Year 1724* (London: 1725); *An Account of the Success of Inoculating the Small Pox in Great Britain, for the Year 1725* (London: 1726); *An Account of the Success of Inoculating the Small Pox in Great Britain, for the Year 1726* (London: 1727).
5. Marie Boas Hall highlighted the role played by the Royal Society in promoting and publicizing correspondence among natural philoso-

phers, especially under the secretaryship of Henry Oldenburg. See Marie Boas Hall, 'The Royal Society's Role in the Diffusion of Information in the Seventeenth Century', *Notes and Records of the Royal Society*, xxviii (1973–4), 173–92.

6. Recent work in the history of science and cultural history more generally has highlighted these issues and suggested ways in which natural philosophers and others attempted to address challenges to authority. See, for example, Steven Shapin and Simon Schaffer, *Leviathan and the Air Pump – Hobbes, Boyle, and the Experimental Life* (Princeton: Princeton University Press, 1986).
7. Shapin raised these issues in the context of experiments and natural history observations which could not be brought to the Royal Society. In these cases, testimony became 'crucial'. See Steven Shapin, 'The House of Experiment in Seventeenth-Century England', *Isis,* lxxix (1988), 373–404. Marie Boas Hall also noted that credibility of reports became an increasingly important issue in the Royal Society with the decline of experimental demonstrations at their meetings. See Hall, *Promoting Experimental Learning – Experiment and the Royal Society 1660–1727* (Cambridge: Cambridge University Press, 1991).
8. Emanuele Timoni, 'An Account, or History, of the Procuring the Small Pox by Incision, or Inoculation; As it Has for Some Time Been Practised at Constantinople', *Philosophical Transactions,* xxix (1714), 72–82; Jacob Pylarini, 'Nova et tuta variolas excitandi per transplantationem methodus; nuper inventa et in usum tracta: qua rite peracta immunia in posterum praeservantur ab hujusmodi contagio corpora', (Venice: 1715), reprinted in *Philosophical Transactions,* xxix (1716), 393–9. See Genevieve Miller, *The Adoption of Inoculation for Smallpox in England and France* (Philadelphia: University of Pennsylvania Press, 1957), 55–63.
9. The history of inoculation in Britain is well-trod historical terrain. Genevieve Miller's excellent comparative study of the adoption of inoculation in England and France remains the benchmark for all subsequent studies; see Miller, *op. cit.* (note 8). More recently, Peter Razzell has called attention to the widespread practice of inoculation in late eighteenth-century Britain, and questioned the exact relations between vaccination and inoculation. Peter Razzell, *The Conquest of Smallpox: The Impact of Inoculation on Smallpox Mortality in Eighteenth Century Britain* (Sussex: Caliban Books, 1977); *idem, Edward Jenner's Cowpox Vaccine: The History of a Medical Myth* (Sussex: Caliban Books, 1977). Deborah Brunton has examined the extent to which inoculation was practised in Scotland: 'Smallpox Inoculation and Demographic Trends in Eighteenth-Century Scotland', *Medical History,* xxxvi (1992), 403–29; and *idem,* 'Pox Britannica: Smallpox Inoculation in Britain, 1727–1830', Ph.D. Dissertation, University of Pennsylvania, 1990. J. R. Smith has focused on smallpox in Essex, see *The Speckled Monster, Smallpox in*

England, 1670–1970, with particular reference to Essex (Chelmsford: Essex Record Office, 1987). Others have looked at the political allegiances of inoculators, providing yet another axis to plot the controversy surrounding inoculation. See Adrian Wilson, 'The politics of medical improvement in early Hanoverian London', in Andrew Cunningham and Roger French (eds), *The Medical Enlightenment of the Eighteenth Century* (Cambridge: Cambridge University Press, 1990), 4–39; and Francis M. Lobo, 'John Haygarth, Smallpox and Religious Dissent in Eighteenth-century England', *ibid.*, 217–53. Finally, Larry Stewart has examined the Royal Society's interest in the use of inoculation in the slave trade; see Stewart, 'The Edge of Utility: Slaves and Smallpox in the Early Eighteenth Century,' *Medical History*, xxix (1985), 54–70.

10. William Wagstaffe, *A Letter to Dr. Freind; Shewing the Danger and Uncertainty of Inoculating the SmallPox* (London:1722), 5.
11. The pamphlet literature on inoculation is extensive and for the most part repetitive. See Miller's book for a bibliography of English and French pamphlets. Miller, *op. cit.* (note 8).
12. Jurin, *op. cit.* (note 4), 214.
13. There are many articles and books which address this theme. For some of the most recent, see Shapin & Schaffer, *op. cit.* (note 6), Michael Hunter, *Establishing the New Science: The Experience of the Early Royal Society* (Woodbridge and Wolfeboro: Boydell and Brewer, 1989); Peter Dear, '*Totius in verba*: Rhetoric and Authority in the Early Royal Society', *Isis*, lxxvii (1985), 145–61; and Larry Stewart, *The Rise of Public Science – Rhetoric, Technology, and Natural Philosophy in Newtonian Britain, 1660–1750* (Cambridge: Cambridge University Press, 1992).
14. Miller highlighted Nettleton's role in suggesting a statistical analysis. See Miller, *op. cit.* (note 8), 111–16.
15. See Nettleton to Jurin, 5 May, 1722, Royal Society *Early Letters* N.1.92; and 'A Letter from Dr Nettleton, Physician at Halifax in Yorkshire, to Dr Whitaker, concerning the Inoculation of the Small Pox', *Philosophical Transactions*, xxxii (1722), 35–48.
16. Nettleton to Jurin, 16 December, 1722, Royal Society *Early Letters* N.1.94.
17. Jurin to Nettleton, 8 January, 1723, Wellcome MS. 6146.
18. See *Philosophical Transactions*, xxxii (1723), no. 378, unnumbered last page; xxxiii (1724), no. 383, unnumbered last page. Jurin altered the invitation in later years as I will discuss below.
19. Jurin, *Account* (1724), unnumbered last page of pamphlet.
20. These letters may be found in the Inoculation Papers, Royal Society, *Classified Papers* XXIII (1–2); Royal Society *Early Letters*; Jurin Correspondence, Library of the Wellcome Institute; and 'Letters relating to Inoculation', Sloane MS 406B, British Library.
21. Jurin, *Account* (1724), 12.

22. The Journal Books of the Royal Society recorded many accounts of inoculation presented at their meetings. See, for example, Royal Society *Journal Books*, XII, 22 March 1722.
23. Nettleton to Jurin, 5 May, 1722, Royal Society *Early Letters* N.1.92.
24. Nettleton to Jurin, 24 January, 1723, Royal Society *Early Letters* N.1.95.
25. Jones to Jurin, 25 April, 1724, Royal Society, *Classified Papers* XXIII(2), no. 17.
26. Oliver to Jurin, 16 February, 1725, Royal Society, *Classified Papers* XXIII(2), no. 53.
27. Jurin to Fuller, 19 February, 1726, Royal Society, *Classified Papers* XXIII(2), no. 5.
28. Jurin to Fuller, 19 February, 1726, Royal Society, *Classified Papers* XXIII(2), no. 5.
29. Jurin to Hepburn, 18 February, 1724, Royal Society, *Classified Papers* XXIII(2), no. 2.
30. Woodhouse to Jurin, 14 February, 1726, Royal Society, *Classified Papers* XXIII(2), no. 89.
31. See, for example, Jurin to Woodhouse, 12 February, 1726; Jurin to Thorold, 30 March, 1727; Royal Society, *Classified Papers* XXIII (2), nos 3 & 14.
32. Jurin to Towgood, 6 April, 1727, Royal Society, *Classified Papers* XXIII(2), no. 15.
33. Hepburn to Jurin, 18 February, 1724; Brady to Jurin, 21 February, 1724; Burges to Jurin, 21 April, 1726; Royal Society, *Classified Papers* XXIII(1), nos 71, 19 & 30.
34. Amyand to Jurin, 16 January, 1724, Royal Society, *Classified Papers* XXIII(1), no. 2.
35. Roy Porter has recently argued that patient confidentiality and privacy depended on class in the nascent medical journalism of the eighteenth century. Reporters' names, however, were frequently published especially in controversial subjects as a guarantee of authenticity. See Porter, 'The Rise of Medical Journalism in Britain to 1800,' in W. F. Bynum, Stephen Lock and Roy Porter (eds), *Medical Journals and Medical Knowledge –Historical Essays* (London: Routledge, 1992), 6–28.
36. Jurin, *Account* (1724), 3.
37. *Ibid.*, 4.
38. Oliver to Jurin, 29 July, 1730, Royal Society *Early Letters* O.2.182.
39. Jurin, *Account* (1724), 17.
40. Jurin published the letters from Amyand and Lady Percivall in his *Account ... for the Year 1725* (1726), 36–53.
41. 'A Copy of the Journall of the Right Honble. the Lady Percivall during the Inoculation of her Son George aged 3 years', Royal Society, *Classified Papers* XXIII(2), no. 62. Reprinted in Jurin, *Account...for the Year 1725* (1726), 38–46.

42. Monro to [Jurin], 14 April, 1726, Royal Society *Classified Papers* XXIII(2), no. 32. Reprinted in Jurin, *Account ... for the Year 1725* (1726), 50–3.
43. *Ibid.*
44. Amyand to Jurin, 26 August, 1725, Royal Society *Classified Papers* XXIII(1), no. 8. Reprinted in Jurin, *Account...for the Year 1725* (1726), 37–8.
45. Jurin, *Account ... for the Year 1725* (1726), 54.
46. Jurin to Nettleton, 31 March, 1726, Royal Society, *Classified Papers* XXIII(2), no. 9.
47. Nettleton to Jurin, 17 November, 1725; Nettleton to Jurin, 26 November, 1725; and Nettleton to Jurin, 22 March, 1726; Royal Society, *Classified Papers* XXIII(2), nos. 38, 39 & 40.
48. Jurin, *Account* (1724), 29.
49. Jurin, 'A Letter to the Learned Dr Caleb Cotesworth,' 217–18.
50. *Ibid.*, 216.
51. John Graunt, *Natural and Political Observations made upon the Bills of Mortality* (London: 1662).
52. Jurin, 'A Letter to the Learned Dr Caleb Cotesworth', 219.
53. Jurin conceded that some infant deaths might be due to smallpox, but went on to argue: '... but then, on the other hand, as it is certain, that of the remaining 614/1000 of Mankind, that are above one or two years of Age, there are great Numbers, that never have the Small Pox, it will I presume be judged to be no unequal Supposition, if I suppose all that are contain'd under the Heads abovemention'd [i.e., infant diseases], to have miss'd that Distemper, when by way of Compensation, I allow all the remainder of Mankind to undergo it; which Concession is so large, that it will abundantly make up for what I assume too much in the former Supposition.' Jurin, 'A Letter to the Learned Dr Caleb Cotesworth', 220.
54. *Ibid.*, 220–1.
55. Dixon to Jurin, 15 February, 1726, Royal Society, *Classified Papers* XXIII(1), no. 49.
56. Lynch to Jurin, 20 January, 1727, Royal Society, *Classified Papers* XXIII(2), no. 25.
57. Beard to Jurin, 9 November, 1726, Royal Society, *Classified Papers* XXIII(1), no. 33.
58. Perrott Williams wrote to Jurin that in Pembroke smallpox 'has entirely ceased above a twelvemonth ago, and I perceive some of the Inhabitants of that Town are (for some reasons to 'emselves best known) very unwilling to have the number of such as lost their Lives by the Small-Pox discover'd, and consequently very industrious to conceal their Names etc.' Williams to Jurin, 23 April, 1724, Royal Society *Early Letters* W.3.132.
59. Jurin, *Account* (1724), 7.
60. Jurin to Beard, 3 December, 1726, Royal Society, *Classified Papers*

XXIII(2), no. 12.

61. Edlin to Jurin, 15 September, 1726, Royal Society, *Classified Papers* XXIII(1), no. 54.
62. Bayly to Jurin, 29 February, 1724, Royal Society, *Classified Papers* XXIII(1), no. 20.
63. Jurin, *Account ... for the Year 1725* (1726), 10–11.
64. Jurin, *Account ... for the Year 1725* (1726).
65. Jurin, *Account ... for the Year 1725* (1726), unnumbered last two pages.
66. William Clinch, *An Historical Essay on the Rise and Progress of the Small-Pox. To Which is Added, a Short Appendix, to Prove, That Inoculation Is No Security from the Natural Small-Pox* (London: 1725).
67. Jurin to Jones, 22 February, 1726, Royal Society, *Classified Papers* XXIII(2), no. 7; also see Jurin, *Account ... for the Year 1725* (1726).
68. Parry to Jurin, 1 March, 1726, Royal Society, *Classified Papers* XXIII(2), no. 64; also see Jurin, *Account ... for the Year 1725* (1726).
69. Jurin to Parry, 5 March, 1726, Royal Society, *Classified Papers* XXIII(2), no. 8; also see Jurin, *Account ... for the Year 1725* (1726).
70. Jones to Parry, 11 March, 1726, Royal Society, *Classified Papers* XXIII(2), no. 20; also see Jurin, *Account ... for the Year 1725* (1726).
71. Parry to Jurin, 13 March, 1726, Royal Society, *Classified Papers* XXIII(2), no. 65.
72. Tomkies to Amyand, 5 September, 1726, Royal Society, *Classified Papers* XXIII(2), no. 74.
73. Benjamin Colman, *A Narrative of the Method and Success of Inoculating the Small-Pox in New England. With a Reply to the Objections Made Against It from Principles of Conscience. In a Letter from a Minister at Boston. To Which Is Now Prefixed an Historical Introduction by Daniel Neal* (London: 1722), 6.
74. Benjamin Colman, *Some Observations on the New Method of Receiving the Small-Pox by Ingrafting or Inoculating* (Boston: 1721), 1.
75. Woodhouse to Jurin, 9 February, 1726, Royal Society, *Classified Papers* XXIII(2), no. 90.
76. Dixon to Jurin, 15 February, 1726, Royal Society, *Classified Papers* XXIII(1), no. 49.
77. Williams to Jurin, 19 March, 1723, Royal Society *Early Letters* W.3.131.
78. Nettleton to Jurin, 31 May, 1725, Royal Society *Early Letters* N.1.98.
79. Edlin to Jurin, 15 September, 1726, Royal Society *Classified Papers* XXIII(1), no. 54.
80. Wagstaffe, *op. cit.* (note 10), 48. Wagstaffe's objections were directed against Arbuthnot's pamphlet, but one can assume he felt similarly about Jurin's approach. See [John Arbuthnot], *Mr. Maitland's Account of Inoculating the Small-Pox vindicated from Dr Wagstaffe's Misrepresentations of That Practice, with Some Remarks on Mr. Massey's Sermon* (London: 1722).

81. Francis Howgrave, *Reasons against the Inoculation of the Small-Pox* (London: 1724), 69.
82. Isaac Massey, *A Short and Plain Account of Inoculation; with Some Remarks on the Main Arguments Made Use of to Recommend That Practice, by Mr. Maitland and Others,* 2nd edn (London: 1723), postscript, 2.
83. *Ibid.*, postscript, 3.
84. *Ibid.*, postscript, 5.
85. Although it should be noted that medical topics occupied a significant position in the Royal Society's affairs from its foundation. See A. Rupert Hall, 'Medicine in the Early Royal Society', in Allen G. Debus (ed.), *Medicine in Seventeenth Century England* (Berkeley: University of California Press, 1974), 421–52; *idem,* 'English Medicine in the Royal Society's Correspondence: 1660–1677', *Medical History,* xv (1971), 11–25; and Roy Porter, 'The Early Royal Society and the Spread of Medical Knowledge', in Roger French and Andrew Wear (eds), *The Medical Revolution of the Seventeenth Century* (Cambridge: Cambridge University Press, 1989), 272–93.
86. Cohen and Cassedy are primarily concerned with developments in North America, and Money in Britain. See Patricia Cline Cohen, *A Calculating People: The Spread of Numeracy in Early America* (Chicago: University of Chicago Press, 1982); Cohen, 'Reckoning with Commerce: Numeracy in Eighteenth-Century America', in John Brewer and Roy Porter (eds), *Consumption and the World of Goods* (London and New York: Routledge, 1993), 320–34; James H. Cassedy, *Demography in Early America — Beginnings of the Statistical Mind, 1600–1800* (Cambridge: Harvard University Press, 1969); John Money, 'Teaching in the Market-Place, or "Caesar adsum jam forte aderat": The Retailing of Knowledge in Provincial England during the Eighteenth Century', in John Brewer and Roy Porter (eds.), *Consumption and the World of Goods* (London and New York: Routledge, 1993), 335–79.
87. See Lorraine J. Daston, *Classical Probability in the Enlightenment* (Princeton: Princeton University Press, 1988); Ian Hacking, *The Emergence of Probability* (Cambridge: Cambridge University Press, 1975); *idem, The Taming of Chance* (Cambridge: Cambridge University Press, 1990); Gerd Gigerenzer, Zeno Swijtink, Theodore Porter, Lorraine Daston, John Beatty, and Lorenz Krüger, *The Empire of Chance – How Probability Changed Science and Everyday Life* (Cambridge: Cambridge University Press, 1989).

13

Methodism and Dr George Cheyne's 'More Enlightening Principles'

David E. Shuttleton

> 'For Christ's sake, my Christian brethren, if you have any regard to the *health* of your souls, shun, as you would the *plague*, these anti-Christian recreations...'
>
> The people, seeing a man of a tolerable appearance thus exalted above the crowd, and preparing to harangue, began to stare, and to enquire of each other what he would be at! As they heard imperfectly the word *health*, and more words of a medicinal tendency, the prevailing opinion was, that a mountebank was going to dispense his medicines for the benefit of mankind: and Tugwell's wallet was supposed to contain the sovereign packet of the learned Doctor. Mr. Wildgoose, however soon undeceived them, by addressing the crowd in the apostolical style; though he had not yet aquired the true *bon ton* or Gospel lingo of Mr. Whitfield [sic] and his associates.
>
> Richard Graves, *The Spiritual Quixote* (1773)

Mockers of early Methodism were quick to equate religious and medical quackery. Field-preachers were caricatured as mountebanks selling instant spiritual panaceas to a gullible populace. The fact that the founders of Methodism promoted preventive asceticism as a means to physical and spiritual *Restoration* or *New Birth*, and took a practical interest in lay-medicine encouraged such satire.[1] In particular John Wesley's career as a medico-religionist might be placed within an established tradition of Pietist medicine which, in its British manifestation, is only now coming under serious scholarly investigation. Jonathan Barry, in his detailed study, 'Piety and the Patient: Medicine and Religion in Eighteenth-Century Bristol', has mapped some of the complex interelationships between forms of Pietism and medical practice in an early Methodist stronghold.[2]

Barry focuses upon the diaries (1751–1801), of the Bristol accountant and amateur healer, William Dyer (b. 1730), who belonged to a loose, somewhat ecumenical circle of educated Pietists active in the Bath-Bristol area during the period of the 1750s to the 1770s, many of whom were close associates of Methodism, if not actual converts. Like Wesley, Dyer became a private practitioner in electrical therapy as a result of studying William Law's Behmenist analogy between fire and divine energy. Consequently he helped to edit the theosophical study *Fire Analysed* (Bristol, 1771), by Law's correspondent, the Bristol rector Richard Symes. Typically, Dyer studied a broad Pietist-theosophical tradition represented by such 'mystics' as Jacob Boehme, Madam Guyon, Baron Marsay, Pierre Poiret and Law, and he assisted in the related editing projects of the evangelical Bristol bookseller Thomas Mills, who printed works like Boehme's *The Way to Christ Discovered and Described* (1775), and *An Address to all Orders of Men Recommending the Works of William Law etc.* (1781). Dyer sympathetically recorded the deaths of two older West Country Pietist physicians, Dr Charles Middleton, the Bristol man-midwife and his famous brother-in-law, the obese Scottish-born dietician, Dr George Cheyne of Bath (1672–1743).

As the most prominent and materially successful medico-religionist of the early Georgian period, Cheyne deserves closer attention as a spiritual father-figure to this movement.[3] Symes had once been Cheyne's medical disciple. More obscure associates were Stephen Penny, who endorsed Cheyne's doctrines in his *Letters on the Fall and Restoration of Mankind* (Bristol 1765), and the Wells physician and Hutchinsonian, Dr John Robertson, a childhood friend of Middleton, who had earlier served George Cheyne as translator of his works into Latin. More notably, the Bath philosopher–physician David Hartley, who had attended his colleague George Cheyne on his deathbed, was also connected to this circle and the influence of Cheyne's Behmenist-Newtonian theology can be felt in the accounts of the relationship between 'Sensory Vibrations', and the theopathic love of God in the *Observations on Man* (1749). But above all, Cheyne's significant role as a key link in this tradition lies in the fact that William Law's own development of a mystical theology had been encouraged by direct contact with Cheyne. The physician not only introduced Law to Boehme's works but also put him in touch with an established network of scholarly Pietists (with a London–Scotland–Continental axis), with whom Cheyne had been closely involved since he began a search for 'more enlightening *Principles*', after a physical and spiritual crisis in 1704–5.[4] Barry is right to describe Cheyne as 'a major figure in this intellectual tradition' (167).

By the 1730s Cheyne had established a major, if controversial medical practice as the leading 'nerve doctor' to the over-consumptive Hanoverian establishment. His practical and witty medico-religious tracts, most notably *An Essay of Health and Long Life* (London and Bath, Strahan and Leake, 1724), and *The Natural Method of Cureing the Diseases of the Body and the Disorders of the Mind* (London, Strahan and Knapton, 1742), with their promotion of a 'Milk and Seed Diet' were controversial bestsellers and, according to Arbuthnot, had caused 'Sects in the *Dietetick Philosophy*'.[5] In a recantatory preface to the former, Cheyne had renounced his 'ungentlemanly' role as defender of the iatro-mathematical theories of his Edinburgh mentor, Dr Archibald Pitcairn, in favour of the spiritual values of 'Naked Faith and Pure Love' which he had absorbed from the inspired outpourings of the French quietist-mystic Madam Jeanne Marie Guyon (1646–1719).[6] Cheyne's freethinking Bristol rival, Dr Thomas Morgan, facetiously noted this professional reorientation in the Preface to his own strictly materialistic *Philosophical Principles of Medicine* (1725):

> A CELEBRATED Member of the Faculty, who, till within these few Years, had been universally allow'd as the greatest Physician in England...rais'd vast Expectations of a new animal Oeconomy; in which the deepest Mysteries of Nature were to be reveal'd, every Particle of Blood measur'd and weigh'd, and all Powers of the minutest Springs and Movements of the animal Machine adjusted, computed and reduced to a mathematical Certainty of fluxionary Geometry.
>
> But this animal Oeconomy never appear'd, and I shall make no reflections upon Theory, because the Doctor seems now to have no great Opinion of Theorys himself; he has, I believe, convinced every body of the Vanity of philosophizing [sic] in Physick. he has found out a better way of rendering mankind immortal, without knowledge of Mathematicks or Mechanism, only by Fasting and Prayer, by subsisting without Meat and Drink, and Living by Faith above the World on the Philosophical Principles of Reveal'd Religion (li–lii).

The last sentence alludes to the fact that Cheyne had first publicly betrayed his unorthodox religious interests in the revisions to his expanded *Philosophical Principles of Religion: Natural and Reveal'd* (London: Strahan, 1715), where he attempts to marry Newtonian physics and Behmenist metaphysics through a notional force of 'spiritual attraction'.

Cheyne's career had always been surrounded by controversy but, as an enthusiastic wit, he gladly embraced martyrdom by the barbed pens of those he dismissed as 'Hackney Scribblers'. It was perhaps inevitable that his name would be invoked in later attacks upon Methodist medical *Enthusiasm.* This vulgar association is nowhere made more blatant than in the sophisticated Fieldingesque comic-romance *The Spiritual Quixote: or the Summer's Ramble of Mr Geoffrey Wildgoose* (1773), by Richard Graves.[7] Significantly, during the years immediately following Cheyne's death, Graves belonged to the intellectual circle of the Bath entrepreneur Ralph Allen in which Cheyne himself had been welcome.[8]

Although begun in 1757, *The Spiritual Quixote* gently satirizes aspects of Methodist activity during the 1730s. In a chapter entitled 'History of a Long-Liver', we meet the Methodist rector, Mr Slicer, a hypochondriacal, valetudinarian, dietary faddist, who entertains his guests with 'the History of Francis Hongo, surnamed Hyppazoli.' Although living to 114,

> Hongo was never sick; his sight, hearing, and intellectual faculties, continued entire unto the last. He would walk seven or eight miles every day. At an hundred, his white hairs are said to have turned black again; and, what is surprizing, having lost all his teeth, at an hundred and ten he cut two large ones in his upper jaw (343).

This parodies Cheyne's admiration for longevists like the Italian, Luigi Cornaro (1475?–1566), author of *Trattato della Vita Sobria* (1558), as part of a broader assault on medical-faddism.[9] Subverting Cheyne's idealized notions of 'Platonick Love', Slicer closes his account with the ironic afterthought that, although 'a man of great merit, wit and honour', Hongo had the minor failing of being 'too greatly attached to the fair sex' and 'had, by his wife and two or three concubines, nine and forty children'. Slicer concludes his story declaring that '*the only way to preserve health, is to eat plain food,* says the Scotchman: *and the only way to destroy it, is to cram in such mixtures as you do in England, since French Cooks have been in vogue.*' But later, in Chapter XVII, (entitled 'Rules for Health'), he warns that whilst health is a great blessing,

> too great a solicitude on that account is not only unworthy a man of sense and a good Christian, but is really destructive of what we are so anxious to preserve...I have read a treatise on sleep, that has kept me awake all night; and studied Dr Cheyne upon *Health and Long Life,* till I brought myself to the brink of *Death* (344–5).

After a youthful attendance at an anatomy class and dabbling in medical books, he had brought himself 'by whims and apprehensions, and by tampering with my own constitution, into a very bad state of health'. A rector present at this conversation remarks:

> It is certainly better to be really ill sometimes than to be so hippish, and perpetually anxious about one's health. A friend of mine, a jolly fellow, finding me in my room with Cheyne's book upon health and Long Life before me, threw it into the fire; partly to cure me of my whims, and partly to repeat extempore:
>
> *I'd scorn the health, such rigid rules must give;*
> *Nor Sacrifice the ends of life, to live* (346).

A schoolteacher leaps to the defence of Slicer's medical whimsicality, and the quixotic hero Wildgoose adds his own approbation of Cheyne's *Regimen*: 'in many cases, even fasting, or an entire abstinence from all kinds of food; this, at least, if made use of at the beginning of a disease, I have always found sufficient to check the progress, or put a stop to most complaints' (346). Elsewhere in the book further attention is drawn to the parallel between Wildgoose's religious and medical unorthodoxy and related claims to universal restoration or cure (358). In his autobiographical *The Invalid with the Means of Enjoying Health, by a Nonagenarian* (1804), Graves was later to remark that he had once put himself in 'a valetudinary state of health' by following Cheyne's ascetic dietary rules (22–6). His fictional satire prompts a consideration of what precisely was the relationship between Cheyne's established promotion of a preventive medical regimen and the ascetic practices of the founding Methodists.

There is evidence that Cheyne's books directly encouraged the Methodist founders to practise a 'Dietick Gospel' and provided a model for their own promotion of 'Primitive Physick', based upon fundamentalist Christian conception of healing as both a physical and spiritual process of lapsarian *Restoration.* Whitefield's famous conversion at Lent 1735, was precipitated by his emulation of Cheyne's ascetic prescriptions. Significantly this was the climax of a period of soul-searching during which Whitefield sought to experience 'the life of God' within, prompted by his reading of William Law and works by the Scottish Neo-Platonist, William Scougall and the quietist Castanzia. Cheyne had found similar solace in spiritual texts, as he explains in his much-cited account of his breakdown, *The Author's Own Case at Large,* which had recently appeared as a conclusion to his study of nervous disorders, *The English Malady* (London: Strahan, 1733).

Whitefield deliberately imitated the austerities Cheyne records adopting in this account. Writing to Wesley at Epworth from Oxford on 1 April, 1735, Whitefield was in a panic concerning the low state of his health which provided 'the Enemy' with room to 'Blaspheme'.[10] He had just borrowed a copy of Cheyne's *Essay of Health* having 'resolved some time agone ... to consult nothing as to my eating or drinking yet but what should be essentially necessary for the preserving of my body in a fit Condition to serve my Master and fellow Christians'. With little time to 'revise him', he used Cheyne's text as a medical bible or oracle, 'providentially finding a place which I think exactly suits my present case & that is the 9th Chapter wherein he treats of persons of weak nerves, all the symptoms he gives of them jointly incurring in me'.[11] Fearing the onset of a chronic distemper, Whitefield described his symptoms in detail, asking Wesley to reread the relevant passage in Cheyne before offering his advice: 'Dr Cheyne I think prescribes such things as Herbs, Milk etc., for Spring which I would very readily come in with, having little or no appetite and hoping such a way would be a means of mortifying me to sensual pleasures and greatly to promote Christian Purity'. Whitefield thought that illness had providentially brought about 'a much better use of my understanding', which allowed him to keep the Devil at bay. His conversion experience followed very shortly afterwards, when physical weakness drove him to bed for seven weeks.[12]

Whilst Cheyne's *Case* provided a model for Whitefield's search after spiritual restoration, Cheyne's essentially mechanistic account of nervous illness reassured Whitefield that his symptoms were in fact merely physical, and as such not indicative in themselves of either diabolic possession or spiritual growth. They were, however, a dangerous distraction to his 'understanding', by which he could consciously keep Satan at bay. At some later stage Whitefield probably met Cheyne, who contributed a rather stingy 'guinea' 'for the Poor of Georgia', when Whitefield set up a pre-embarcation fund in 1738.[13]

At least three of Cheyne's books formed part of John Wesley's reading during his formative years at Oxford, when his experimental interest in dietary regimens began.[14] On his 68th birthday, he attributed his longevity to a youthful adherence to Cheyne's principles.[15] At an unknown date, Cheyne had personally encouraged Wesley to keep to a strict regimen which he had been tempted to abandoned as offensively over-enthusiastic.[16] In his journal for 12 March, 1742 Wesley records: 'I read part of Dr Cheyne's *Natural Method of Cureing Diseases*, of which I cannot but observe it is one of the most ingenious books which I ever saw. But what epicure will ever regard it? for the man talks against good eating and drinking?' (II, 534).

John Wesley's endorsement of Cheyne's medical doctrines took a practical turn during his stay in America and as part of his mission to the poor in 1746, when he established free dispensaries at The

Foundery, Upper Moorfields and at Bristol. Wesley acknowledged his debt in *Primitive Physick; or an Easy and Natural Method of Curing Most Diseases* (1747), which concludes with 'a few plain, easy Rules, chiefly transcribed from Dr *Cheyne*'.[17] Echoing Cheyne, Wesley's preface talks of the uncorrupted, immortal nature of the pre-lapsarian angelic bodies of men, and endorses Cheyne's account of medical history as a decline into unnecessarily complex theories. According to Wesley, Drs Sydenham, Dover and, latterly, Cheyne were rare exceptions who, amidst great hostility from the profession, returned to basic remedies. Wesley's 'poor-man's' compendium was undoubtedly the most widely read medical book of the late eighteenth century and it served to democratize the preventive doctrines that Cheyne had previously advocated amongst his educated middle- and upper-class clientele.[18] As we have seen, Graves frequently equates dietary faddism with Methodist enthusiasm and this association is supported in fact. A fascinating 'List of some Names and the Places of Abode of persons in whose Minds the Light of God had Arisen, or is Graciously Rising', compiled by the Pietist Ralph Mather in 1775, contains numerous entries like the following:

> Carrickfergus – E. Pendril, shoemaker, a married man, who under great persecution lives in continence, and abstinence from animal food...
>
> Belfast – William Forde, Hercules Lane a poor man, he is not as solid as E.P. but teachable, and lives on roots and water...
>
> Bolton – W. Winkbridge, fifteen years in purification...[19]

John Wesley also took a keen intellectual interest in Cheyne's early attempt to counter rationalist scepticism with a theology of 'naked faith and pure love'.[20] We do not have his reaction to the unorthodox *Discourses* published as the second part of Cheyne's otherwise practical *Essay on Regimen* (London, Strahan and Rivington, 1740), which endorse the heresy of Universal Salvation, but we do know that at Oxford in 1726, Wesley read the revised 'Behmenist' version of Cheyne's *Philosophical Principles*.[21]

There is no overt evidence for Cheyne having had any direct involvement with the Oxford Holy Club. However, the physician was a frequent vistor to Oxford in the early 1730s, when both his son John and his half-brother William were attending St Mary's Hall.[22] Cheyne was on intimate terms with both the College's Jacobite principal, Dr William King and King's guests, Cheyne's old patron George Baillie of Jerviswood and his wife, the songstress Grisell, all of whom were self-confessed 'disciples' of Cheyne's 'Dietick Gospel'.[23] But by the 1740s close connections existed between the Wesley and Cheyne families. After being cured *gratis* of a feverish cold in 1740, Charles Wesley became an intimate friend of Cheyne's brother-in-law, Dr John Middleton of Bristol.[24] When Middleton died, Charles Wesley composed a memorial hymn testifying to the physician's piety. Middleton was reportedly a death bed convert to Methodism. He died in the arms of his friend, Cheyne's translator, Dr John Robertson, who subsequently corresponded with the Wesleys.[25]

Wesley's biographers are probably correct in assuming that it was Cheyne whom he visited on foot from Bristol during the hard frost of December 1741: 'I walked over to Bath, and had a conversation of several hours with one who had lived above seventy, and studied divinity above thirty years; yet remission of sins was quite a new doctrine to him. But I trust God will write it on his heart.'[26] His failure to name Cheyne and the general tone, suggests Wesley's disappointment at not making an immediate convert out of the pious old doctor (we shall return to the question of Cheyne's 'conversion' shortly). In the early 1730s Cheyne began to find other patients who equated his medico-religious doctrines with conversion to the New Faith.

In 1753, when a feverish Sarah Wesley was receiving Dr Middleton's fatherly attentions, she was also visited by Selina Hastings, the Countess of Huntingdon (1707–91), one of Methodism's first aristocratic patrons.[27] Significantly, it had been during a serious bout of ill health that Selina had converted to the New Faith. Her friend Lord Bateman, the nervous dedicatee of *The English Malady* had introduced her to Cheyne, who probably correctly attributed her numerous 'nervous' complaints to being constantly weakened by repeated childbearing.[28] Throughout the 1730s she was an adherent to Cheyne's precepts and he sent her many reassurances that 'in spite of sneer, puzzle, fright and terror', she must persevere in the regimen:[29]

> I extremely approve and rejoice at your ladyship's courage in your diet, not to make you a hugeous compliment. Do you know many ladies of your rank, quality, youth, and necessary high living, that has sense, virtue, or indeed faculties capable of a conviction, resolution, and courage to enter upon such a course of self-denial for these poor disregarded low things (such as they are commonly reckoned), of good spirits, cheerfulness, health, and long-life: and pray what is all the grandeur and glory of the world without them (*Huntingdon,* 10).

Although he feared that she would abandon his regimen, on the whole his genial irony worked. Bateman, a model patient, reported that he had found her 'gay spirituous and lively on milk and vege-tables'. In 1733, she adopted a rigorous 'Milk and Seed' diet. Cheyne remarked that 'it is particular and inconvenient in the world, and all man and womenkind will be up in arms against me, and your ladyship will be often told you are killing yourself by Dr Cheyne's whims' ... 'if I could cure my patients with burgundy and ham pie, I might be cried up to the skies' (28; 41). As he predicted, when she suffered an attack of 'Hysteric Colic' in 1734, the London physicians blamed Cheyne's methods.

Throughout 1733 Cheyne was urging Lady Huntingdon (suffering from certain post-natal complications which she was too bashful to describe in her letters), to visit Bristol, via Bath, in order to benefit from water-treatment and personal consultations with both himself and Dr Middleton (33–4). In 1735 she was delivered of what Cheyne welcomed as a 'fine vegetable child'. After a lapse, in February 1737, Cheyne was congratulating her on returning to 'the simplicity of the dietetical Ghospel [sic]' and reprovingly cites the example of Bateman, who does not 'apostatize nor hunt new medicines' (58), Whilst there is a playful tone in Cheyne's use of this sectarian vocabulary, none the less his sincere Pietist aims suggest many parallels with the religious injunctions of Methodism. This is particularly evident in his advice that the Countess should use her intuition as a guide: 'For Nature and your feeling will point it out. Providence and its sovereign has got you in his power, and you must only attend to him, and he will bring you by your feelings to the condition he wants you to be in; the cross is his school and it will teach you true wisdom' (50). Cheyne might easily be talking about the New Faith, rather than merely faith in his 'dietetical Ghospel'. It illustrates the affective basis of his mature medico-religious philosophy, and the validity his sympathetic doctrine of nervous sensibility gave to feelings, moreover a woman's feelings, as a valid test of moral truth. Inevitably, satirists equated Lady Huntingdon's medical faddism with her religious unorthodoxies. Richard Graves caricatures an aristocratic convert, Lady Sherwood, in *The Spiritual Quixote:* 'she listened with the same attention to the enthusiastic doctrines of these itinerant Preachers, as a person labouring under an hypochondriacal distemper does to the extravagant pretensions of a Mountebank' (174). This is almost certainly a satiric portrait of Lady Huntingdon, or perhaps Cheyne's other Bath patient, Lady Cox, another Methodist convert.

Cheyne does not discuss doctrinal issues in his extant letters to Lady Huntingdon, but she reveals her deep respect for her physician's piety in writing to her husband from Bath in December 1741, when she reports that after dining with Cheyne and his wife, she had spent the rest of the evening, 'in the most pious and religious conversation, a thing hard to be found here'.[30] A few days later she wrote: 'to-day Dr Cheyne has been sitting with me and has been talking like an old apostle. He really has the most refined notions of the true spiritual religion I almost ever met with. The people of Bath says I have made him a Methodist, but indeed I receive much light and comfort from his conversation'.[31] In the light of this accumulation of evidence for Cheyne's influence upon the founders of Methodism, we might ask whether the Bath gossips were correct in assuming that Cheyne became a convert. Charles Mullett, asking himself the same question in 1940, points to what seems like a slighting remark in a letter of Cheyne's to his patient and printer, Samuel Richardson, in which he asks if the novelist has read William Law's *Appeal to All that Doubt the Gospel* (1740), adding that 'the Methodists should get it by heart'.[32] Cheyne's mature opinion regarding Methodism has in fact survived, buried in John Keble's dense *Life of the Right Reverend Father in God Thomas Wilson, D. D., Lord Bishop of Sodor and Man* (Oxford, 1863), but this is best presented within the context of a brief account of Cheyne's relations with the Wilson family.[33]

Keble's biography reveals that Cheyne was a friend of both the Bishop (1663–1755), and his son of the same name (rector of St Stephen's Walbroke 1737–84). As an outspoken opponent of hard-drinking, Cheyne was one of the 'several physicians' who were consulted by the younger Wilson over the writing of his influential temperance tract *Distilled Spirituous Liquors, the Bane of the Nation* (1736). Bishop Wilson recorded Cheyne in the Mortuary List as 'a most excellent religious physician and philosopher: for whose excellent works I and many more stand indebted'.[34] Cheyne had written to the Bishop's son on 9 March, 1740 that he was glad to hear, with the announcement of his father's tract, *The Indian Instructed*, that 'the good worthy Bishop of Man, continues an honour to human nature, and a faithful dispenser of the words of the holy Jesus'.[35] 'Some months later', Cheyne warmly acknowledged the receipt of the work in question: 'I esteem it much, for its justness, solidity, and propriety for the end proposed ... I gave a copy to good Mr Jones, who is the source and great promoter of the Welch [siç] schools'.[36] Wilson's popular *Essay Towards an Instruction for the Indians* (1740), (17 editions by 1802), dedicated to the Trustees of the Colony of Georgia, was motivated, as its preface reveals, by a millennialist concern with the conversion of the Indians (considered remnants of the Tribe of Israel).[37] Cheyne took a practical interest in these missionary endeavours, but had little joy when he tried to distribute the tract amongst the Bristol dealers to the West Indies: 'alas! they are most of them pirates and Madagascar men'.[38] Similar efforts amongst the 'Jamaica traders' were equally fruitless, the Spanish War having thrown the West Indian merchant fleet into a state of perpetual alarm. In the face of these hindrances to his zealous attempts to speed on the millennium, Cheyne reflected resignedly upon the progress of the 'Divine Restoration':

> We do our best, and wait God's time, and seize only the moments of eternity ... I hope, though the nation, especially those of the two extremes, the highest and the greatest, and the lowest and most abject, be extremely ignorant, corrupted, and vicious, yet there is the dawning of some good spirit abroad among the middling rank; and that even the Methodists, though novices, indiscreet and precipitate, may be sent to move the waters, to bring some to hearken to the gentle, still voice, which in time may lead them into solid truth, if the evil spirit do not creep in, as it has ever done in all these specious pretensions and divisions. But the times and seasons are in the hands of the Father. 'What is that to thee? Follow thou Me?.'. Depend on it, whatever be your or my outward state of existence, you shall, and all your relatives, possess the heart and all the most tender and amiable affections and actions of mine ... (Keble, I, 924–5).

As Cheyne's most overt extant comment on the contemporary state of Britain this reveals his cynical view of the aristocracy, tainted by luxury and vice, and equal despair at the depravity of what he thought were the insensitive labouring classes. It was in the rising 'middling-classes' that he saw hope of spiritual restoration. Cheyne placed his long-held hopes for moral recovery in men like his pious printer, Samuel Richardson, who epitomized the principles of frugality, restraint and cultivated sensibility which Cheyne advocated in his medico-religious works.[39] Though sympathetic, Cheyne clearly had misgivings about the socially disruptive effects of Methodist *Enthusiasm*.

Cheyne's early years in late seventeenth-century Scotland had convinced him that sectarian dissent discredited Christianity, creating damaging, sometimes violent social divisions. At the time of his own religious reawakening, he had observed several members of the circle of Episcopalian 'mystics', who he considered his 'Spiritual friends', abandon their outwardly conformist 'internal religion', for the agitations of the French or Camisard Prophets, a radical Protestant sect whose ecstatic mission to Britain, beginning in 1706, was characterized by public displays of shouting, dancing, nudity, and claims of miraculous healings, prophesies, resurrections and sudden conversions.[40] When the

Prophets arrived, several of Cheyne's predominantly Scottish circle had already identified themselves with the patiently restrained millenarian hopes of the Philadelphians (the English Behmenists), amongst whom the Camisards found early converts. When Methodist converts made similar claims to miracles and prophecy over two decades later, critics were quick to make comparisons with the Camisard Prophets. John Wesley disapproved of the extravagant claims of his followers, but in Bristol he made converts amongst a small group of second-generation Prophets. Cheyne (or Middleton), was probably the physician who first informed Wesley of the activities of the original Prophets, and in particular that of Cheyne's intimate patient, the Scottish Pietist Andrew Cunningham of Barnes (d. 1715). Cunningham become a leading convert in 1709, after a certain Fifeshire convert, Lady Abden employed her child as a medium to reveal knowledge of private conversations which had taken place earlier at Bath between Cunningham and Cheyne.[41]

All the fragmentary evidence indicates that from the outset, Cheyne endorsed the verdicts of those amongst his quietist associates, notably Andrew (later Chevalier) Ramsay, the London Pietist physician Dr James Keith, and their spiritual mentors, Dr George Garden, Dr Francis Lee and Pierre Poiret, who all repudiated the Camisards (and Cunningham), as either deluded or ill and who choose to distance themselves from such anarchic social activities.[42] The detailed work of Hillel Schwartz on the history of the Prophets has done much to enlarge our understanding of the distinctions and connections between the Pietist sects with whom Cheyne had contact.[43] In so doing, Schwartz plots a move amongst British Pietists towards an introverted, quietist millenarianism by the second decade of the eighteenth century which absorbed the more radical ethos of the Prophets.[44] This shift is particularly important for an understanding of the role of mysticism in Cheyne's later career, as the psychological obsession with mental calm and stability ('recollection'), informing this reactionary tradition came to underscore his influential doctrines of nervous sensibility. Cheyne shared his mystical-millenarianism with other outwardly conformist scholarly 'seekers' whose sentimental mysticism fused the Augustinian tradition informing the quietism of Guyon with the Behmenist absorption of Hermetic and Neo-Platonic concepts of correspondence (or as Cheyne termed it 'Divine Analogy), in a politically cautious, patient, introverted ethos of the 'Restoration of all Things'.[45]

The distinction between this quietist millenarianism and the 'enthusiastic sensibility' of the Camisards was usefully defined back in 1943 by J. L. Davis in an article revealing entitled *Mystical versus*

Enthusiastic Sensibility.[46] Davis argues that 'there are adequate grounds for making a distinction between Mysticism and Enthusiasm as historical types of Christian sensibility' (301). The mystical type is associated primarily with St Augustine and Neo-Platonism, (with which Cheyne was deeply engaged), whereas that of the enthusiast was often identified with the tradition of Montanus, (as in Francis Lee's overtly anti-Camisard, *History of Montanism,* printed in George Hickes edition of *The Spirit of Enthusiasm Exorcised* (4th edition, London, 1710)). Both traditions 'involved the conviction that the individual might know God as a presence through Christ or the Holy Ghost, and that this knowledge was a mode of complete experience that enlisted and transformed every faculty, including sense-perception' (302). The two types of sensibility differ in their conception of how this knowledge is achieved and its communicative or charismatic content. For the mystics, to whom Cheyne turned, this knowledge came about through, what Davis tentatively terms, 'regenerative gradualism' involving a slow advance through various stages of spiritual awareness (awakening, purgation, illumination, 'the dark night of the soul' and union). In contrast, enthusiasts like the Camisards (and later the Methodists), saw no need for initiation, purification, mortification or self-doubt, but claimed that Divine Inspiration comes suddenly to the unprepared, with profound bodily changes such as sudden cures, and other hysteric symptoms, in a process of what Davis terms 'inspirational automatism'. Cheyne embraced the mystic rather than enthusiastic tradition; a distinction vital to any understanding of his apparently paradoxical career as unorthodox religionist and fashionable Hanoverian physician. By the early 1730s, when Cheyne had reached a socially enabling compromise between private Pietism and material success as a fashionable, best-selling 'nerve-doctor', he was suspicious of another outbreak of anarchic evangelical activity.

It is in this context that we should read Cheyne's description of the Methodists as 'novices'. The inspired writers admired by this older Pietist movement, like Bourignon and Guyon, laid down strict Augustinian rules regarding noviateship into the spiritual life, which only gradually led towards illuminated states of *Recollection.* There is evidence that Cheyne already subscribed to this doctrine at the time of his spiritual reawakening. In 1708, for example, when his well-meaning friend Andrew Ramsay, withdrew himself to a remote Bourignonist community on the Banffshire coast, Cheyne endorsed the view of their mutual friend Dr Keith that 'soltitude and retirement and mechanism paid sometimes strange pranks with such people' and he politely reminded him of Cassian's warnings about the dangers of 'spiritual pride'.[47] Discussing Cheyne's 'conversion', Professor G. S. Rousseau overlooks the fact that in the 1733 account, Cheyne dates his first major revelatory recovery to 1709–10 (not 1706 when the Camisards arrived), and moreover, in so doing Cheyne also deliberately rejects an over-enthusiastic interpretation of his recovery as miraculous cure:

> I found so wonderful a Change in my whole Man, as *Spirits, Chearfulness, Strength* and *Appetite*, by it, that I thought it *Enchantment* and could scarce believe I was myself; and had I been much *Enthusiastically* given, would have accounted it *Miraculous*, being naturally one of these *Quick Thinkers*, who have a great Sensibility either of Pleasure or Pain ... from that Time forward I encreas'd in *Spirits, Strength, Appetite* and *Gaiety* (*English Malady*, 340–1).

In an *Essay on Regimen* (1740), Cheyne warns at length against spiritual self-delusion and endorses the cautious quietist attitude to spiritual noviateship:

> The *Operations* and Influences of the Divine *Spirit*, or *Grace* and spiritual Aid and assistance, are *Secret and Imperceptible*; and are always to be suspected, when they are *impetuous, sensible* and acting only by *Fits* and *Starts*, as the gross Macin [sic] is *in* or *out* of *Tune*, and as the animal Functions play *easily* or *labour*, especially in *young unexperienced* Persons, who have not been *tried* and *purified* in the School of the *Cross;* for these uncommon and *extraordinary*, or even *perceptible* Operations of the *Divine Spirit*, seldom happen *pure, sincere* and *unmixt;* but to the long and severely *Tried* and *Purified*, and when the Passions, Appetites, and *Spiritual Humours* are moderated, calm'd and subdued, in the Decline of Life spent in due Retirement, and proper Silence; not in the *Storm* and *Tempest*, but in the *still calm Voice*, does the Divine *Spirit* speak; and a truely humble, and enlighten'd Person, ought to suspect himself, *get above*, and pass over every Impulse, *Sweetening* or *Glance* of Light that comes not thus accompanied. Children, Beginners, and Noviciats in the *Spiritual Life*, are often gratified with such *sugarings* for their Encouragement; but Bread is for grown person, which is got by the *sweat* of *the Brow*, and bearing the Cross; and a prudent staid Person will have too great a regard for the Purity and Dignity of the *Divine Spirit*, to bring him down, to account for all the *mechanical* and *animal* operations of his *volatile* and various *Imagination* (339).

This was almost certainly written with the activities of Methodist field-preachers in mind. Everything in Cheyne's extant writings suggests that he diagnosed any sudden behavioural changes as simply the symptoms of bodily dysfunction. The weakening effects of a constitutional predisposition to nervous sensibility could indirectly serve to guard an individual against the errors of the voluptuary, but nervous symptoms are essentially mechanistic, and not to be interpreted as, in themselves, evidence of spiritual enlightenment.

Until his departure for America in 1735, John Wesley was under William Law's spiritual guidance, but upon his return, he rapidly became estranged from Law's increasingly mystical theology. It was too coldly philosophical for both Wesleys who believed that restoration to a state of grace should be a dynamically transforming experience, reflected in an outward dramatic show of emotions.[48] The Richardson correspondence confirms that Cheyne, well-informed of this estrangement, sided with Law's intellectual theosophical-Pietism. This rift closely parallels the earlier reaction of English and Scottish quietists to the Camisards. It provides the context in which we should read Cheyne's notable statements advocating 'common-sense' and social conformity in the Preface to *An Essay on Regimen* (1740), and its identification serves to resolve what earlier commentators have regarded as the ambiguous relationship between Cheyne's private unorthodoxy and outward conformity. Moreover, it enables us to understand how Cheyne's numerous medico-religious 'Disciples' were able to distinguish between a positive concept of nervous sensibility, and the so-called symptoms of enthusiasm which free-thinking or more orthodox critics could all too easily interpret as signs of madness.

Acknowledgement

I am grateful to Roy Porter for his helpful comments on the earlier draft of this paper.

Notes

1. David Hampton, *Methodism and Politics in British Society* 1750–1850 (Hutchinson, 1984), 28–9.
2. *Patients and Practitioners: Lay Perceptions of Medicine in Pre-industrial Society,* Roy Porter (ed.), (Cambridge: Cambridge University Press, 1985), 145–77. Continental Pietist-medicine has received more attention: see three related essays by Johanna Geyer-Kordesch and the editors, in *The Medical Enlightenment of the Eighteenth Century* Andrew Cunningham and Roger French (eds), (Cambridge: Cambridge University Press, 1990).
3. The present essay is derived from my study, *'My Own Crazy Carcase': The Life and Works of Dr George Cheyne (1672–1743),* (unpublished Ph.D. thesis, Edinburgh University, 1992), which presents a substantial amount of fresh research into primary sources. For an important account of Cheyne's role as medico-religionist with which I am not in entire agreement, see G. S. Rousseau 'Mysticism and

Millenarianism: "Immortal Doctor Cheyne"', in *Millenarianism and Messianism in English Literature and Thought 1650–1800 Clark Library Lectures,* edited by Richard H. Popkin (Berkeley etc., Brill, 1988), 81–126; Cheyne's early career as a 'Tory Newtonian' is examined in Anita Guerrini, 'James Keill, George Cheyne, and Newtonian Physiology, 1690–1740', *Journal of the History of Biology,* xviii, no. 12 (Summer, 1985), 247–66 and 'The Tory Newtonians: Gregory, Pitcairne and their Circle', *Journal of British Studies,* xxv (July, 1986), 288–311.

4. 'Dr Cheyne incidentally influenced Law more than any living man, having been, as Law himself told Byrom *the providential occasion of his meeting or knowing of Jacob Boehme, by a book which the Doctor mentioned to him in a letter, Which book mentioned Behmen'* (J. H. Overton, *William Law: Non-juror and Mystic* (1881), 92). The recommended book Baron Wolf von Metternicht's *Fides et Ratio Collatae* (Amsterdam, 1708), a theosophical rebuttal of Locke, by a Continental associate of Cheyne's patron Alexander, Lord Forbes. This work influenced Cheyne's revisions to his *Philosophical Principles* (1715) (Francis Okely, *Memoirs of Behmen* (1780), 105n. and Stephen Hobhouse, '*Fides et Ratio*': *the Book that Introduced Jacob Boehme to William Law* (extracted from *The Journal of Theological Studies,* 1936). Cheyne describes his nervous breakdown in his famous 'The Author's Own Case', in *The English Malady* (London and Bath, 1733) (facsimile reprint, Tavistock Classics in the History of Psychiatry, Routledge, 1991, with an introduction by Roy Porter). Cheyne's Pietist connections, first mapped by G. S. Rousseau, are substantially clarified in my thesis. Key figures were Lord Deskford, Lord Forbes of Pitsligo and George Garden in Scotland, Dr Keith and Revd John Heylyn in London, Pierre Poiret in Holland and Chevalier Ramsay in France.
5. Arbuthnot, *An Essay Concerning the Nature of Aliments* (London: 1731), preface.
6. M. de la Bédoyere, *The Archbishop and the Lady: the story of Fénelon and Madame Guyon* (London: 1956).
7. Quotations are from the Oxford University Press edition by C. Whibley (Oxford: 1926).
8. Benjamin Boyce, *The Benevolent Man: A Life of Ralph Allen of Bath* (Harvard: 1967).
9. Cheyne often cites Cornaro alongside the Jesuit Leonard Lessius (1554–1623). Cheyne's promotion probably prompted publication of *Hygiasticon: or the Means of Health and Long Life written originally in Latin by Leonard Lessius. Now rendered into English, by T. S. Smith. whereunto is annex'd Cornaro's Treatise of the Benefits of a Sober Life* (1742).
10. Unpublished letter, Whitefield Papers, Methodist Archive, John Rylands Library, University of Manchester.

11. Revealingly, beneath Whitefield's crossing out, his original words read, 'but incidentally dipped in a place'.
12. Arnold Dallimore, *George Whitefield* (1970), I, 75–7.
13. L. Tyerman, *Life of Whitefield* (1876), I, 106 (Cheyne's patient Lady Cox contributed £50).
14. V. H. H. Green, *The Young Mr Wesley* (1961), Appendix I, 305–19. Wesley wrote, 'for six or seven and twenty years I had made Anatomy and Physic the diversion of my leisure hours'. On 1 November, 1724 he wrote to his mother in praise of Cheyne's *Essay of Health,* and noted that Cheyne's assertion that health required temperance and exercise was 'much cried down by the physicians' (*The Letters of the Rev. John Wesley* (1931), II, 307; I, 11 (hereafter '*Letters*').
15. 'When I grew up, in consequence of reading Dr Cheyne, I chose to eat sparingly, and drink water. This was another great means of continuing my health, till I was seven-and-twenty.' *The Journal of the Rev. John Wesley* (1909), V, 373 (hereafter '*Journal*'). Familiar with Cheyne's theory of fevers, John Wesley sought his guidance in November 1734, when stricken with smallpox, he took to his bed for the first time in over 35 years, upon the advice of Cheyne's brother-in-law (*Letters,* I, 359).
16. Wesley writes to Gibson, Bishop of London, in 1747, to answer charges that his asceticism has the 'appearances of an uncommon sanctity, in order to captivate the people', and explains that he had actually returned to wine and meat rather than 'make my brother to offend', but 'Dr Cheyne advised me to leave them off again, assuring me *Till you do, you will never be free from fevers.* And since I have taken his advice, I have been free (blessed be to God) from all bodily disorders (I continued this about 2 years)' (*Letters,* II, 285–6).
17. John Wesley, *Primitive Physick ...* (1747), 29–30.
18. At the time of Wesley's death in 1791 it had reached its 23rd edition. In America, where Methodism rapidly took root, many editions had appeared by the same date and it remained popular on both sides of the Atlantic well into the next century.
19. William Walton, *Notes and Materials for an Adequate Biography of... William Law* (privately printed, 1854), 595.
20. Richard Brantley, *Locke, Wesley and the Method of English Romanticism* (1984) examines Wesley's debt to Pietism in resisting Locke's empirical epistemology and notes the significance of Wesley's exposure to Cheyne's *Philosophical Principles* (Chapter 1 *passim,* f. 1; and 237–8).
21. Green, *op. cit.* (note 14), 306: Wesley read the third edition of 1726 (identical to that of 1715).
22. *Alumni Oxoniensis,* J. Foster (ed.), (Oxford: 1888), I, 246.
23. George Cheyne, *An Historical Character of the Honourable George Baillie Esq.* (1738), printed by Samuel Richardson for private distribution; Marchmont letterbooks, Scottish Records Office, GD

158/1257; Baillie's exemplary 'Case History' appears anonymously in *The English Malady*, 275.

24. *The Journal of the Rev. Charles Wesley* (1846), I, 248 (hereafter '*Journal')*. Middleton respected Wesley who, in July 1744, recorded passing 'two hours in Christian conference and prayer with Dr M., and the church in his house' (*Journal*, II, 38). On other occasions he talks of being received very 'cordially' at Middleton's house. In February 1750, Charles sought Middleton's help when his pregnant wife was caught in a thunderstorm, but an entry of two days later is tragically brief: 'Sat., Feb. 3rd. She miscarried' (*Ibid.*, II, 67). Three years later, when Sarah Wesley was seriously ill with smallpox, her husband noted that, 'Dr Middleton has been a father to her' (*Ibid.*, II, 100). I am indebted to Jonathan Barry's study (cited earlier), for some references concerning Middleton's circle.
25. *On the Death of Dr Middleton, Dec. 16th, 1760* (*Journal*, II, 36–64), by Charles Wesley? A long poem published in the *Armenian Magazine* of 1783 (445; 502; 507), also treats of Middleton's deathbed Methodist conversion.
26. *Journal*, II, 517.
27. Her youthful piety was fostered by her sisters-in-law, Ladies Betty and Margaret Hastings, who converted after hearing the preaching of the Moravian Minister, Benjamin Ingham (1712–72), an original member of the Oxford Holy Club. See Anon, *The Life and Times of Selina, Countess of Huntingdon*, 2 vols (1839, 1840); Cheyne's letters to the Countess (1732–9), in the Huntington Library, were published by C. F. Mullett as *The Letters of Dr George Cheyne to the Countess of Huntingdon* (San Marino: 1940), (hereafter, '*Huntingdon*').
28. No precise date for her conversion, but by the late 1730s, she had become intimate with the Wesleys and she was an original member of the first official Methodist Society at Fetter Lane in 1739. She appointed Whitefield her household chaplain in 1748, and used her aristocratic privilege to support a distinctly Calvinist branch of the Methodist movement (the 'Huntingdon Connection').
29. *Huntingdon*, 48.
30. *Report of the Manuscripts of the late Reginald Rawdon Hastings Esq.*, (1934), 32–3, (hereafter *'HMC Hastings*').
31. *Ibid.*, 33.
32. *Ibid*, vii, and *Cheyne to Samuel Richardson*, 88.
33. 2 parts in 1, being Volume 1 of *The Works of Thomas Wilson*, 7 vols (1847–63), hereafter 'Keble'.
34. *Ibid.*, I, 923.
35. Keble's account relied upon 'an ample and curious store of letters to and from Dr Wilson, his son', including several letters of Cheyne's from which he prints brief extracts. I traced this collection of manuscripts to the collection of Keble College Library, Oxford, but

the present librarian informs me that, although listed in the inventory, the relevant bundles 'disappeared' in the 1960s!

36. Keble, I, 923–4. Griffith Jones (1683–1761), a Welsh evangelical Anglican divine involved in the S.P.G.F.P. who established a number of charity schools throughout Wales from 1730 onwards and increasingly identified with the Methodists. A Welsh translation of Wilson's book appeared at Llundain in 1774 (*DNB*, X, 991–2).
37. General James Oglethorpe, met Bishop Wilson in 1735 and suggested the need for such a work in the colony where he had taken Whitefield, and both John and Charles Wesley (his personal secretary), to act as spiritual leaders. Wilson's book was a response to his interest in the activities of Oglethorpe and the S.P.G.F.P.. Wilson also become interested in the Moravians after meeting Count Zinzendorf in 1737.
38. Keble, I, 923 (Cheyne to Wilson, 13 August, 1740).
39. Cheyne's initiation of Richardson as his medical disciple is recorded in *The Letters of Dr George Cheyne to Samuel Richardson (1733–1743)*, edited with an introduction by Charles F. Mullett (Columbia, University of Missouri, 1943).
40. Hillel Schwartz, *The French Prophets: the History of a Millenarian Group in Eighteenth-century England* (Berkeley: UCLA, 1980). I thank Dr Schwartz for his assistance in the early days of my research.
41. G. D. Henderson (ed.), *Mystics of the North East including i. Letters of James Keith M.D. and others to Lord Deskford: ii Correspondence Between Dr George Garden and James Cunningham* (Third Spalding Society, Aberdeen, 1934).
42. Cheyne and others to Andrew Michael Ramsay, 1708–10 (National Library of Scotland, Acc. 4796, 26b) and Francis Lee see his *State of the Philadelphian Society* (1697), 10. Fuller evidence discussed in detail in Chapter 3 of my thesis.
43. Schwartz, *op. cit.* (note 40), especially 202 f; 288 f.
44. *Ibid.*, ch. 5.
45. At the time of his death Cheyne was seeking Samuel Richardson's help in publishing a translation of the works of the Franco-German theosopher Baron Marsay whose 'Mystical and Literal Explication of J. Christ to St John the Apostle', opens with prefatorial remarks upon the 'New Birth' or 'Work of Regeneration'. Although Revelation has an 'external' historical meaning, 'it is likewise the whole *Mystic Divinity*, or an account of the ways which *J. Christ* conduct every soul wherein he designs to reveal ... himself and to re-establish his Kingdom'. Revelation 'is therefore a Recitat of what J. Christ operates in that Soul, and of the various States thro' which she must pass in order to her Renovation; what must happen to her and what she must experience from the first step of her conversion to god until her entire re-union with him, or until her regeneration, whereby she again becomes a new Creature, the Temple where God dwells, the

New Jerusalem' (extracted from ms translation which belonged to Cheyne's Pietist associate Lord Forbes: Scottish Records Office, GD 12, 20, Items 16–17, I, 16).

46. *Journal of the History of Ideas,* vi (1943), 301–19. This essay is indispensable for distinguishing the temper of Cheyne's 'mysticism'.
47. National Library of Scotland, Acc. 4796.
48. See Charles Wesley's negative response to William Law's *Grounds and Reasons for Christian Regeneration, or the New Birth Offered to the Consideration of Christians and Deists* (1739), where he concludes that 'his knowledge of the new birth is mostly theory' (*Journal,* I, 191). John Wesley's temperamental and doctrinal differences with Cheyne's philosophical Pietism may be inferred from his detailed reply to Cheyne's disciple Dr John Robertson in response to a present of an annotated copy of Andrew Ramsay's *Philosophical Principles* in 1753 (*Letters,* I, 107–9). There are parallels between Ramsay's *magnum opus* and Cheyne's mature 'Philosophical Discourses' of 1740, in part the result of personal contact. John Wesley also criticises mysticism in a long formal letter to Law (*Letters,* III, 332–70).

14

Anti-Lockean Enlightenment?: Mind and Body in Early Eighteenth-Century English Medicine

Akihito Suzuki

Introduction

The Enlightenment was marked by an optimism about improving the mankind and a belief in the malleability of the human mind.[1] Here the influence of Locke, as an intellectual backbone of the belief, was enormous.[2] In his *Essay concerning Human Understanding* (1690), Locke rejected the doctrine of innate ideas and instead put forth the model of the mind as a *tabula rasa*, gradually equipped with ideas acquired via senses.[3] Philosophers on both sides of the Channel – Hume, Hartley, Priestley, Condillac, Charles Bonnet, and others – were fascinated with the task of tracing the step-by-step development and moulding of the mind and its faculties and powers in response to stimuli from the external world: Hume's causal judgement, Hartley's and Priestley's association of ideas, and Condillac's and Bonnet's statue.[4] The idea of the malleable mind was not discussed as a philosophical topic of purely intellectual interest, in accordance with the Enlightenment enthusiasm for changing society by putting intellectual ideas into practice – Locke himself applied his epistemology to his writings on the education of children.[5] Towards the end of the century, calls for radical reformation became rampant, with C.A. Helvétius, the Baron d'Holbach, Jeremy Bentham and Pierre Cabanis vigorously preaching the idea of shaping and adapting the human mind into more desirable forms.[6]

As the cases of Priestley, La Mettrie, Helvétius, d'Holbach and Cabanis well exemplify, the Enlightenment drive to recast the mind has often been associated with materialism and radical social reform. By eliminating the transcendental and otherworldly soul provided with innate faculties, the philosophers put forth the model of the human being as a sensible machine receptive to, and moulded by, environmental controls and sensations from outside.[7] In order to improve man's mind and to maximize human happiness, therefore, one should set up a rationally designed environment with its physical, psychological, social, and political factors carefully calculated to achieve those ends. The calls for social and political reform, the attacks against the institutions of the *ancien régime*, and the schemes for remodelling prisons, schools, hospitals, and factories were thus underpinned by the new 'science of man', a power/knowledge aiming at achieving circumstances for the correct socialization of malleable man.[8] As has been pointed out, *inter alia*, by Michel Foucault, medicine played a significant role in this materialistic science of man and in the reformist schemes for setting up the new social environment as a well-designed factory of human beings.[9]

Caution is necessary here. As is evident from the figures mentioned above, the alliance between medicine, Lockean philosophy of the mind, materialism, the 'science of man', and radical social reform was a phenomenon of the *late* eighteenth century.[10] English medical psychology and its relation to Locke during the *early* Enlightenment has been neglected, and historians tend to project the late Enlightenment marriage of Lockean philosophy and medicine on to the early Enlightenment.[11] Michel Foucault refers to Locke several times as one of the backbones of psychiatry in the whole 'l'âge classique' without producing any tangible evidences, and Roy Porter does not substantiate his claim that Lockean philosophy of mind was influential on medical psychology and psychiatry '*throughout* [my italics] the eighteenth century'.[12] Indeed, the chronology of the relation between medicine and Lockean psychology tells a different story. In Hunter and Macalpine's *Three Hundred Years of Psychiatry*, there is an entry from Locke's own *Essay* published in 1690, and the next time that Locke's name appears in the book is in the entry for David Hartley's *Observations*, published more than half a century later.[13] The fact is that there were very few, if any, medical writings in the earlier half of the century which explicitly embraced Locke's psychology, in sharp contrast to the late eighteenth and early nineteenth centuries, when doctors such as William Cullen, Thomas Arnold, Alexander Crichton and Philippe Pinel incorporated the psychology of Locke and Locke-inspired philosophers.[14]

Given the absence of Lockeanism, how was early eighteenth-century English medical psychology formulated then? The aim of the present paper is to show that during the early eighteenth century the relation between medical psychology and Lockeanism was quite different from the happy alliance that existed in the late

Enlightenment, and medical discourse on the mind in the earlier Enlightenment was framed within a socio-cultural and ideological setting quite distinct from the later radical and reformist one. First, I will show that medical psychology in England in the early eighteenth century was overtly *anti*-Lockean. Relying on contemporary metaphysical writings which repudiated Locke, many eminent physicians at that time explicitly criticized Locke's secularized understanding of the mind, and set up a model of the human mind which was other-worldly and was quite different from, or even diametrically opposite to, Locke's formulation. They did so, largely because they wanted to refute monistic materialism and defend the Christian religion by promoting a rigorously dualistic notion of the mind-body. Unlike the later *philosophes* and the figures of Margaret Jacob's 'radical Enlightenment', they were by no means irreligious and materialistic unbelievers who sought alternatives to Christianity.[15]

They were, nevertheless, rightly called children of the Enlightenment, for they championed belief in the malleability of the mind as confidently as the later materialistic thinkers. They vigorously maintained that emotional disturbances, which tormented many English people at that time, had somatic and organic causes and hence should be treated medically. They also preached that the moral and intellectual powers of man could be enhanced by the art of medicine, through taking care of the body, rather than through religious and spiritual means. In the sense that they provided a secularized alternative to the religious discipline of the mind, their discourse was congruent with our understanding of the Enlightenment as the process of secularization.[16] Medical writings on the mind and its disturbances in the early eighteenth century, therefore, represent another version of the Enlightenment belief in the malleability of the human mind: despite the differences, both early and late eighteenth-century medical psychology subscribed to the belief in non-religious means to remould the human mind.

Moreover, the socio-cultural settings of the two versions of the medical discourses on the mind's plasticity were quite distinct. I will argue that English medical psychology in the early eighteenth century was preached and practised within a cultural and commercial site whose major codes were politeness, refinement of taste, civility and élitist distinction, rather than scientific, anti-establishment, reformist, populist and sometimes democratic values. On the basis of surplus wealth, the urbane well-to-do both in London and in provincial towns employed their riches to achieve cultural distinction from vulgar country bumpkins and unrefined boorish squires, by investing in cultural apparel such as dress, belongings, accomplishments, manners and behaviour, and, most importantly, learning – the cultural package propagated in extremely successful journals like the *Tatler* and *The Spectator*.[17] The Third Earl of Shaftesbury gave a moral philosophical and political sanction to this sometimes flippant pursuit of politeness by showing that politeness and sociability were the bases of liberty and civic values.[18]

Since this 'polite Enlightenment' was much more concerned with verbal, literary and artistic refinement than with pursuit of scientific knowledge, historians of science and medicine have long neglected it, or even regarded it as an obstacle to the progress of science, industry and medicine.[19] Recently, however, some historians such as G. S. Rousseau and Roy Porter have stressed that science and medicine were a part of the programme for cultural refinement and the progress of politeness.[20] Following their lead, I shall put the medical psychology of George Cheyne – one of the most popular medical writers and the most ardent opponent of the Lockean understanding of the mind – in the context of the polite Enlightenment *à la* Shaftesbury and Addison and Steele. I will try to demonstrate that Cheyne invested substantial energy in shaping the literary style of his discourse according to the taste of the gentle and genteel audience/ patients, and that his medical psychology incorporated some of the cultural codes of the polite Enlightenment.

The present essay will discuss the topics delineated above. In the first section I will examine anti-Lockeanism of early and mid-century medical and metaphysical writings. The second section will discuss the promotion of the bodily interpretation of mental phenomena, such as emotional disorders and moral and intellectual capacity. There, particular attention will be paid to the advancing of an alternative to religious and spiritual discipline of the mind. The third section will examine the socio-cultural setting of the medical discourse of Cheyne, and will contextualize his bodily interpretations of mental phenomena in the cultural codes of the polite Enlightenment.

Reactions to Locke: Dualism and Transcendental Pneumatology

The strongest opposition to Locke in the eighteenth century was centred at the thinking-matter hypothesis. The controversy had its origin in Locke's carefully composed passage in his *Essay*, which said that it is intelligible that God could have 'superadded' the power of thinking to matter.[21] Soon after Locke made the suggestion, there rose around him a coterie of thinking materialists, who were at the same time deistic, free-thinking and sometimes freemasonic, e.g.

Anthony Collins, John Toland and Samuel Bold.[22] Outside the circle, some obscure writers such as William Coward, Henry Layton and Samuel Strutt were active in developing materialistic arguments.[23] Locke and the Locke-inspired materialists triggered a storm of protest from such eminent figures as Edward Stillingfleet, Bishop of Worcester and Richard Bentley, one of the Boyle Lecturers. In his *Psychologia*, John Broughton launched an attack against the 'partisans of Spinoza, Hobbs, Le Clerc, L-k, and Toland'. Andrew Baxter published several books to refute the materialists from the 1730s, some of which went through several editions.[24] The core of their arguments was that God cannot provide matter with the power of thinking without destroying the nature of the matter, hence, thinking matter is a logical absurdity God would never create.

Some issues related to the problem of diseases of the mind popped into this controversy over thinking matter. Indeed, madness had posed a metaphysical problem since Lucretius' polemics. In his *De rerum natura*, Lucretius observed that the soul, though it is alleged to be immaterial, immortal and imperishable, loses its power in madness. From the observation he deduced that the soul is actually just material. He added another twist to his materialist challenge, by drawing attention to the cure of madness: if the soul were immaterial, how would you explain everyday medical practices which cure madness by somatic methods like purging and medication?[25] Confronted with the revival of Lucretius, physicians and metaphysicians in the sixteenth and seventeenth centuries were desperate to refute the materialist contention.[26] The same pattern of the materialist use of madness versus the orthodox re-interpretation of mental diseases appeared in the eighteenth century: William Coward employed the same Lucretian polemic, and Broughton, Baxter and John Balignac denied the materialist interpretation of madness.[27] Baxter was so annoyed at the 'modern sceptic' (almost certainly he thought of Coward here) who quoted Lucretius' polemics, and was afraid that 'this objection is so plausible, that the generality of men allow it to be matter of fact'.[28]

Against the assault on the immateriality of the soul based on the case of madness, metaphysicians in the mid-eighteenth century replied with a very rigorous version of dualism, which enabled them to claim that disturbances of reason did not demonstrate corruptibility and materiality of the soul. They denied the materialists' claim that madness damages the essential part of the soul, and instead maintained that what is damaged during madness is only *apparent* mental operations, with hidden and *real* powers of the soul being intact even in raging madness. Accordingly, they developed a scheme of psychology which rigidly distinguished two categories of the powers of the soul: 1) our mental operations in this world, during the soul's union with the body, and 2) the immaterial substance's original powers, which become manifest only after its separation from the body. The original and real powers were vastly greater, for while they permeated through the body, they were diminished because of the *impediment* provided by the body:

> The more it [the soul] is disengaged from matter, ... the more capable it is to perform its most exalted operations, and consequently, by an absolute separation, it is so far from perishing, that it ascends to its perfection.[29]

In other words, the soul is endowed with original and innate supreme powers, which are the hidden but ultimate cause of our apparent mental operations. This is the diametrically opposite position to the Lockean model of the mind as a *tabula rasa*, building up its own powers from infancy to maturity in response to the external stimuli via bodily means.[30]

Early eighteenth-century physicians largely adopted the non-Lockean model of psychology when they talked about the human mind and its disorders. Since madness and physicians' capacity to cure the disease were at issue, they had good reason to show great concern in refuting the materialists. Like the metaphysicians examined above, Cheyne argued the intactness of the original and real powers of the soul:

> The radical qualities of ... intelligence may be invariable in the rank and degree proper to such a species of spiritual nature, whatever machine or bodily organ it be cloathed with. Only it cannot exert its elicit or exterior acts without a proper machine.[31]

Nicholas Robinson repeated the same argument, by arguing that the soul 'under the severest symptoms of the most raging madness, ... is the same mind, the same self, the same ray of divinity, that almighty God infused, when he form'd it a living soul'.[32]

The physicians and metaphysicians shared the model of the mind endowed with innate powers, as well as the model of madness. Indeed, physicians sometimes employed more religious, metaphysical, and mystical language.[33] Cheyne maintained that man's soul is a 'diminutive angel shut up in a flesh prison or vehicle'; the immaterial substances are 'miniatures, effluxes, emanations, infinitesimals, or infinitely small sparkles' of God that is the 'infinite source of living, intelligence, action, perfection and happiness'.[34] The body-prison, argued Cheyne, is an impediment to the free exercise of the original, pre-lapsarian, and paradisiacal powers of the soul, the image of God in us:

> In this our own lapsed state, our gross and earthly prisons were designed by infinite Wisdom, to curb, concentrate, and restrain the exalted functions of the radical and intellectual faculties.[35]

Again Robinson expressed the same sentiment, arguing that the body blocke'd the innate and semi-divine powers of the soul:

> These little spots of Earth, human machines, to which we are chain'd, ... are the causes why we cannot discover the nature of this spiritual being, and why its moving power is so greatly suspended in its action: but were it once unfettered from the bondage of these shackles, it would naturally rise, and takes its seat in the proper *ubi* of this immense theatre, ordain'd the happy mansion of spirits, by the sovereign director of the universe.[36]

Early eighteenth-century medical psychology thus maintained: the matter or the body cannot think; the soul is endowed with original powers to perform our mental operations; and the body is the impediment that diminishes the original powers.

This scheme of pneumatology adopted by many early eighteenth-century physicians and metaphysicians was at odds with the fundamental tenets of Locke's understanding of the mind. Besides opposing the thinking-matter hypothesis, physicians expressed dissatisfaction at the more essential part of Locke's tactics of his *Essay*, i.e., avoiding 'physical consideration' of the soul.[37] The task Locke imposed on himself in the work was to examine the operations of the human mind in this world, without recourse to either the nature of the immaterial substance or to the physiology of the body. Locke thus established this-worldly considerations of the mind as a free-standing genre of discourse.[38] The scheme of pneumatology which stated that all apparent workings of our mind were just a diminished shadow of the other-worldly, semi-divine, and by definition undetectable innate powers of the soul was a quite alien viewpoint to Locke's.

Accordingly, the physicians criticized Locke for not paying proper attention to the other-worldly nature of the soul. Cheyne wrote:

> Locke considered man, and his faculties, not indeed in their already reprobated and hellish estate, but as he really now is, in the world, a composition of moral and natural good and evil: and this state he has very farely and justly represented as far as it goes. But then, either having no notion, or at least no regard, to his higher faculties, which in natural and lapsed man, lye buried under the rubbish of his present corruption and sensuality.[39]

Robinson made a similar charge against Locke, with the added twist of incorporating refutations of Locke's argument about personal identity.[40] Robinson criticized Locke for confusing other-worldly and this-worldly aspects of the mind, that is, 'person, a real subsisting principle', and 'consciousness, only an affection of that principle, depending on the regular exercise of the corporeal organs'. Another way to put it was, Robinson argued, that Locke failed to distinguish 'the action of intelligent beings from their spiritual essence'.[41]

Early eighteenth-century physicians were, therefore, firmly against Locke's programme for the study of the human mind. Major components of Lockean philosophy, i.e., his suggestion of the possibility of thinking matter, the model of the mind as a *tabula rasa*, and the limit of the discourse to this-worldly mental operations, were all denied by the leading physicians, who embraced rigorous dualism (with no power of thinking in matter), the innate and original powers of the soul, and the significance of other-worldly aspects of the soul. Unlike medical psychology in the late eighteenth century, that in the early eighteenth century was marked by anti-Lockeanism.

The Bodily Interpretation of Mental Phenomena

There was, however, another side of this overtly spiritual understanding of the problem of the soul/mind. Paradoxically, the scheme developed an almost exclusively bodily interpretation of the operations and mis-operations of the mind, since the dualistic position logically led to the idea that all the actual operations of the mind depended on bodily organs, in the sense that they were *limited* by the body. Since every mental operation was interactive and exercised through the body, the influence of the body prevailed, both in its healthy and diseased states. As the soul's original powers were something given by God and beyond the reach of human intervention, the only site where one could intervene to improve the mental operations was the body.

Moreover, as the physicians and metaphysicians embraced the premise that the hidden power of the soul is unchangeable throughout the life of an individual and is equal in different individuals, they were led to conclude that the only variable factor was the body. Accordingly, the differences between the intelligent powers of different individuals were explained in exclusively somatic terms. Developing what might be termed a neurophysiology of genius, Cheyne argued that what made the difference between Newton and a village idiot were the different compositions of their bodies, especially of intellectual organs: 'what men call a genius, or a man of fine natural parts, a hero, or a philosopher is much owing to the perfection of the machin or vehicle and its spiritual and ethereal organs.' An anonymous poem entitled *An Essay on the Soul of Man* (1744) echoes the idea:

> The soul, althou' in human kind the same,
> Yet various seems, in every various frame,
> The model of the fabric, where it dwells;
> Tis wrong, or right; it fails, or it excells;

Robinson joined the chorus, by maintaining that 'the differences between an idiot and the most enlarg'd understanding ... arise from the different mechanical affections of matter and motion', for 'their souls are the same'.[42]

Likewise, the doctors advised that to improve your own mental powers, you must take care of the body: 'the perfection ... of the intellectual faculties', argued Cheyne, depended on the 'soundness and health of the bodily machin', i.e. 'proper organs, springs, ropes, and pipes': Robinson wrote that mental capability did 'depend upon the power of its faculties, whose exercise are the more conspicuous, the more the finest fibres of the brain, in which they lie enveloped'.[43] Cheyne almost said that if one follows a proper diet, one can be a Newton, for men of great intelligence 'maintained their superiority of parts, their penetration, attention, just and close thinking, by extreme temperance'.[44] The notion of the coarse body as the impediment to the free exercise of the soul's hidden power is lurking behind the temperance and the thin diet prescribed to improve one's mind: slender, scant, thin, delicate fibres make acute mind, and gross and fat ones obstruct thinking. In a word, the less the body, the more perfect the mind. Making the bodily impediment smaller was the only possible way to enhance your mental powers.

Even when Cheyne distinguished the moral and the intellectual powers of the mind and argued that the former could improve the latter, he thought that the one could improve the other only via the body:

> The restoration [of intellectual faculties] must be brought about by the culture of the moral qualities, which perfect and develop the natural ones, and thereby purify and sublime the [bodily] vehicle, extend and form intellectual organs.[45]

In other words, the moral power could 'mend and improve the bodily health by temperance and abstinence, and consequently rectify and tune the organs of the intellectual faculties'.[46] Moreover, moral virtue itself was a product of bodily health: 'calmness, serenity, chearfulness and common sense, and an esteem and love of virtue ... are the constant attendants, and only infallible symptoms of perfect bodily health.'[47]

The importance of the body for the improvement of the mental state was even more remarkable when the physicians talked about mental disturbance and its cure. Especially significant was 'the spleen', an enigmatic and amorphous disease of the eighteenth century.[48] Although they disagreed over the aetiology of the disease, there was a unanimous agreement among eighteenth-century physicians that it was a bodily-caused disease. Indeed, they were engaged in a sort of militant attack against the opposing view, scornfully denying that the symptoms of the spleen such as whims, inconstancy, and despair were the *maladies imaginaires* of hard-to-please malcontents. In a letter to Samuel Richardson, Cheyne rectified the novelist's erroneous notion of the spleen:

> You have quite a wrong notion about the hyp, as in truth all but sensible physicians have. We call the hyp every distemper attended with lowness of spirits, whether it be flatulence from indigestion, wind cholic, head-pains, or an relaxed state of the nerves ... so that the hyp is only a short expression for any kind of nervous disorders.[49]

John Hill, too, maintained that splenetic depression was a real disease, although he located it in the blood instead of the nerves.[50] The bodily interpretation of the emotional disorder was not a product of such and such medical theories, but rather a sweeping assumption that every change in mental state must be accompanied by a corresponding change in the body.[51]

Hypochondriacs were not the only target of the somatization of mental disturbances. The physicians included a lot of other mental disturbances, many of which were related to religious issues. Echoing Robert Burton's and Henry More's attacks on the 'enthusiasts' in the seventeenth century, early eighteenth-century physicians diagnosed undesirable over-zealous religious believers as bodily disordered.[52] Robinson maintained that Methodists and French Prophets were mad because of their bodily disorder.[53] Not only the over-religious, but also the non-religious were regarded as bodily disordered. As if echoing *The Spectator* which wrote that the infidels and atheists 'are made up of pride, spleen and cavil', Cheyne thought that a disturbing free-thinking libertine was actually disturbed in his body: 'he is in a bad state of health, under a dangerous bodily disease, or under a perpetual mal-regimen'; Robinson included 'atheistical madness' in his list of bodily-caused mental disorders.[54] Undesirable religious mental states were thus provided with somatic underpinning.

The progress of somatization represented the expansion of the realm of medicine, if compared with the opinion held a century before. Late sixteenth- and early seventeenth-century physicians like Bright and du Laurens were eager to maintain that there were two sorts of mental disturbances, one being caused by bodily diseases, the other purely mental one with no accompanying organic disorder. Hence there must be two distinctive sets of treatment for each type of mental disturbance: Bright wrote that medicine can do nothing to mitigate the pain of the wounded conscience; Laurens wrote 'I goe not about to redresse this deformitie [of purely spiritual mental disorder], I leave the discourse for the learned divines.'[55] In sharp contrast, Blackmore wrote that religious melancholy was a bodily disease and hence a problem for physicians rather than for priests: sufferers from the disease 'must more depend upon the art of the physician, and the force of medicine than the skill and reasonings of the casuist, for their recovery'. Cheyne wrote that bodily regimen is much more important than religious and mental instruction in the case of emotional disturbances:

> different improvements from education, philosophy, or religion, may make some small odds in the behaviour of different persons under these disorders. But this depends much upon the degrees of distemper, and the original frame and make of the body.[56]

The realm of the body and of medicine actually expanded. Early Georgian medical writers no longer admitted 'purely mental' disturbances, neither did they explicitly admit that any mental disturbances should be left in the hands of divines. Instead, they claimed that the whole field of mental disturbances was theirs.

This does not mean, however, that the doctors examined above were infidels, anti-Christians, or materialistic reductionists like La Mettrie or d'Holbach: indeed, as I have examined above, they were active in refuting materialism, buttressing Christianity, and promoting the anti-Lockean and transcendental understanding of the soul.[57] Neither did contemporary clergymen find the medicalization of mental disturbance a particular threat. One can indeed detect their readiness to accept the somatic view of certain sorts of emotional disorders. Lewis Southcomb cited Cheyne and admitted that it was so difficult to recognize a bodily-caused depression that both clergymen and laymen had been deceived into believing that the complaints were mere fancy and whims: Benjamin Fawcett, a dissenting minister, expressed the view that 'I am the more desirous to avail myself of the judgment of the best writers in medicine, because it is very difficult to convince persons afflicted with melancholy, that their distemper arises from the body, and is from thence communicated to the mind.'[58] No antagonism is found here between the two professions. In general, the religious and the medical were in agreement as to how to treat mental disturbances, as well as regarding schemes of pneumatology.

Science in Polite Culture: Cheyne's Medical Discourse in the Luxury Market

I have looked at the intellectual content of medical psychology in the early eighteenth century, and have argued that the concentration on the body was a consequence of their rigorous version of dualism. Now I will turn to the socio-cultural setting of medical psychology and clarify its function in eighteenth-century culture by examining the case of George Cheyne, one of the most successful writers of medical advice for a lay audience.

Cheyne has been regarded as the epitome of early Georgian fashionable doctors, with a flourishing practice among the noble and eminent: he was active mainly at Bath, the most fashionable spa resort of the eighteenth century, and many of his books went through numerous editions and translations.[59] The key to Cheyne's success lay, I will show below, in his effective use of his medical expertise and his reconciliation of scientific and literary culture, based on the keen grasp of the codes of the polite Enlightenment.

In general, natural philosophy and fine literature, or, the scientific Enlightenment *à la* Newton and the cultural Enlightenment *à la* Addison and Steele and Shaftesbury went hand in hand.[60] There are, however, numerous signs which suggest that tension existed between natural philosophy and literary culture: many literary figures hurled merciless satires to the Royal Society, Addison writing that the fellows of the Royal Society 'seem to be in a confederacy against men of polite genius'.[61] Given the existence of the tension, the alliance between science and politeness was not something given, but was something to be achieved. Algarotti's *Sir Isaac Newton's Philosophy Explained for the Use of the Ladies* said that 'it was extremely difficult to recivilize this savage philosophy.'[62]

Cheyne was well aware that mere scientific knowledge was not always in high demand when people sought medical advice and bought medical books.[63] At the time that he started publishing medical books for lay readers, he was himself disillusioned at the pursuit of rigorous scientific knowledge and mathematical medicine *à la* Archibald Pitcairn, for which he had been famous, or notorious, around 1700.[64] In his *Essay of Health and Long Life* (1724), he wrote that although mathematical knowledge might help invention and mechanical arts, it would do more harm than good; it does not 'rectify the will, sweaten the temper, or mend the heart' and it often leaves 'a stiffness, positiveness, and sufficiency' in the mind of the readers. In a word, it would make arrogant, ill-mannered and unsociable people.[65] Accordingly, Cheyne tactfully adopted the strategy of selling his rhetorical skill and suave persuasion, instead of scientific expertise expressed in esoteric jargon.[66] Criticizing the austere and often harsh style of the other medical advice books, he claimed that he had achieved a more refined one:

> when they come (which is rarely to be found among them) to give the reasons and philosophy of their directions, they have not the perspicuity and natural way of convincing the ingenious, sickly, and tender sufferers, so necessary to make them cheerfully and readily undergo such severe restraints; which I take to be by far the most difficult part of such a work, and which I have laboured with my utmost power to supply.[67]

To fashion a piece of medical advice suitable for genteel sufferers, one must make sure that its language would kindly invite sufferers to enter the treatment. Likewise, in his *Essay on Regimen*, he announced his major aim in the work was to entertain and amuse the reader. In so doing, Cheyne sacrificed the value of scientific rigour: although 'the stiff, rigid, and precise' men would not like the work, for such people would surely 'censure my conjectures and sentiments as dangerous and presumptuous', he valued entertainment more than correct scientific knowledge.[68]

When Cheyne incorporated medical expertise into his books, he did so mainly to titillate his clientele and audience, rather than to impose scientific authority. The role of medical science as premium is most evident in his *Essay of Health and Long Life*. According to his own account, the book was written as a guide for health at the request of Sir Joseph Jekyll (1663–1738). Although initially Cheyne simply put down only a bunch of rules, he was afraid that blunt precepts would be too coarse to be offered to his client:

> it [is] not respect enough to his good taste and capacity to judge of the reasons of things, to prescribe him bare and dry directions in matters of so great moment. I added therefore the philosophical account and reasons of these rules, which made up the bulk of the chapters themselves.[69]

He was quite right in so thinking, particularly because the rules he put down in the book turned out to be regarded as 'primitive'. John Wesley praised Cheyne and incorporated the precepts verbatim in his *Primitive Physic*, an aggressively anti-intellectual, anti-theoretical and populist medical advice manuals intended explicitly for the poor.[70] In order to make the rules a respectful offering, Cheyne felt obliged to add a flavour of distinction to the book by including his scientific learning.

In Cheyne's works, therefore, scientific expertise functioned as a device to distance them from cheap and unlearned how-tos, and rhetorical and literary values made the books more agreeable readings than blunt and dry-as-dust scientific books. The twofold values made his advice into a luxury item merchandised in a market for medical books, by adding something that is not neccesary from simply practical point of view. Just as the well-to-do displayed their distinction by attaching neo-classical Palladian façades to their houses, genteel valetudinarians differentiated themselves by purchasing guides for healthy living with natural philosophical theory and suave rhetoric.[71] Cheyne might even have calculated the effect of emulation and competition for status: his books must have enticed those who were aspiring to look like civilized gentlemen with scientific learning and literary taste.[72]

The role of the scientific Enlightenment and the polite Enlightenment in Cheyne's medical advice books lay, therefore, in the manufacture of a piece of luxurious discourse for an up-market readership. In so doing, Cheyne was adopting the values of the cultural hegemony of the flourishing and progressive élite of the English urban renaissance: Cheyne was more concerned with making a cultural distinction between the élite and the plebs than with reforming society or challenging the establishment with the aid of a rational and scientific world-view.[73] The environment in which Cheyne exercised his power/knowledge did not, therefore, square with the programme of the progress of scientific knowledge, nor with the later 'science of man', accompanied with the programme of reform from above. Cheyne assumed the role of a fellow-sufferer and a fellow-gentleman, offering learned, polite and sympathetic medical advice with attached cultural values.

Michael MacDonald has correctly contextualized the progress of the somatic interpretation of mental disorders into the cultural setting of the polite Enlightenment. Polite culture then was increasingly looking askance at the naked and too violent display of religiosity, especially that of Catholics and Puritans. Accordingly, fashionable doctors and their genteel and enlightened patients were departing from the 'spiritual physick', which decoded mental disturbances as residing in the spiritual realm of man, and prescribed repentance and humble submission to God's mercy.[74] The body became more desirable means for intervention into the mind. Psychological means such as confession of one's misdeeds, probing into the conscience of the miserable sinners, and the imposition of close examination into one's own mind in search of God's message, were becoming regarded as culturally irrelevant ways to take care of one's mind.[75] The social site where the other-worldly, spiritual and psychological methods of treating the mental disturbances remained practised was not the venue where the polite Enlightenment flourished. Driven out of the learned sphere, psychological treatment was marginalized into the popular and 'vulgar' province, from which the élite culture was increasingly distancing itself.[76] The doctors then were fighting the battle against the view that said the spleen was mental, which they found 'vulgar', 'ignorant' and 'cruel'.[77]

Moreover, as Roy Porter has suggested, within the power-relation between doctors/medical authors and patients/readers examined above, it must have been hardly possible for a doctor to tell his patient that he had a bad mind.[78] Unlike the relations between clerics and the congregations, between teachers and the pupils and between the late-century reformers and the target of the reform, the relation between Cheyne and his genteel patients/audience does not seem to have allowed the doctor to say that the patient had a defective personality and the doctor would hammer it into a correct form. The mind was, therefore, an untouchable zone for polite doctors, and the body was turned into a culturally correct site to act on the mind.

Given the congruity between élite cultural values and Cheyne's medical psychology, one is tempted to look at Cheyne's medical discourse as a symbolic politics of the cultural hegemony of the élite over the plebs.[79] Just as the soul was the noble and superior part and the body was coarse and ignoble part in the microcosm of man, they were respectively the principles of the higher and lower sorts of people in the macrocosm of state. Cheyne expressed the view that there are two sorts of people, i.e., 'those whose eminence consists chiefly in their heads, faculties, and spiritual nature' and 'those whose great use and design is to excell in the exercise and use of their bodies', or, 'those who govern, and those who are governed'.[80] The soul, therefore, represented the élite, and the body stood for the manual workers or the plebs. Cheyne's medical psychology consisted in the government of the body and turning it into a nice instrument:

> Our bodies ... cannot brought into absolute subjection and obedience; but we may readily bring them to the present docility and subjection we have of the domestic animals; by timeously bridling, trammelling and disciplining them, i.e., by feeding them cooly and sparingly, giving them due air, exercise and cleanness, and physicking them properly when they grow rampant, rebellious, or obstreperous.[81]

Here Cheyne was talking about mild discipline, without recourse to coarse and violent forces, which squared with the general strategy of the cultural hegemony of the eighteenth century.[82] The body was thus a site of symbolic politics of the government of the lower sort, and by disciplining one's body, I would like tentatively to argue, the Enlightenment cultural élite were reproducing their role in the society.

Conclusion: Two Enlightenments?

The point I want to emphasize again is that the doctors' bodily interpretation of mental phenomena in the early eighteenth century followed a quite distinct pattern from the later 'science of man'. It was largely a product of overtly anti-Lockean and other-worldly characterization of the soul/mind. Since the original and innate powers of the soul were put in a transcendental realm, the only possible site one could act on the mind was the body. The anti-Lockean pneumatology and the belief in the malleability of the mind through bodily means went hand in hand during the early Enlightenment in England. Although I am by no means devaluating Locke's influence on Enlightenment thought, the case I have advanced above shows that Locke was not an open-sesame for the belief that man's mind is perfectible through secular and natural means.

The cultural and ideological settings of the two versions of belief in the mind's malleability were distinct, too. As is evident from the model of polite and sympathetic medical advice as a luxury item manufactured according to the taste of the civilized *beau monde*, the early eighteenth-century medical disciplining of the mind via body did not square with the late-century models of scientific reforms and the schemes of control over the bodies of the plebeian masses.[83] Although Cheyne's keen grasp of the codes of the polite and literary culture was somewhat exceptional, there is much evidence that shows that eighteenth-century doctors followed a similar pattern of incorporating polite and sympathetic values.[84]

One is, therefore, tempted to say that there were two versions of Enlightenment ideal of improving the mind through bodily means: one is based on the Lockean model of the mind as a *tabula rasa*, materialistic, anti-religious, radical reformist, populist and scientific; the other is anti-Lockean, anti-materialist, dualistic, innatist, friendly to Christianity, élitist and aiming at cultural refinement sometimes at the expense of scientific values. It is, however, questionable whether there was a highly marked and drastic watershed between the early and the late Enlightenment beliefs in the malleability of the mind. Moreover, we are now having so fragmented picture of the Enlightenment that we are in danger of losing sight of it.[85] An attempt to trace the shift in intellectual and socio-cultural settings, to correlate the two versions of medical psychology, and to contextualize them in a single unit with the continuities and changes clearly articulated seems to be wanting.

Notes

1. See John Passmore, *The Perfectibility of Man* (London: Duckworth, 1970), 190–211; R. V. Sampson, *Progress in the Age of Reason* (London: Heinemann, 1956), 39–66.
2. Locke's influence on the Enlightenment was so enormous and multi-faced that no full-range survey has been done. See Roland Hall and Roger Woolhouse, *80 Years of Locke Scholarship* (Edinburgh: Edinburgh U.P., 1983).
3. John Locke, *An Essay concerning Human Understanding,* (ed.) with an introduction by Peter H. Nidditch (Oxford: Clarendon Press, 1975), book 1. The best intellectual historical account of Locke's rejection of the doctrine of innate ideas remains John Yolton, *John Locke and the Way of Ideas* (Oxford: Clarendon Press, 1956).
4. Ernst Cassirer, *The Philosophy of the Enlightenment* (Princeton: Princeton U.P., 1951 & 1979), 93–133.
5. *The Educational Writings of John Locke*, James L. Axtell (ed.), (Cambridge: Cambridge U.P., 1968).
6. Elie Halévy, *The Growth of Philosophic Radicalism* (1928; London: Faber & Faber, 1972); Simon Schaffer, 'States of Mind: Enlightenment and Natural Philosophy', in *The Languages of Psyche: Mind and Body in Enlightenment Thought,* G.S. Rousseau (ed.), (Los Angeles: University of California Press, 1990), 233–90; Martin S. Staum, *Cabanis: Enlightenment and Medical Philosophy in the French Revolution* (Princeton: Princeton U.P., 1980); Alan C. Kors, *D'Holbach's Coterie: an Enlightenment in Paris* (Princeton: Princeton U.P., 1976).
7. L. J. Jordanova, 'Earth Science and Environmental Medicine: the Synthesis of the Late Enlightenment', in *Images of the Earth: Essays in the History of the Environmental Sciences, idem,* and Roy Porter (Chalfont St Giles: BSHS, 1979), 119–46; Sergio Moravia, 'The Enlightenment and the Sciences of Man', *History of Science*, xviii (1980), 247–68; Clarence J. Glacken, *Traces on the Rhodian Shore* (Berkeley: University of California Press, 1967), 551–622.

8. Michael Ignatieff, *A Just Measure of Pain: the Penitentiary in the Industrial Revolution 1750–1850* (Harmondsworth: Penguin, 1989), 44–79; Schaffer, *op. cit.* (note 6); Michel Foucault, *Discipline and Punish: the Birth of the Prison*, trans. by Alan Sheridan (London: Allen Lane, 1977: Harmondsworth: Penguin, 1979).
9. Michel Foucault, 'The Politics of Health in the Eighteenth Century', in *The Foucault Reader*, Paul Rabinow (ed.), (Harmondsworth: Penguin, 1984), 273–89; Staum, *op. cit.* (note 6); Ignatieff, *op. cit.* (note 8), 58–62; Roy Porter, 'Was There a Medical Enlightenment in Eighteenth-Century England?', *British Journal of Eighteenth Century Studies*, v (1982), 49–63.
10. For a re-assessment of the idea of the year 1750 as the watershed from the 'lost half a century of British medicine' to the age of great reformists, see Adrian Wilson, 'The Politics of Medical Improvement in Early Hanoverian London', in *The Medical Enlightenment of the Eighteenth Century*, Andrew Cunningham and Roger French (eds), (Cambridge: Cambridge U.P., 1990), 4–39.
11. In the present paper, I use the term 'psychology' to mean knowledge of the mind or soul, with no implication of similarity with what we understand by the word. A good historical study of eighteenth-century 'psychology' is still wanting. Informative and helpful over-views are given in G. S. Rousseau, 'Psychology', in *The Ferment of Knowledge*, *idem* and Roy Porter (eds), (Cambridge: Cambridge U.P, 1980), 143–210; Christopher Fox, 'Introduction. Defining Eighteenth-Century Psychology: Some Problems and Perspectives', in *Psychology and Literature in the Eighteenth Century*, Christopher Fox (ed.), (New York: AMS Press, 1987), 1–22.
12. Michel Foucault, *Histoire de la folie à l'âge classique*, 2nd edn (Paris: Éditions Gallimard, 1972), 213, 228, 368; Roy Porter, *Mind-Forg'd Manacles: a History of Madness in England from the Restoration to the Regency* (London: the Athlone Press, 1987), 187–95.
13. Richard Hunter and Ida Macalpine, *Three Hundred Years of Psychiatry* (London: Oxford U.P., 1963), 236–9 & 379–82. John Hollings, *The State of Human Nature Delineated, as Delivered in a Latin Oration before the President and Fellows of the College of Physicians 1734* (London: T. Roberts *et.al.*, 1734), 10 is the only favourable reference to Locke in the context of medical psychology.
14. Porter, *op. cit.* (note 12), 191–3; Dora B. Weiner, 'Mind and Body in the Clinic: Philippe Pinel, Alexander Crichton, Dominique Esquirol, and the Birth of Psychiatry', in *The Languages of Psyche: Mind and Body in Enlightenment Thought*, G. S. Rousseau (ed.), (Los Angeles: University of California Press, 1990), 331–402; Akihito Suzuki, 'Mind and Its Disease in Enlightenment British Medicine', Ph.Dissertation, University of London, 1992, ch. 6.
15. Peter Gay, *The Enlightenment: an Interpretation*, 2 vols (New York: Vintage, 1966–9); Margaret C. Jacob, *The Radical Enlightenment:*

Pantheists, Freemasons and Republicans (London: George Allen & Unwin, 1981).

16. Gay, *op. cit.* (note 15), Vol. 1. See, however, Carl Becker, *The Heavenly City of the Eighteenth-Century Philosophers* (New Haven: Yale U.P., 1932).
17. J. H. Plumb, 'The Public, Literature and the Arts in the Eighteenth Century', in *The Triumph of Culture: Eighteenth-Century Perspective,* Paul Fritz and David Williams (eds), (Toronto: A. M. Hakkert Ltd., 1972), 27–48; *idem, The Commercialization of Leisure in Eighteenth-Century England* (University of Reading, 1973); Peter Borsay, *The English Urban Renaissance: Culture and Society in the Provincial Towns 1660–1770* (Oxford: Clarendon Press, 1989), 225–7 & 263; Paul Langford, *A Polite and Commercial People* (Oxford: Clarendon Press, 1989), 59–121; *The Spectator,* 5 vols, D.F. Bond, (ed.), (Oxford: Clarendon Press, 1965), Vol.1, 'Introduction'; Roy Porter, 'The Enlightenment in England', in *The Enlightenment in National Context, Idem* and Mikulás Teich (eds), (Cambridge: Cambridge U.P., 1981), 1–18.
18. Lawrence Klein, 'The Third Earl of Shaftesbury and the Progress of Politeness', *Eighteenth-Century Studies,* xviii (1984–5), 186–214; *idem,* 'Liberty, Manners, and Politeness in Early Eighteenth-Century England', *The Historical Journal,* xxxii (1989), 583–605.
19. As for the 'two cultures' view, see, for instance, Arnold Thackray, 'Natural Knowledge in Cultural Context: the Manchester Model', *American Historical Review,* lxxix (1974), 672–709.
20. G. S. Rousseau, 'Science Books and Their Readers in the Eighteenth Century', in *Books and Their Readers in Eighteenth-Century England,* Isabel Rivers (ed.), (Leicester U.P., 1982), 197–255; *idem,* 'Sinews of Science, Medicine, and Art during the Enlightenment', *Eighteenth-Century Studies,* xxvi (1992), 77–96; Roy Porter, 'Science, Provincial Culture and Public Opinion in Enlightenment England', *British Journal for Eighteenth-Century Studies,* iii (1980), 20–46.
21. Locke, *op. cit.* (note 3), 4.3.6. John W. Yolton, *Thinking Matter: Materialism in Eighteenth-Century Britain* (Oxford: Blackwell, 1983).
22. *Ibid.*, 38–42; James O'Higgins, *Anthony Collins: the Man and His Works* (Hague: Martinus Nijhof, 1970); Jacob, *op. cit.* (note 15), *passim.*
23. William Coward, *Second Thoughts concerning Human Soul,* (London: R. Basset, 1702); *idem, The Grand Essay* (London: P. G., 1704). [Samuel Strutt?], *A Philosophical Enquiry into the Physical Spring of Human Actions, and the Immediate Cause* (London: J. Peck, 1732). For Strutt and his pantheistical circle, see Jacob, *op. cit.* (note 15), 174. For Leyton, Yolton, *op. cit.* (note 21), 36–9.
24. Yolton, *op. cit.* (note 3); *idem, op. cit.* (note 21), John Broughton; *Psychologia: or an Account of the Nature of the Rational Soul* (London: T. Bennet, 1703), 139; Andrew Baxter, *An Enquiry into the Nature*

of the Human Soul, 2nd edn 2 vols. (London: for the Author, 1737).

25. Lucretius, *De rerum natura libri sex*, 3 vols, Cyril Bailey (trans. and ed.), (Oxford: Clarendon Press, 1947), Vol.1, 325–9.
26. Timothy Bright, *A Treatise of Melancholie*, (London: Thomas Vautrollier, 1586), 'Epistle Dedicatory' & 188; André du Laurens, *A Discourse of the Preservation of the Sight: of Melancholike Diseases; of Rheumes, and of Old Age*, Richard Surphlet (trans.), (London: for Ralph Iacson, 1599), 81–2; Henry More, *A Collection of Several Philosophical Writings of Dr Henry More*, 2 vols (London: William Morden, 1662; rept New York: Garland Publishing, 1978), Vol.2, *The Immortality of the Soul*, 207. John Henry, 'The Matter of Souls: Medical Theory and Theology in Seventeenth-Century England', in *The Medical Revolution of the Seventeenth Century*, eds. by Roger French and Andrew Wear (Cambridge: Cambridge U.P., 1989), 87–113, interestingly connects this highly intellectual concern of physicians with the popular perception of physician as atheist.
27. Coward, *Second Thoughts*, (note 23), 133; *idem*, *The Grand Essay (note 23)*, 1–2 & 223–6; Broughton, *op. cit.* (note 24), 199–200; John Balignac, *An Essay Founded upon Arguments Natural and Moral, Proving the Immortality of the Soul* (London: L. Gilliver, 1730), 28–9.
28. Baxter, *op. cit.* (note 14), Vol. 1, 382–3 & 386.
29. Balignac, *op. cit.* (note 27), 30. See also Baxter, *op. cit.* (note 24), Vol. 1, 248 & 257.
30. For a later criticism of Hartley's Lockean scheme from the dualistic point of view, *Letters on Materialism and Hartley's Theory of the Human Mind, Addressed to Dr Priestley* (London: G. Robinson *et.al.*, 1776).
31. George Cheyne, *An Essay on Regimen, together with Five Discourses, Medical, Moral and Philosophical* (London: C. Rivington, 1740), 159.
32. Nicholas Robinson, *A New System of the Spleen, Vapours and Hypochondriack Melancholy* (London: A. Bettesworth,1729), 33–4.
33. For the mystical components of Cheyne's life and writings, see G. S. Rousseau, 'Mysticism and Millenarianism: "Immortal Dr Cheyne"', in *Millenarianism and Messianism in English Literature and Thought 1650–1800*, R. H. Popkin (ed.), (Leiden: E. J. Brill, 1988), 81–126. Later in his life, Robinson conceived of a large work with a tinge of Christian mysticism, *The Christian Philosopher...In Twelve Books* (London, 1741). Only two of them seem to have been published.
34. Cheyne, *op. cit.* (note 31), 120, and *idem*, *The Natural Method of Curing the Diseases of the Body, and the Disorders of the Mind Depending on the Body* (London: Geo. Strahan, 1742), 79. See also Robert Eberwein, 'Samuel Johnson, George Cheyne, and the "Cone of Being"', *Journal of the History of Ideas*, xxxvi (1975), 153–8.
35. Cheyne, *op. cit.* (note 31), 166. See also *idem*, *Philosophical Principles of Religion: Natural and Revealed* (London: George Strahan, 1715), 160–1.
36. Robinson, *op. cit.* (note 32), 29–30. See also Richard Blackmore, 'An

Essay upon the Immortality of the Soul', in *Essays upon Several Subjects*, 2 vols. (London: E. Curll *et al.*, 1716), Vol. 1, 297 & 350; William Smith, *A Dissertation upon the Nerves* (London: for the Author, 1768), 5–6; *A Dissertation upon the Nervous System to Show Its Influence upon the Soul* ([London]: for the Author, 1780), 49–51.

37. Robinson, *op. cit.* (note 32), 51–2; Malcolm Flemyng, *A New Critical Examination of an Important Passage in Mr. Locke's Essay on Human Understanding* (London: Jacob Robinson, 1751).
38. Locke, *op. cit.* (note 3), 1.1.2.
39. Cheyne, *Philosophical Principles* (note 35), 114–15.
40. For Locke's idea of personal identity and his critics, see Sylvana Tomaselli, 'The First Person: Descartes, Locke and Mind-Body Dualism', *History of Science*, xxii (1984), 185–205; B. C. Tennant, 'The Anglican Response to Locke's Theory of Personal Identity', *Journal of the History of Ideas*, xliii (1982), 73–90; Christopher Fox, 'Locke and the Scriblerians', *Eighteenth-Century Studies*, xvi (1982), 1–25.
41. Robinson, *op. cit.* (note 32), 36–8 & 40. A similar criticism was raised by Joseph Butler, *The Works of Joseph Butler*, 3 vols (Oxford: Clarendon Press, 1896), Vol. 1, 387–96. For Butler's idea on personal identity, see Terence Penelhum, *Butler* (London: Routledge & Kegan Paul, 1985), 113–46.
42. Cheyne, *op. cit.* (note 31), 164 & 166. Robinson, *An Essay on the Soul of Man* (London: Jacob Robinson, 1744), 3 & 34. See also Richard Blackmore, *A Treatise of the Spleen and Vapours: or Hypochondriacal and Hysterical Affection...* (London: J. Pemberton, 1725), 256–7.
43. Cheyne, *op. cit.* (note 31), 161 & 166; Robinson, *op. cit.* (note 32), 31. Optimism about improving the mind by somatic means had been expressed by Descartes in his *Discourse on Method.* See *The Philosophical Writings of Descartes*, 3 vols, John Cottingham *et al.* (eds), (Cambridge: Cambridge U.P., 1985–91), Vol. 1, 143.
44. Cheyne, *The Natural Method* (note 34), 82.
45. Cheyne, *op. cit.* (note 31), 167.
46. *Ibid.*, 165–66. His advice to the Countess of Huntingdon tells the same assumption. See Cheyne, *The Letters of Dr George Cheyne to the Countess of Huntingdon*, Charles F. Mullett (ed.), (San Marino, Calif.: Huntingdon Library, 1940), 10.
47. Cheyne, *The Natural Method*, (note 34), 84–85.
48. The literature on the spleen is vast. See, *inter alia*, Roy Porter, 'The Rage of Party: a Glorious Revolution in English Psychiatry?' *Medical History*, xxviii (1983), 35–50.
49. Cheyne, *The Letters of George Cheyne to Samuel Richardson (1733–1743)*, Charles F. Mullett (ed.), (Columbia: University of Missouri Press, 1943), 108. See also Robinson, *op. cit.* (note 34), 175; Sir John Midriff [pseud.], *Observations on the Spleen and Vapours*

(London: J. Roberts, 1721), 9; Roy Porter, *op. cit.* (note 12), 57; *idem*, 'Divided Selves and Psychiatric Medicine', *Cycnos*, vi (1990), 95–106.

50. John Hill, *Hypochondriasis: a Practical Treatise on the Nature and Cure of that Disorder* (London: for the Author, 1766), 3 As for Hill, see G. S. Rousseau, 'John Hill, Universal Genius *manqué*: Remarks on His Life and Times, with a Checklist of His Works', in *The Renaissance Man in the Eighteenth Century*, J. A. Leo Lemry and G.S. Rousseau (eds), (Los Angeles: William Andrews Clark Memorial Library, 1978), 45–129.
51. Robinson, *op. cit.* (note 32), 176–8; Cheyne, *The Natural Method* (note 34), 78.
52. The literature on the medical and pseudo-medical attack on 'enthusiasm' is vast. See, *inter alia*, Michael Heyd, 'The Reaction to Enthusiasm in the Seventeenth Century: towards an Integrative Approach', *Journal of Modern History*, liii(1981), 258–80.
53. Robinson, *op. cit.* (note 32), 246–7. For French Prophets, see Hillel Schwartz, *Knaves, Fools, Madmen, and that Subtile Effluvium: a Study of the Opposition to the French Prophets in England, 1706–1710* (Gainesville, Florida: The University Press of Florida, 1978).
54. Addison and Steele, *The Spectator*, no. 381; Cheyne, *The Natural Method* (note 34), 84; Robinson, *op. cit.* (note 32), 239–40 & 246–7.
55. Bright, *op. cit.* (note 26), 'Epistle Dedicatory' & 194; du Laurens, *op. cit.* (note 26), 81. See also John Abernethy, *A Christian and Heavenly Treatise: Containing Physicke for the Soule* (London: Robert Allot, 1630), 54; Levinus Lemnius, *The Secret Miracles of Nature: in Four Books* (London: by Jo. Streater, 1658), 63–5.
56. Blackmore, *op. cit.* (note 45), 160; George Cheyne, *The English Malady* (1733; rept. with introduction by Roy Porter, London: Routledge, 1991), 2.
57. Blackmore defended immortality of the soul and attacked atheists and Arians; Cheyne was very pious and found by the Countess of Huntingdon (who was a Methodist) to have 'the most refined notions of the true spiritual religion I almost ever met with'. See Blackmore, *op. cit.* (note 36), Vol. 1, 291–356 & Vol. 2, 1–166; Cheyne, *The Letters ... to the Countess of Huntingdon*, viii.
58. Lewis Southcomb, *Peace of Mind and Health of Body United* (London: M. Cooper, 1750), 15 & 26; Benjamin Fawcett, *Observations on the Nature, Causes and Cure of Melancholy: Especially of That Which is Commonly Called Religious Melancholy* (Shrewsbury: J. Eddows, 1780), 3.
59. Roy Porter, 'Introduction' to Cheyne, *op. cit.* (note 56), gives the most perceptive account of Cheyne's life and ideas. For an extensive literature on Cheyne, see the works cited *ibid*, notes 20 & 21.
60. Rousseau, *op. cit.* (note 20), Porter, *op. cit.* (note 20).
61. *The Tatler*, no.236, quoted in Rousseau, 'Science Books and their

Readers', 202.

62. *Sir Isaac Newton's Philosophy Explained for the Use of the Ladies*, (London: E. Cave, 1739), author's preface, v–vi. See also Klein, 'The Third Earl of Shaftesbury and the Progress of Politeness', 201–203; Rousseau, 'Science Books and their Readers'.
63. Dorothy Porter and Roy Porter, *Patient's Progress: Doctors and Doctoring in Eighteenth-Century England* (Oxford: Polity Press, 1989).
64. The iatro-mathematical phase of Cheyne's life is nicely discussed in Anita Guerrini, 'Isaac Newton, George Cheyne and the *Principia Medicinae*', in French & Wear *op. cit.* (note 26), 222–45.
65. Cheyne, *An Essay of Health and Long Life* (London: George Strahan, 1724), v–vi.
66. The stress on physician's linguistic skill as a curative device is discussed in Porter and Porter, *op. cit.* (note 63), 141–2.
67. Cheyne, *op. cit.* (note 65), xvii.
68. Cheyne, *op. cit.* (note 31), iv–v.
69. Cheyne, *An Essay of Health and Long Life*, xi–xii.
70. John Wesley, *Primitive Physick* (London: Thomas Trye, 1747), 'The Preface', xiii & xix–xxiv. A. Wesley Hill, *John Wesley among the Physicians* (London: The Epworth Press, 1958). See also Cheyne, *op. cit.* (note 56), 'Preface', iii, where he complains about some people's (probably he meant Beau Nash) perception of the precepts as uncivilized.
71. The cheapest almanacs at the bottom end of the market have been perceptively analysed in Mary E. Fissell, 'Readers. Texts, and Contexts: Vernacular Medical Works in Early Modern England', in *The Popularization of Medicine 1650–1850*, Roy Porter (ed.), (London: Routledge, 1992), 72–96.
72. The effect of competition is discussed in Borsay, *op. cit.* (note 17), 223–56.
73. *Ibid.*, 284–308; E. P. Thompson, 'Patrician Society, Plebeian Culture', *Journal of Social History*, vii (1974), 382–405.
74. Michael MacDonald, 'Religion, Social Change, and Psychological Healing in England, 1600–1800', in *The Church and Healing*, W. J. Sheils (ed.), (Oxford: Basil Blackwell, 1982), 101–25. See, however, Porter, *op. cit.* (note 12), 56–7.
75. See Johanna Geyer-Kordesch, 'Cultural Habits of Illness: the Enlightened and the Pious in Eighteenth-Century Germany', in *Patients and Practioners: Lay Perceptions of Medicine in Pre-Industrial Society*, Roy Porter (ed.), (Cambridge: Cambridge U.P., 1985), 177–204; Jeremy Gregory, 'Anglicanism and the Arts: Religion, Culture and Politics in the Eighteenth Century', in *Culture, Politics, and Society in Britain, 1660–1800*, Jeremy Black and Jeremy Gregory (eds), (Manchester: Manchester U.P., 1991), 82–109.
76. MacDonald, 'Religion, Social Change, and Psychological Healing' (note 47).

77. Cheyne, *op. cit.* (note 56), 117, Hill, *op. cit.* (note 50), 3.
78. Porter, *op. cit.* (note 12), 55–61; *idem*, 'Bodies of Thought: Thoughts about the Body in Eighteenth-Century England', in *Interpretation and Cultural History*, Joan H. Pittock and Andrew Wear (eds), (London: Macmillan, 1992), 82–108, 88–95.
79. Eighteenth-century symbolic politics of cultural hegemony has been discussed in Thompson, 'Patrician Society, Plebeian Culture'. Eighteenth-century body as a symbolic site of politics is perceptively discussed in Porter, 'Bodies of Thought' (note 78) . See also Akihito Suzuki, '"A Duumvirate of Rulers within Us": Politics and Medical Pneumatology in Restoration England', in *The Restoration Mind*, G. Marshall (ed.), (Newark: University of Delaware Press, forthcoming).
80. Cheyne, *The Natural Method*, 82.
81. *Ibid.*, 87.
82. Thompson, 'Patrician Society, Plebeian Culture'.
83. See Porter, 'Bodies of Thought' (note 78), 89–90.
84. See Porter and Porter, *op. cit.* (note 63), *passim.*
85. J. V. Golinski, 'Science *in* the Enlightenment', Review of Thomas L. Hankins, *Science and the Enlightenment. History of Science*, xxvi (1986), 411–24.

15

An Enlightenment Science? Surgery and the Royal Society[1]

Philip Wilson

Historians typically claim that British surgical 'science' began with John Hunter. D'Arcy Power, for instance, identified Hunter as the individual who 'made surgery a science' by basing it upon experiments.[2] Few, however, go so far as Ralph Major's acknowledgement that any pre-Hunterian 'science' of surgery existed. Major claimed that Hunter 'found surgery an operative science; ... [and] made it a physiological science as well'.[3] L. S. Jacyna has argued that our image of the 'science' of surgery that Hunter is frequently described as 'founding' was not the eighteenth-century view of science at all. Rather, Jacyna claimed this image originated in the early nineteenth century when surgeons were struggling for their profession to gain the status which 'medical science' had achieved.[4]

A quick perusal of eighteenth-century English surgical literature produces many examples of pre-Hunterian surgeons describing their surgery as a 'science'. William Salmon referred to 'Professors' of the 'Science' of surgery in the dedication of his *Ars Chirurgica* (1698). He claimed that the methods of practice he described 'agree[d] with the Principles of the Science [of Chirurgery], and the Safety and Health of the Patient'.[5] Royal Naval surgeon, James Handley, argued in 1733 that the bone-setters had proved to be a 'scandal to all [the] Science' of surgery.[6] Eleven years later, the eminent London surgeon Charles Bernard was cited as having compared surgical writers with those in the 'other learned Arts and Sciences'.[7] Little attention, however, has been directed towards discerning what specifically comprised the 'science' of surgery that Bernard and the other authors discussed. Were there attempts before Hunter's to explicitly establish an experimentally-based 'science' of surgery in England? Or, as Christopher Lawrence has claimed, was there merely an eighteenth-century 'change of emphasis' in defining surgery as a science rather than an art – a change Lawrence argues would have been 'unremarkable to English readers'?[8]

This chapter explores the depiction of surgery as a 'science' in Enlightenment England. I discuss what contemporary surgical authors communicated as the 'science' of surgery. As London's Royal Society provides an exemplary model of England's 'scientific community', I have limited my investigation to the reports by surgeons or about 'surgical' conditions which appeared in the Society's *Philosophical Transactions.* I further confine my research to the period of reports between the death of Royal Society President, Sir Isaac Newton in 1727 and the election of Sir Joseph Banks to the same position in 1778. Compared to the scholarly interest devoted to the early years of the Society, little research has focused on the Society's activities during the mid eighteenth century. Thus, this chapter meets the challenge of exploring this historical 'valley of darkness'.[9] I also discuss several probable reasons why some surgeons chose to define their work as a 'science'. Among the reasons I explore is the surgeons's contemporary attempt to display a more 'professional' image by modelling their practice as a science. I then analyse the content of the surgical writings to ascertain which components of the 'science' they described arose from the 'scientific enterprise' of the Enlightenment and which stemmed from the earlier Baconian model of science. From this analysis, we begin to gain a better understanding of the contemporary expression, the 'science of surgery'.

Surgical Reporting to the Royal Society

Between 1727 and 1778, 220 reports by surgeons or about 'surgical' conditions appeared in the*Philosophical Transactions.*[10] Just over half of these conditions were similar to those described in contemporary surgical texts. For example, this periodical contained multiple accounts of treatments of bladder and kidney stones (34 reports), fractures and dislocations (17), methods for stopping haemorrhage (11), repairing hernias and ruptures (11), excising tumours (10), couching cataracts, curing skin diseases and treating ascites (6 each). The *Philosophical Transactions* also contained single reports on 68 other disorders typically discussed in surgical writings. Surgeons also described the anatomy of rattlesnakes, ostriches, and viviparous eels, the heat production in animals and vegetables, the causes of animal and human monstrosities, and commented on the human remains exhumed from ancient burial sites and the illnesses attending the consumption of poisonous fish in the South Seas. These topics rarely received any mention in contemporary surgical texts.

Figure 1: Surgical Reports in Philosophical Transactions

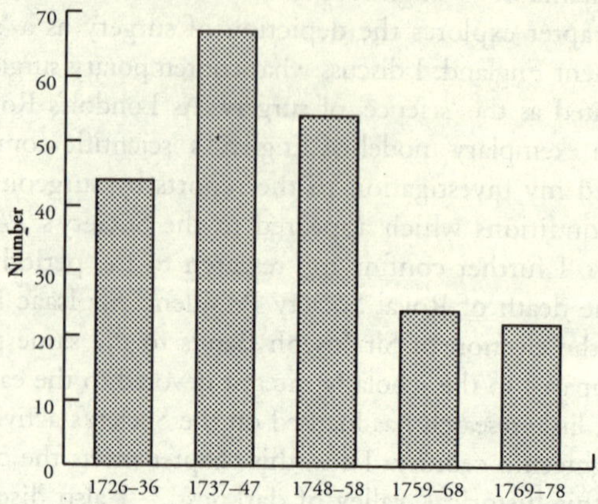

Figure 1 shows that the number of reports of surgical conditions published during the two latter decades of the period under examination had significantly declined from that of the preceding 30 years.[11] Most probably, this decline represents the Society's 1752 change of policy regarding the publication of the *Transactions.* At this time, a 'Committee of Papers' was formed among the Society's Fellowship to take full responsibility of selecting which of the papers delivered before the Society were 'proper to be printed'. Prior to this, the Society had appointed one of its secretaries to select and edit the publications. This change of policy resulted in a 'Committee' of reviewers whose collective scrutiny reduced the number of reports which were subsequently published in their *Transactions.*[12]

Contemporary accounts describe bladder stones as among the most common ailments for which many eighteenth-century Londoners called upon surgeons. Some surgeons had developed a virtual specialty in 'cutting for the stone' (i.e., lithotomy). In addition to surgical treatment, hundreds of 'proven' remedies were advertised in contemporary medical writings and domestic manuals, each proffering particular solvents to 'cure' those afflicted with this disorder. By mid-century, a massive literature had been amassed on this subject.[13] Joseph Warner, surgeon to Guy's Hospital and Fellow of the Royal Society (F.R.S.), proclaimed that the 'circumstances' of the causes and treatments of this disorder were, 'in general so well known, and so much alike, as to render few [new] cases ... worthy of communication'.[14] Given the vast literature on the stone already available, the continued reporting of information on this disorder in the *Philosophical Transactions* begs further inquiry.

One noteworthy contribution came from John Douglas, one of London's premier lithotomists. Douglas was surgeon to the Westminster Infirmary and an F.R.S. His local fame stemmed, in part, through his success with a particular technique. Specifically, Douglas promoted the removal of bladder stones by making a large incision into the pubic region of the lower abdomen (the 'high operation'). Another locally-renowned lithotomist and F.R.S., William Cheselden, argued that this method, the '*Lithotomia Douglassiana*', put patients in much more danger than his own method of making a small incision in the lateral perineal region (the 'lateral operation'). By mid-century, Cheselden's method had gained international renown. Douglas, however, never publicly acknowledged Cheselden's demonstrated success, but rather continued to seek alternative techniques to improve upon Cheselden. His contribution to the 1727/8 *Philosophical Transactions* is suggestive of a quest to secure operations for patients who are unable to 'submit to any of the great Operations of the Stone with tolerable hopes of success' due to their 'great Age, [or] bad Habit'. He argued that by making an artificial fistulae in the perineum, patients themselves could, by passing an 'Oiled Probe' through this opening, 'push the Stone back', thereby allowing them to 'make Water'. Otherwise, he argued, this 'urge' could not be relieved 'with out the Ceremony of sending for, and staying in misery till a surgeon comes to pass the Catheter'.[15] He also argued that by adopting his modified technique, surgeons could enhance their reputation as competent 'cutters' of the stone.

The eminent surgical authors, Lorenz Heister and Claude-Nicolas Le Cat also used the *Philosophical Transactions* to promote improvements in their well-known lithotomy techniques. A less well-known surgeon, John Mudge, proposed a different method to the Royal Society which, he claimed, would improve the success of the 'lateral method' of lithotomy. He asked that his description be 'laid before the Society; and if it be thought to deserve it', he urged them to 'communicate' this method 'to the Public in their *Transactions*'.[16] Thus, this periodical provided both renowned and relatively unknown surgeons publicity of their recommendations in improving the surgical art. Some, like Mudge, appear to have deferred judgement about the usefulness of particular surgical methods to the Fellowship of the Royal Society.

Most reports of operations for the stone in the *Philosophical Transactions* describe particular cases which their authors deemed were 'remarkable' or 'very extraordinary'. Joseph Warner, for example, claimed that his removal of an 'irregular piece of bone' together with a stone from Elizabeth England's bladder was of 'singular, and perhaps unparallel'd circumstance', and thereby, worthy of communicating.[17] He deemed a later case to be of 'extraordinary' merit as it showed practical advice 'contrary to the received opinion'. This case recounted a surgeon's judgement of a patient in which, upon finding one rough stone in the patient's bladder, he looked no further for more stones. The surgeon had assumed, what Warner claimed was the 'maxim laid down by the ... best received Writers ... in surgery', that if a patient had multiple stones, they are all likely to be smooth due to constant frictional contact. However, when this patient 'relapse[d] into the like disorder ... a short time after the healing of their wounds', Warner was called upon to 'oblige' the patient to 'submit to a second operation'. In this operation, several stones were removed. Warner argued that this second surgery was avoidable if the first surgeon had been more thorough in his work. He deemed this case worthy of reporting as it 'may prove of the greatest consequence to the future ease and welfare' of patients.[18]

Warner continued to relate cases of his successful surgical treatments for the stone to *Philosophical Transactions'* readers. He explained that, although many of the procedures he described were well known, 'when matters of fact, however common in themselves, are so circumstanced, as to assume extraordinary appearances, the uncommon phaenomena accompanying such facts, when capable of being pointed out, will, I believe, be always considered by the Royal Society, as a sufficient apology for the freedom of the[ir] communication.'[19] But identifying just what Warner deemed 'remarkable' about the shapes and sizes of these stones is difficult, for many of these cases are strikingly similar to case reports in the contemporary literature. This similarity leads me to wonder whether Warner was displaying the case or his own surgical prowess as the more extraordinary feature.

Stopping the flow of blood after surgery, often the initial test of a surgeon's post-operative technique, was also a common theme of surgical reports in the *Philosophical Transactions*. Cautery irons and tourniquets had long been used to achieve this means. These procedures, however, were not without risk. *Philosophical Transactions'* reports suggest that in the eighteenth century there was a growing preference for the use of styptics instead of or in addition to the abovementioned forms of haemostasis.

Experiments to evaluate the efficacy of styptics designed to

'Improve' the control of haemorrhage were discussed in earlier volumes of the *Philosophical Transactions.* In 1693, surgeon – anatomist William Cowper had reported his investigations into the efficacy of John Colbatch's styptic powder. Cowper argued that the success of Colbatch's styptic on animals was not found when applied to humans.[20] Sixty years later, experiments testing the efficacy of another styptic, the agaric (or fungus) of oak, in both animal and human subjects, were reported to the Royal Society.

During the eighteenth century French surgeons appear to have initiated investigations as to which styptics were the most effective, the least caustic and the most humanitarian methods in controlling excessive blood loss. Pierre Dionis, for instance, displayed cautery irons to his students more 'to excite horror with regard to their cruelty, than to advise their use'.[21] M. Faget's 1752 report in the *Philosophical Transactions* described M. Brossard's success in Paris from the use of the agaric of oak in stopping haemorrhages in patients. 'This application', he argued, 'exceeds every thing, which has hitherto been produced by the operation of our hands' (i.e., cautery and ligature).[22] By the following year, three English surgeons, Samuel Sharp, Joseph Warner and Benjamin Gooch, all Fellows of the Royal Society, responded to this claim with 'Experiments' and case evidence in support of the Frenchman. Surgeons James Ford and William Thornhill added several cases in succeeding years which attested to their own successful use of this agaric as a styptic. Thornhill claimed he was 'surprised' that 'any objections are made to ... [its] use' . He speculated that the 'true reason of its not being used in general practice proceeds from a narrow selfish way of thinking', but claimed himself 'well satisfied, [that] it is the best medicine in all the materia medica yet discovered for that purpose'.[23]

If surgical 'experiments' are defined as the accounts of treatments which explicitly compared the efficacy of one method or medication with another, then besides the eleven reports on the use of the agaric, there were few *Philosophical Transactions* reports which described surgical 'experiments'. The data gathered in Figure 2 show that reports of surgical experiments comprised a relatively small percentage (between 0–27%) of the surgical reports published during this period. Instead, between 63–89% of the surgical reports presented detailed descriptions of 'extraordinary' observations which surgeons had encountered during their course of practice. My calculated percentage of 'experimental' surgical reports is consistent with Charles Bazerman's study of a broader range of *Philosophical Transactions* reports from this period. Bazerman claimed that experimental articles comprised only

5–20% of the articles in each of the first 80 volumes of this periodical.[24] Figure 2. also indicates that the percentage of surgical experiments was significantly greater during the 1769–78 period than in any of the previous four periods.

Figure 2: Content of Surgical Reports

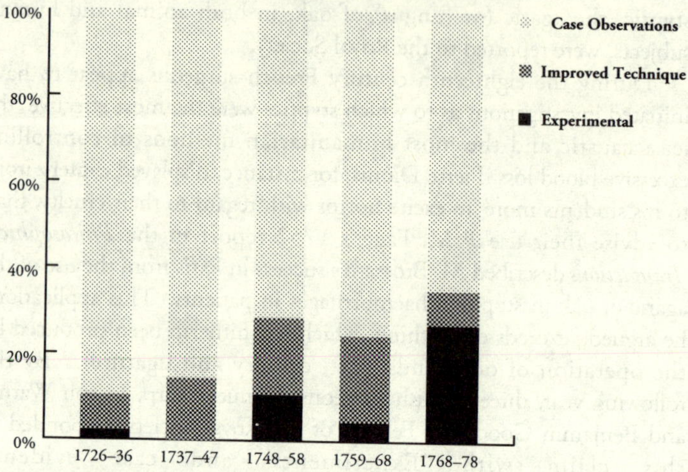

A third type of surgical report appears in the *Philosophical Transactions* – reports which described particular 'improvements' or 'advancements' in surgical technique. For example, Claudius Amyand promoted the 'laying open' of a carious bone as a 'better way' than amputation in 'stopping the Progress of the Evil' caries.[25] Truro surgeon Christopher Warrick reported his 'Improvement of the Practice of Tapping' a patient with ascites in 1744.[26] Archibald Cleland, surgeon to General Wade's Regiment of Horse, presented evidence for the efficacy of his newly designed needles for operating on the eye and ear.[27] Claude-Nicolas Le Cat described a series on 'new invented instruments' to extirpate tumours out of the surgeon's reach, to treat gangrene, hernias, hydrocephalus, and 'to improve the manner of cutting ... and shorten [the time expended in] the Operation' of lithotomy.[28] He also devised a machine resembling 'a hammock' hooked up to a pulley mechanism to lift immobilized patients from their bed in order to apply medications or dressing on their back or posterior side.[29] (See Figure 3.) Samuel Sharp described a 'new method' of couching cataracts whereby he claimed 'Mons. Daviel's operation will be very much shorten'd, the patient will suffer less pain, and every skilful operator will be equal to the undertaking'.[30] The surgeon–anatomist, John Hunter, promoted a new technique for resuscitating 'drowned' victims.[31]

Figure 3

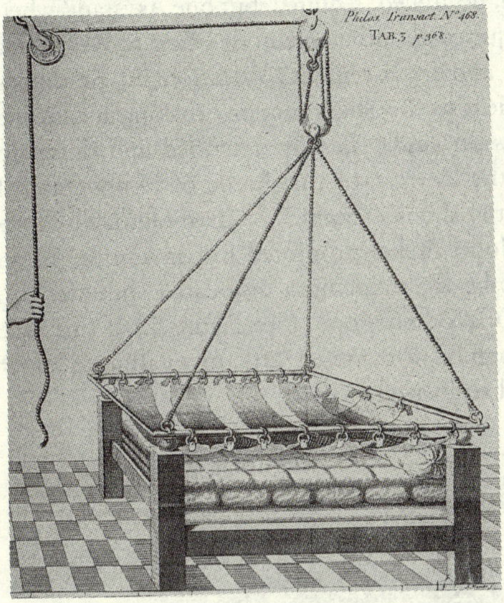

Nicolas-Claude Le Cat's 'Machine for dressing and curing Patients, who are very unwieldy, and are under the Surgeon's Hands for some Ailment on the Back, the *Os Sacrum,* &c. Or are apprehensive of it', *Phil. Trans. Roy. Soc.*, 42 (1742–43), Tab. 3, 368.

Aside from bladder stones, the second most common surgical condition for which *Philosophical Transactions'* authors introduced new or modified techniques was the treatment of dislocated or fractured bones. The early eighteenth-century surgical case records of one London practitioner, Daniel Turner, describe fractures as among the most common disorders for which patients called upon surgeons. Turner claimed that in 'more than 20 Years' of surgical practice, he 'seldom had fewer than four or five [patients with fractures] of one kind or another, at once under ... [his] Inspection.'[32] A contemporary report of St Thomas's Hospital surgical practice corroborates Turner's claim of the common occurrence of fractures.[33]

Philosophical Transactions' reports between 1741 and 1743 contain seven cases describing 'improved' methods to care for patients with fractured or dislocated bones. Surgeon Henry Ettrick discussed and illustrated his 'new Invention' for reducing fractures of the thigh. His invention involved the attachment of an axle and a 'toothed' wheel to the end of a patient's bed which, when strapped to the patient's lower leg, could extend the patient's leg by turning the wheel. (See Figure 4.) This method, he argued, required 'but one Assistant' whereas the many assistants required by other methods often prove, he claimed, 'most troublesome and inconvenient'. Additionally, he designed a bed to 'swing and yield to the Ship's motion', making his invention useful at sea as well as on land.[34] Le Cat described and illustrated his modifications of the 'defects' of the 'Ambe of Hippocrates' for reducing luxations of the shoulder joint.[35] St Bartholomew's Hospital Surgeon and F.R.S., John Freke, promoted his 'invention' of a much more 'portable' Ambe for reducing a dislocated shoulder in the number following Le Cat's description. (See Figure 5.) If this 'Machine' is not portable, he argued, it mattered 'little to an afflicted Patient Ten Miles off, how good an Instrument it is'.[36]

Figure 4

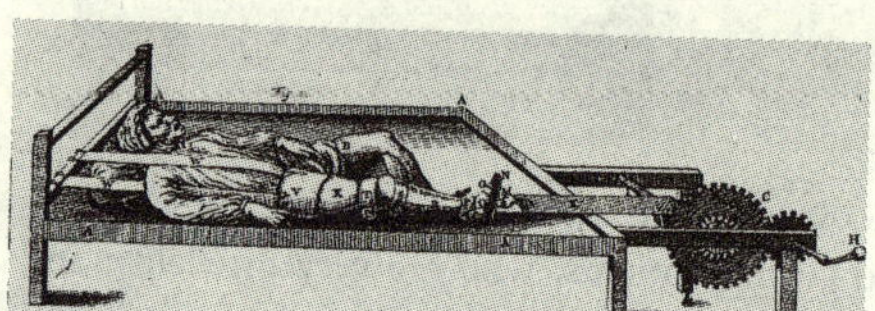

Henry Ettrick's 'Machine for reducing Fractures of the Thigh', *Phil. Trans. Roy Soc.*, 41 (1739–41), Tab. 2, 566.

From the time of its foundation, much of the 'business' of the Royal Society had utilitarian ends. For example, reports describing practical applications of science to agriculture and industry had, according to Peter Mathias, 'as much or more [space] devoted to them as any other'.[37] Although many surgeons were employed to maintain the health and strength of England's naval and military personnel, the *Philosophical Transactions* did not explicitly address the utilitarian view of surgeons upholding England's national and economic power. Nor were the surgical reports explicitly designed to instruct surgeons in their practice, in the manner of contemporary surgical texts by Daniel Turner, John Atkins, George Smith, Alexander Stuart, Samuel Sharp and Perivcal Pott. It is indeed unlikely that many readers of the *Philosophical Transactions* were practising surgeons. What, then, was the reason for reporting the experiences of surgical practice to a group of non-surgical readers?

Figure 5

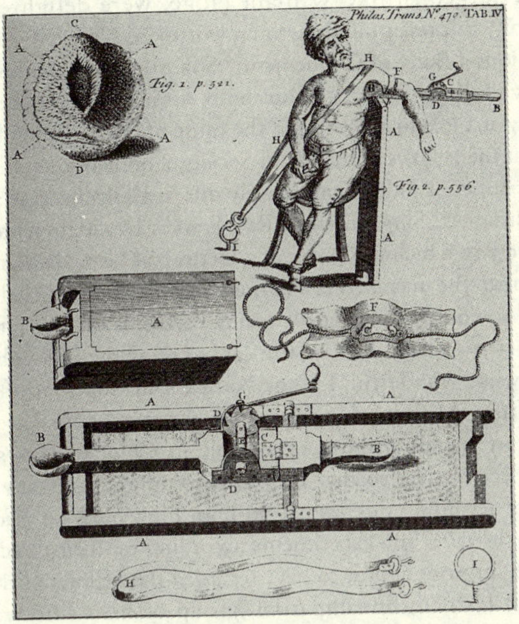

John Frele's 'Instrument for reducing a dislocated shoulder', *Phil. Trans. Roy. Soc.*, 42 (1742–43), Tab. 4, Fig. 2, 556.

Why Surgeons Wrote to the Royal Society

Surgeons appear to have offered reports to the Royal Society for a variety of stated reasons. Some were interested in sharing their knowledge of remarkable incidents they had encountered in practice or at dissection. Robert Home, late surgeon to the Thirtieth Regiment of Foot, and surgeon at Kingston upon Hull, described the treatment of a patient whose flexor tendon of his thumb had accidently been 'torn out'. He noted that although several comparable cases appeared in the *Mémoires de l'Academie Royale de Chirurgie* 'no observations of a similar nature [had appeared] in the *Philosophical Transactions*'.[38] The Manchester surgeon, Charles White described 'the first operation of the kind' whereby although the head of the humerus (i.e., the end of the upper arm bone which contributes to the shoulder joint) was detached from the rest of the bone, the 'entire motion' of the patient's arm had been preserved. Relating this case in the *Philosophical Transactions* might, White argued, 'possibly conduce the improvement of the art'.[39]

Other surgeons, like William Fidge, were delighted at the 'Opportunity of presenting something worthy of Notice to so Learned and Ingenious a Body of Gentlemen.'[40] Still others sought advice from the Society's Fellows. Thomas Woolcomb, for instance, claimed that he was 'wholly at a loss to account for' the cause of one patient's death. He desired that the Fellows of the Royal Society, a body of men he deemed as holding 'superior judgement', review this 'remarkable' case and offer their conclusions.[41] Surgeon and F.R.S. Francis Drake presented a case to the Society in which the bones of a foetus had been 'discharged thro an ulcer near the navel'. He claimed this case contained 'several Particulars' he could not 'reconcile to any natural laws'. But rather than seek the Society's advice, he used this case to show the Fellowship 'most evidently what wonderful Things Nature can do'.[42] James Bate, a surgeon from Maryland, reported his remarkable case of the 'extraordinary metamorphosis observable in Colonel Barnes's negro woman' to the Society so that they might communicate any 'further experiments' regarding this woman to him. He would 'be glad', so he claimed, to 'execute' any experiments according to 'their directions'.[43] Thus, some surgeons appear to have regarded the Fellows of the Royal Society as a learned, but impartial, group of men who were well enough informed about the 'human condition' to comment upon their own practice. The Society's occasional suggestions as to particular surgico-anatomical experiments is evidenced by Oxford anatomist F. Nicholls' report of his study of an aneurism he claimed to have performed 'by Order of the Society'.[44]

Some investigators discussed 'discoveries' they had made during animal or human dissections. Charles Price, for example, communicated his findings of the 'villi' of the stomach in animal dissections 'in Hopes that the Analogy between [animal] ... and human subjects may lead us into a more perfect Knowledge of our own structure'.[45] Claudius Amyand, in 1737/8, reported his dissection findings of an obstructed biliary duct which bore, he claimed, a 'Conformity ... with what he previously reported to the Society', thereby using this periodical to validate his previous work.[46] John Ranby added 'some material Observations' which, he claimed, 'had escaped my Notice in ... [a] former Dissection' he had reported.[47]

Other surgeons reported their findings or experiences which corroborated those of their local and Continental colleagues. St Bartholomew's surgeon, Edward Nourse, described a dissection of a foetus which had been delivered via the anus as similar to what M. Littre had described in the *Mémoires de l'Academie Royale des Sciences* in

Paris.[48] Another report 'confirm[ed] the Great Boerhaave's Opinion, that the Seat of the Lues Venerea is in the Membrana adiposa'.[49] And in several instances contributors abstracted or extracted accounts from foreign writers to show specific similarities to their own findings.

A few surgeons used the *Philosophical Transactions* to express their opposition to other surgeons' techniques or claims. Edward Nourse and George Bell gathered evidence to convince readers of the inefficacy of Mrs Stephens's medicinal 'Cure for the Stone'.[50] Thomas Hope denounced the flamboyant Chevalier Taylor's claims of curing cataracts.[51] And Charles White described his success in reducing a patient's dislocated 'thigh bone', an operation he claimed Boerhaave had argued was useless because the head of the femur was always broken off. White argued that this was not always the case, and attempted to overthrow 'Boerhaave's weight with the generality of the profession.'[52] Newcastle surgeon, James Bent, described a case which 'proves' not only that the above operation Charles White reported to the Society was 'practicable' and 'adviseable' [sic], but 'points out the nature of Mr. White's mistake' as well.[53]

Another possible motivation for contributing surgical reports to the Royal Society must not go unmentioned. As the Society was recognized, by many, as a body of learned gentlemen and scholars, some contributors may have aspired to display themselves as scholarly as much or more than to promote any particular surgical technique. At the time, it was quite unusual for surgeons, apprentice-trained craftsmen, to prepare any written reports, let alone reports before one of London's most august gatherings of gentlemen and scholars. Rather, most of the reports before the Royal Society came from men who shared a similar university education to the natural philosophers, physicians and antiquaries who comprised the vast majority of the Society's Fellowship.

Submitting case reports before the Royal Society was one way to elevate oneself among the ranks of surgeons. For a few, it appears to have been part of their 'grooming' for eventual election into the Society's Fellowship. Between the Society's founding in 1660 and 1700, only six surgeons were admitted into the Fellowship.[54] Of these apprentice-trained practitioners, one had the Royal patronage of Charles II and James II and three others had the backing of Hans Sloane, Secretary to the Society. As the Society operated under what has been called an 'informal network of influence and dependency', with candidacy for Fellowship depending very much upon whom you knew, contributing reports, particularly reports of memorable or 'remarkable' phenomena was one way for surgeons to gain exposure amongst the Society's Fellows.[55] Still, by the mid eighteenth century, the electing members of the Society continued to view surgeons in general, with very few exceptions, as unworthy of Fellowship status.[56]

Only 15 of the 69 surgeons who contributed *Philosophical Transactions* reports between 1727 and 1778 were Fellows of the Royal Society.[57] Of the English members of this group, two were Sergeant-Surgeons to the Monarch, and ten served as surgeons to hospitals in London and Westminster. These hospital surgeons included John Belchier, Joseph Warner, Samuel Sharp and John Hunter from Guys, John Freke, Edward Nourse, and Percival Pott from St Bartholomew's, John Douglas and Henry Watson from the Westminster Infirmary, and William Cheselden from St Thomas's. This finding in the *Philosophical Transactions* suggests that hospital surgeons had, by mid-century, selectively gained a status above that which Fellows of the Royal Society deemed of surgeons in the navy, military or in private practice. The Royal Society's recognition of hospital surgeons supports work, like that of Susan Lawrence, which demonstrates the growing significance of the hospital as a teaching institution in London during the Enlightenment.[58] However, a thorough investigation of the contemporary surgical practice and training within these hospitals is wanting.

Apart from the authors' individual motivations for publishing their work in the *Philosophical Transactions*, there was also, during the second half of the eighteenth century, a general movement among many surgeons in London's Company of Surgeons to elevate the status of surgery. For over two centuries London surgeons had been combined with the barbers in a single Barber–Surgeons' Company. In 1745 the surgeons officially distanced their association with the barbers by separating from the old company and forming a single Company of Surgeons. As Thomas Touchit described of surgeons in the 1740s, they saw themselves as an 'improved Body' which could no longer 'bear to see their Name drag[ged] heavily on ... that of the Barbers'. In 1745, they successfully 'sued out a kind of legal Divorce from their unworthy Yokemates, whose Razors ... have no Right or Pretence to the rank with the Lancets'.[59]

Among the reasons surgeons sought to separate their practice from that of the barbers was to establish surgery as more of a learned or 'professional' following. Identifying what specifically constituted the 'professions' of Enlightenment England remains an active area of investigation. Geoffrey Holmes considers that in addition to the clerics, lawyers and physicians, many 'nascent professional occupations' existed in Augustan England. By 'nascent professional occupation',

Holmes meant all of the 'organizational structure' which upheld three basic characteristics: providing a vocation for the whole of a man's working life, undergoing a long and carefully regulated course of training in that vocation, and working in a vocation through which men offered services to their community.[60] Paula Backsheider has described that holding the status of a 'professional' in Daniel Defoe's London 'told' contemporaries that he was 'a person with some power' and, more particularly, that he did not have to earn a living by working with his hands.[61]

General historical accounts lead us to believe that most physicians during the eighteenth century distinguished their types of practice from the more manual practice of surgery. Surgery was literally a handicraft. To begin casting off this handicraft image, some surgeons sought to reconstruct the image of surgery as more of a learned or scholarly following. One way for surgeons to create this more 'professional' image was to display their knowledge of the practice like recognized experts or scholars did in other fields, particularly that of medicine. John Ranby and William Cheselden, two of the primary draftsmen of the 1745 surgeons' petition, displayed their scholarship in surgery through multiple contributions to the *Philosophical Transactions.* The Society recognized their knowledgeable, scholarly contributions and their attempt to reform the status of surgery by electing them into their Fellowship. These reformists exemplified Thomas Chevalier's claim that if surgery was to be enhanced, its practitioners required the 'usual encouragements of rank and fortune' like those who 'devote themselves to ... the vigour and perfection of any science'.[62]

The background of the authors contributing reports of surgical matters to the *Philosophical Transactions* changed throughout the half-century examined in this chapter. Whereas only 29% of these reports were written by surgeons in the 1726–36 period, 92% of the reports from 1769–78 were written by surgeons. (See Figure 6). During the earlier period, physicians contributed many of the reports of surgical conditions. Although the overall number of surgical reports diminished in the later volumes of this periodical, as shown in Figure 1, the increasing representation of surgeons as authors of the surgical reports (Figure 6) suggests their attempt to become officially recognized as the experts in their field. By the late eighteenth century, surgeons had gained the Royal Society 'Committee on Paper's' recognition as the principal commentators or authorities on the art and science of surgery for the readership of the *Philosophical Transactions.*

Figure 6: Authors of Surgical Reports

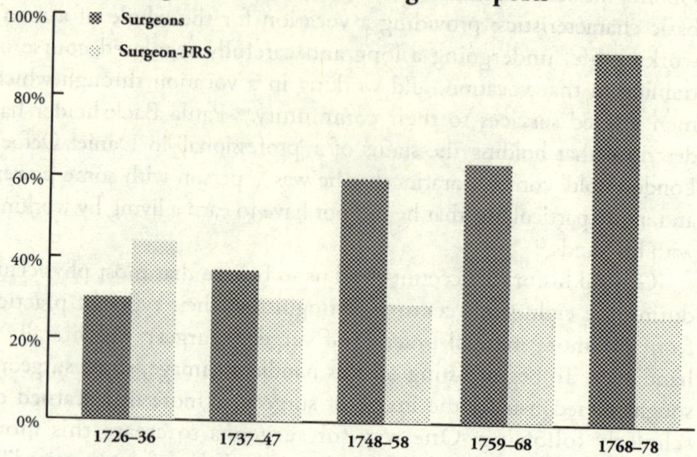

A Baconian or an Enlightenment Science of Surgery?

It might seem appropriate to look at the content of the mid-eighteenth-century surgical reports in the *Philosophical Transactions* only within the context of the Enlightenment. But the Royal Society had, from its institution, embodied a Baconian-based science. In order to determine whether the developing science of surgery owed more to the Baconian model or to Enlightenment thinking, the surgical reports will be considered in each of these contexts separately.

Bacon's seventeenth-century model for the organization of science and the design of scientific inquiry had a long-lasting influence in England. It has been convincingly argued that the interactive environment within the Royal Society was designed after Bacon's description of a utopian 'college of experience', a college which encouraged discussion and collaboration between investigators.[63] Royal Society meetings principally consisted of listening to reports about and discussing the conclusions of the Fellows' experiences with various natural phenomena. According to Peter Dear's work on the Society's form of reporting, the Society's Fellowship considered both the observations of and experiments with these phenomena as experience. *Philosophical Transactions'* accounts of these reports were written, Dear claimed, from the viewpoint of the observer and, by convention, they contained details of the time, place, and participants or witnesses of a particular experience.[64] Steven Shapin has argued that the elaborate narrative details in the reports were rhetorically construed so as to 'give the impression of verisimilitude', compelling the Fellows to accept the reported details as 'matters of fact'.[65] This rhetorical device was particularly useful, he claimed, when there were no actual witnesses of an event. Thus, the narrative itself acted as a corroborative substitute for witnesses to substantiate the observer's claims.

The majority of the surgical reports printed in the *Philosophical Transactions* were of the narrative style. They were typically short, single-author reports on a particular theme, attributes which were characteristic of contemporary scientific literature.[66] Figure 2 shows that between 63–89% of the surgical reports in the *Philosophical Transactions* recounted particular observations from what the authors' deemed to be 'remarkable' cases. This high percentage suggests that the use of detailed narratives, a form which Dear and Shapin have shown extended back as far as Robert Boyle's reports to the Society, remained a dominant form of reporting into the Society's second century.

By reporting these cases to the Royal Society rather than privately printing them in texts of surgery, the authors subjected themselves to feedback, either supportive, neutral or critical, from the Fellows. This self-subjection exemplifies what Dear claimed to be 'cooperative inquiry', a trait which he argued was symbolic of the Society's Baconian pursuit of science.[67] Few surgical reports, however, appear to have sparked controversy. Rather, the authors' appeal to the Royal Society appears to have enhanced both the credibility of their claims and their image as competent, learned surgeons. Their reports in the *Philosophical Transactions* were frequently cited in contemporary surgical literature as being the most recent, authoritative information on particular surgical conditions.

Recognizing surgeons as being knowledgeable about their practice is consistent with one of the definitions of science provided by Samuel Johnson, one of England's pre-eminent Enlightenment figures. Johnson, in his 1755 *Dictionary*, defined the term science as '1. Knowledge. 2. Certainty grounded on demonstration. 3. Art attained by precepts, or built on principles. 4. Any art or species of knowledge. 5. One of the seven liberal arts.' This definition conformed, in part, with the contemporary pursuits of London's 'scientific' society, the Royal Society. Fellows of the Royal Society had, for instance, designed experiments to demonstrate their knowledge of mechanics. They also predicted, with certainty, the action of chemicals, magnets and electricity. Other Fellows described the principles of the art of navigation and ballooning in their correspondence. And from its

1660 foundation, the Royal Society had, as Thomas Sprat described, served to foster 'the Improving of Natural Knowledge'.

Depicting 'science' in England as a dedicated pursuit of improving natural knowledge is most commonly traced to Bacon's writings. Indeed, all of the 'sciences' developed in England might claim that their methods were founded upon Baconian origins. Thus, it would not be unexpected to find proponents of a 'science' of surgery espousing some Baconian ideas in their writings. However, I have not uncovered sufficient evidence to allow me to claim that the authors of the surgical reports in the *Philosophical Transactions* were specifically arguing that the 'science' of surgery should be based upon the Baconian model. Rather, they were merely conforming to the Society's method of reporting.

The surgical reports do, however, exemplify several aspects of the 'scientific enterprise' of the Enlightenment. Specifically, they demonstrate the cosmopolitan feature of Enlightenment science, the contemporary attempts of 'scientists' to delve into greater and wider fields of enquiry, and the general critical acumen of the Enlightened age. These three currents of the Enlightenment are individually examined below.

Anglo-French relations during the Enlightenment have been described as ranging from 'Natural and Necessary Enemies' to France's admiration of and 'cultural borrowing' from the English.[68] This diversity of opinion is also found in contemporary surgical writing. Early in the century, many surgical authors expressed sentiments of mutual Anglo-Franco disdain. St Andre translated Rene-Jacques-Croissant de Garengeot's *Traité des Operations de Chirurgie* to share the 'Happiness' he received from witnessing 'eminent Masters' in Paris; the city in which, he argued, the surgical art was 'daily improved' more than anywhere else in Europe.[69] One contemporary English surgical author found such French claims unwarranted. 'France produce[d no] better Surgeons than Great Britain', so Royal Naval surgeon James Handley declared. If the French showed any 'more Experience' in treating wounds, it was only those 'in their Back parts', for they were, he mused, 'so much used to run away'.[70]

Later, however, the English began to show greater admiration of French surgical technique. The cosmopolitan spirit or 'universality' of surgery during the Enlightenment was clearly expressed by J. Sparrow, an English surgeon and translator of many French writings. In his 1739 translation of Henri-François Le Dran's *Observations de Chirurgie,* Sparrow argued that '[al]though we ... [might] have a political Objection to [some] Nation', we should 'embrace the

Sciences of that Nation for our own Advantage'. Since 'Arts and Sciences are cultivated with the View of a general Benefit to our Fellow Creatures', he claimed, 'I hope we are too much *Englishmen* to imagine that we cannot improve by them, since they are so generous as to acknowledge [that] they have improved by us.'[71]

The mid-century surgical reports before the Royal Society denote similar admiration for French surgery. The most vivid example of the influence of French ideas about surgical practice upon the Fellowship of the Royal Society came from Claude-Nicolas Le Cat. Le Cat, Professor and Demonstrator Royal in Anatomy and Surgery, and perpetual Secretary to the Academie des Sciences in Rouen, contributed 19 reports to the Royal Society which were published in the *Philosophical Transactions* between 1739 and 1767. No English author contributed anywhere near this number of surgical reports, the closest being Joseph Warner with ten reports.[72] Why was there such a disproportionate number of reports from a Frenchman in an English periodical?

French surgery, particularly the practice in Paris, was revered by many Englishmen. London surgeons cited the virtual surgical 'profession' in Paris as an imitable model in their 1745 petition to dissolve the Barber–Surgeons' Company of London. Two years prior to this petition, French surgery had, according to a Declaration by Louis XV, become recognized as an 'art scavant' and a 'vrage science'.[73] Francois Quesney, Secretary of the Académie Royale de Chirurgie, described French surgery as being organized according to an 'inductive' scientific method; a method which, according to Toby Gelfand, distinguished French surgical science from the 'speculative reasoning' of physicians and the 'purely empirical' work of the barbers.[74] The Academie, Quesney claimed, functioned to compile and interpret the observations of surgical experience.[75] This model, indicative of the inductive scientific method whereby data is gathered and incorporated into general principles, owed its origin to England's Francis Bacon. The surgical reports in the *Philosophical Transactions* suggest that as least some English surgeons were also thinking in terms of a similar science-based surgery. Thus, what historians have typically described as the English attempts to emulate French surgery may, in fact, have been, at least in part, the English relying upon their own Baconian methods.

Another French influence upon the development of English surgery has attracted the attention of historians. In a 1746 advertisement in the *London Evening Post*, William Hunter claimed that students who attended his lectures on the operations of surgery would also have the 'opportunity of learning the Art of Dissection ... in the same manner as at Paris'.[76] In addition to Hunter's highly attended instructive dissections at his Great Windmill Street school, reports in the *Philosophical Transactions* suggest that private dissections were frequently performed in London. Detailed accounts of 39 dissections appeared in the 52 years of *Philosophical Transactions'* reports I have examined. One report from the volume covering 1739–41 begins with the claim that 'As the frequent Dissection of Morbid Bodies tends greatly to ascertain the Diagnostic and Prognostic of Diseases, ... The following may be of some Use in Practice.'[77] Other dissection reports emphasize a different utilitarian goal – the importance of visualizing the anatomy that was of particular concern to surgical operations. These two aims of dissection suggest that what Andrew Cunningham stipulated as different 'kinds' of anatomy in the seventeenth century remained in existence in the eighteenth century as well.[78] The first 'kind' of anatomy cited above, by Dr John Huxham, was more of a 'medical' anatomy whereas the second 'kind' conforms more to what may be called a 'surgical' anatomy.

The human body, as Barbara Stafford claimed, represented the 'ultimate visual compendium' to an era of encyclopaedists. Its visible whole was known to be composed of invisible, dissimilar parts.[79] Knowledge of these otherwise invisible parts was attainable, to a limited extent, through surgical operations and, more broadly, through post-mortem dissection. The widespread use of dissection as a form of surgical education appears to have been a product of Enlightenment thinking. Basing surgical know-how upon the principles of anatomy gained from dissection strengthened the image of and legitimated surgery as a science. According to Samuel Johnson, science was an art built upon principles. Finding accounts of the extensive use of dissection in both French and English surgical writings suggests that there were attempts to contrive universal principles of surgery, principles which, like the principles of gravitation, knew no national boundaries.

One way to avoid any misinterpretation of the anatomically based surgical principles among the readers of the *Philosophical Transactions* was through the use of illustration. By reinforcing the written text with illustration, the authors could identify unmistakably which anatomical features were considered crucial to their surgical report. Plymouth Dock surgeon John Cagua provided two illustrated plates, one of five bone fragments, and another of the external view of the head of a patient with a fractured skull whom he claimed to have 'cured'.[80] Le Cat offered illustrations of both his patient, Catherine Guilmatre, and her 'incomplete hernia' upon which he operated.[81] Perhaps the most explicit illustration of a surgical 'kind' of anatomy is found in London surgeon, Jonathan Wathen's plate of a method he used to clear an obstructed Eustachian tube to restore hearing. (See Figure 7.) In this figure, Wathen illustrated the operator's hand holding a syringe with which he injected a mixture of *mel rosarum* and water into the Eustachian tube of a midsagittal section of a human skull.[82] This representation of a surgeon 'operating' upon a post-mortem specimen, quite rare among contemporary surgical illustrations, vividly reinforces the pedagogical aspect of Walthen's report.

More commonly, surgeons illustrated the procedures they had found most useful in 'improving' the art or science of surgery. This objective of the surgeons conforms to the depiction of the Royal Society's 'reformist enterprise' as dedicated to 'improving the manual arts'. [83] As discussed above, the surgeons' campaign for improvement was likely associated with contemporary movements to enhance the status of surgery in England. However, not all of the suggested surgical improvements came from the most active figures of the Company of surgeons. Henry Ettrick, Archibald Cleland, Christopher Warrick and William Sharp, for example, each contributed reports to the Society, but were not propelled to the professional status of their contemporaries including John Ranby, Claudius Amyand, Samuel Sharp, Benjamin Gooch, and John Hunter. The motivations of these lesser-known surgeons to present ideas for 'improving' the practice of surgery may be seen as examples of the critical acumen of the age. Specifically, the authors had developed specific practical surgical techniques through which they could overcome the errors and inefficient practices of earlier eras. Their offerings of 'a vision of Progress and improvement' were also characteristic of what Margaret Jacob has termed the 'English scientific culture' of the eighteenth century.[84]

Throughout the mid eighteenth century, the *Philosophical Transactions* effectively remained a clearinghouse of new information which might be of interest to its readers, many of whom were men of 'science'. I have shown that the 220 reports of surgical conditions which appeared in the *Philosophical Transactions* between 1727 and 1778 are indicators that at least some contemporary surgeons were actively engaged in the Society's 'scientific' enterprise. The reporting of surgical information in a publication devoted to science is one indication that the information may be regarded as scientific. More to the point, however, the surgeons contributing these reports were participating in the same activity which contemporaries regarded as science: gathering incidences of 'remarkable' phenomena; critically assessing their observations of these phenomena; at times, attempting to reproduce these phenomena through trial and error experimentation; and reporting these experiences to a wide audience of intellectuals in order to broaden the base of general knowledge. Indeed, for these practitioners, an emerging view of a 'science' of surgery, based to a small extent on Baconian tradition, and, to a greater extent on Enlightenment ideas of science, existed in England before the contributions of John Hunter.

Notes

1. I am grateful for Christopher Lawrence's comments on an earlier draft of this chapter. Additionally, I appreciate Susan Gold's and James Edmonson's invaluable assistance in providing full citations for several references unavailable to me in the Pacific Basin. Mahalo also to the staff of the Thomas Hale Hamilton Library at the University of Hawaii at Manoa and to Janice Wilson for providing me access to the Charles S. Judd, Jr., History of Medicine Collection at the Hawaii Medical Library, Honolulu.
2. D'A. Power, 'The Evolution of Surgery in London', *St. Bartholomew's Hospital Journal*, xix (1912), 91.
3. R. H. Major, *A History of Medicine* (Springfield, Illinois: Charles C. Thomas, 1954), Vol. 2, 606.
4. L. S. Jacyna, 'Images of John Hunter in the Nineteenth Century', *History of Science*, xxi (1983), 85–108.
5. W. Salmon, *Ars Chirurgica. A Compendium of the Theory and Practice of Chirurgery* (London: J. Dawkes, 1698), dedication.
6. J. Handley, *Colloquia Chyurgica: or, The Whole Art of Surgery*, 4th edn (London: A. Bettesworth & C. Hitch, 1733), preface.
7. J. Freind, *The History of Physick* (London: J. Walthoe, 1744), v.1, 215.
8. C. J. Lawrence, 'Democratic, Divine, and Heroic: The History and Historiography of Surgery', in C. Lawrence (ed.) *Surgical Theory, Medical Practice: Studies in the History of Surgery* (London: Routledge, 1992), 6, 36, fn. 36.
9. David P. Miller has begun to explore this period of the Royal Society's activities. See his "Into the Valley of Darkness': Reflections on the Royal Society in the Eighteenth Century', *History of Science*, xxvii (1989),155–66. For a discussion of the medical articles which appeared in early volumes of the *Philosophical Transactions*, see R. Porter's 'The Early Royal Society and the Spread of Medical Knowledge' in R. French and A. Wear (eds), *The Medical Revolution of the Seventeenth Century* (Cambridge: Cambridge University Press, 1989), 272–93.
10. *An Index to the Anatomical, Medical, Chirurgical, and Physiological Papers, Contained in the Transactions of the Royal Society of London from the Commencement of that Work to the End of the Year 1817, Chronologically and Alphabetically Arranged* (London:J. Davy for J. Callow, 1818), remains an indispensable, though incomplete, guide

into searching the surgical literature published in the *Philosophical Transactions.*

11. An inconsistency in the number of years included in each volume of the *Transactions* before mid-century makes dividing the time-scale into precise decades difficult. Thus, the first three groupings of years in this and later figures actually represent 11 years rather than a decade. This slight variation does not, however, significantly alter the graphical representation of the data.
12. H. Lyons, *The Royal Society 1660–1940. A History of its Administration under its Charters* (Cambridge: Cambridge University Press, 1944),178–9.
13. I have previously discussed much of the contemporary literature on the stone in my 'Acquiring Surgical Know-How: Occupational and Lay Instruction in Early Eighteenth-Century London' in R. Porter (ed.), *The Popularization of Medicine* (London: Routledge, 1992), especially 53–60.
14. J. Warner, 'Case of a Piece of Bone, Together with a Stone, in the Bladder Successfully Extracted' *Philosophical Transactions of the Royal Society of London,* xlvii (1751–2), 475. Henceforth, abbreviated *Phil. Trans. Roy. Soc.* and titles of the reports abbreviated as in the *Index* (fn 7).
15. J. Douglas, 'Two Chirurgical Questions (Relative to the Stone) Stated, and Answered', *Phil. Trans. Roy. Soc.*, xxxv (1727– 8), 318–19.
16. J. Mudge, 'Proposal for Removing the Only Real Defect in the Lateral Operation for the Stone', *Phil. Trans. Roy. Soc.*, xlvi (1749–50), 24.
17. Warner, *op. cit.* (note 14), 475– 7.
18. J. Warner, 'Remarkable Instance of Four Rough Stones Found in the Bladder', *Phil. Trans. Roy. Soc.*, l (1757–8), 579.
19. J. Warner, 'Account of Two Stones of Remarkable Shape and Size Firmly Lodged in the Urethra and Successfully Cut Out', *Phil. Trans. Roy. Soc.*, li (1759–60), 304.
20. W. Cowper, 'Experiments made with Colbatch's Styptic', *Phil. Trans. Roy. Soc.*, xvii (1693), 42–4. Harold Cook has lucidly analysed the controversy which arose over these experiments in 'Sir John Colbatch and Augustan Medicine: Experimentalism, Character and Entrepreneuralism', *Annals of Science,* xlvii (1990), 475–505.
21. P. Dionis, *Cours d'operations de chirurgie, demontrees au Jardin royal* (Paris: L. d'Houry ,1707), 704–5, as cited by O. H. Wangensteen and S. D. Wangensteen in *The Rise of Surgery. From Empiric Craft to Scientific Discipline* (Folkestone, Kent:William Dawson & Sons, 1978), 23.
22. M. Faget, 'Remarks on the Use, &c. of the Styptic, &c. (Agaric of Oak)', *Phil. Trans. Roy. Soc.*, xlvii (1751–2), 563.
23. W. Thornhill, 'Account of the Success of the Agaric in Amputations',

Phil. Trans. Roy. Soc., xlix (1755–6), 264.

24. C. Bazerman, *Shaping Written Knowledge. The Genre and Activity of the Experimental Article in Science* (Madison, Wisconsin: University of Wisconsin Press, 1988), 65. Frederic L. Holmes has addressed the historiographical limitations of our understanding of experimentally derived knowledge in 'Do we Understand Historically How Experimental Knowledge is Acquired?', *History of Science*, 30 (1992), 119–36.
25. C. Amyand, 'Some Observations on the Spina Ventosa', *Phil. Trans. Roy. Soc.*, xliv (1746–7), 193– 211.
26. C. Warrick, 'Improvement in the Practice of Tapping', *Phil. Trans. Roy. Soc.*, xliii (1744–5), 12–19.
27. A. Cleland, 'Needles for Operations on the Eyes, and Instruments for (Diseases of) the Ear', *Phil. Trans. Roy. Soc.*, xli (1739–41), 844–51.
28. C.-N. Le Cat, 'Concerning the Cure of Dry Gangrenes with a Description of a New Invented Instrument for the Extirpation of Tumours out of the Reach of the Surgeon's Fingers', *Phil. Trans. Roy. Soc.*, xlvi (1749-50), 80–5, , 72–80; *Ibid.*, 'On Herniae', *Phil. Trans. Roy. Soc.*, xlvii (1751– 52), 324–9; Ibid., 'New Trocart [sic] for the Puncture in the Hydrocephalus', *Phil. Trans, Roy. Soc.*, xlvii (1751–52), 267–72; and Ibid., 'Operation of Lithotomy on Women', *Phil. Trans. Roy. Soc.*, xlvi (1749–50), 97–100.
29. *Idem*, 'Description of a Machine for Dressing Patients for Ailments on the Back', *Phil. Trans. Roy. Soc.*, xlii (1742–3), 364–9.
30. S. Sharp, 'Description of a New Method of Opening the Cornea, &c. to Extract the Crystaline [sic] Humour', *Phil. Trans. Roy. Soc.*, xlviii (1753–4), 161.
31. J. Hunter, 'Proposals for the Recovery of People Apparently Drowned', *Phil. Trans. Roy. Soc.*, lxvi (1776), 412–5.
32. D. Turner, *The Art of Surgery* (London: C. Rivington, J. Lacy and J. Clarke, 1725), Vol. 2, 127.
33. The Medical Library, St Thomas's Campus, United Medical and Dental Schools, 'Charles Oxley Notebook, Case Notes of Surgical Patients Admitted to St Thomas's Hospital, 1725–26', MS.S2.a.6. I have used this manuscript as the basis of my '"Sacred Sanctuaries for the Sick": Surgery at St Thomas's Hospital, 1725–26', *London Journal*, xvii (1992), 36–53.
34. H. Ettrick, 'Description and Draught of a Machine for Reducing Fractures of the Thigh', *Phil. Trans. Roy. Soc.*, xli (1739–41), 562–8.
35. C.- N. Le Cat, 'Ambe of Hippocrates Rectified', *Phil. Trans. Roy. Soc.*, xlii (1742– 3), 387–403.
36. J. Freke, 'Invention of a New Ambe for Reducing a Dislocated Shoulder', *Phil. Trans. Roy. Soc.*, xlii (1742–3), 556.
37. P. Mathias, 'Who Unbound Prometheus? Science and Technical Change, 1600–1800' in A. E. Musson (ed.) *Science, Technology and Economic Growth in the Eighteenth Century* (London: Methuen,

1972), 77.

38. R. Home, 'Account of the Case of the First Joint of the Thumb, with the Flexor Tendon in its Whole Extent Torn Off', *Phil. Trans. Roy. Soc.*, l (1757–8), 617.
39. C. White, 'Account of a Case Where the Head of the Os Humeri was Sawed Off, &c. and the Motion of the Limb Preserved', *Phil. Trans. Roy. Soc.*, lix (1769), 39–46.
40. W. Fidge, 'Account of a Stone Taken Out of the Bladder of a Dog, with a Piece of Dog's-grass in the Centre', *Phil. Trans. Roy. Soc.*, xliv (1746–7), 336.
41. T. Woolcomb, 'Fatal Case of Gun-shot Wound in Boy', *Phil. Trans. Roy. Soc.*,l x (1770), 94–9.
42. F. Drake, 'Account of the Bones of a Foetus Discharged Through an Ulcer Near the Navel', *Phil. Trans. Roy. Soc.*, xlv (1748), 121–3.
43. J. Bate, 'Account of the Remarkable Alteration of Colour in a Negro Woman', *Phil. Trans. Roy. Soc.*, li (1759–60), 175–8.
44. F. Nicholls, 'Observations on Aneurisms in General, and on the Foregoing in Particular', *Phil. Trans. Roy. Soc.*, xxxv (1727–8), 440–4.
45. C. Price, 'Of the Villi of the Stomach of Oxen, and the Expansion of the Cuticle Through the Ductus Alimentalis', *Phil. Trans. Roy. Soc.*, xxxv (1727–8), 532.
46. C. Amyand, 'Obstruction of the Biliary Ducts, and an Imposthumation of the Gall-bladder, Discharging Upwards of Eighteen Quarts of Bilious Matter in Twenty-five Days, Without Apparent Defect in the Animal Functions', *Phil. Trans. Roy. Soc.*, xl (1737–8), 317–25.
47. J. Ranby, 'Some Material Observations upon Dissecting an Ostrich', *Phil. Trans. Roy. Soc.*, xxxvi (1729–30), 275–6.
48. E. Nourse, 'Preternatural Delivery of a Foetus by Anus', Together with an Examination of the Parts', *Phil. Trans. Roy. Soc.*, xxxvi (1729–30), 435– 40.
49. J. Huxham, 'Extraordinary Venereal Disease', *Phil. Trans. Roy. Soc.*, xli (1739– 40), 667.
50. E. Nourse, 'Stones Found in Bags Formed by a Dilatation of the Coats of the Bladder', *Phil. Trans. Roy. Soc.*, xlii (1742–3), 11–14, and G. Bell, 'Nephritic Case, with a Rupture', *Phil. Trans. Roy. Soc.*, xlii (1742–3), 54–6.
51. T. Hope, 'Concerning Daviel's Method of Couching', *Phil. Trans. Roy. Soc.*, xlvii (1751–2),530–3.
52. C. White, 'Account of a Complete Luxation of the Thigh Bone in an Adult', *Phil. Trans. Roy. Soc.*, li (1759–60), 678.
53. J. Bent, 'Account of a Woman Enjoying the Use of her Right Arm After the Head of the Os Humeri was Cut Away', *Phil. Trans. Roy. Soc.*, lxiv (1773–4), 353.
54. James du Moulin, Master of Surgery to Charles II and James II (1667); John Beaumont, Somerset surgeon and naturalist (1685);

Charles Bernard, later Sergeant Surgeon to Queen Anne (1696); William Cowper (1699); Paul Buissiere, Huguenot surgeon (1699); and James Cunningham, surgeon to the East India Company (1699). Michael Hunter provided information about all Fellows elected prior to 1700 in his *The Royal Society and its Fellows 1660– 1700* (Buckinghamshire: British Society for the History of Science, 1982).

55. T. Davis, 'The Ark in the Flames: Science, Language and Education in Seventeenth-Century England', in A. E. Benjamin, G. N. Cantor, and J. R. R. Christie (eds). *The Figural and the Literal: Problems of Language in the History of Science and Philosophy, 1630–1800* (Manchester: Manchester University Press, 1978), 94.
56. Having surveyed the certificates which eighteenth-century Royal Society Fellows presented which stated their recommendation of candidates for Fellowship, Margaret Jacob concluded, without explanation, that 'In general, surgeons did not fare well in the voting process.' M. C. Jacob, 'Scientific Culture in the Early English Enlightenment: Mechanisms, Industry, and Gentlemanly Facts' in A. C. Kors and P. J. Korshin (eds) *Anticipations of the Enlightenment in England, France, and Germany* (Philadelphia: University of Pennsylvania Press, 1987), 161, fn. 47.
57. The surgeons who were elected F.R.S. were John Ranby, William Cheselden, John Douglas, Claudius Amyand, Vincent Bacon, Francis Drake, John Freke, Claude-Nicholas Le Cat, Edward Nourse, John Belchier, Joseph Warner, Samuel Sharp, Percival Pott, Henry Watson and John Hunter. As a point of comparison, there was a total of 125 Fellows in 1700, 301 in 1740, and 460 in 1780 according to H. Lyons (fn. 9), *The Royal Society 1660–1940*, 125, 165.
58. S. Lawrence, 'Science and Medicine at the London Hospitals. The Development of Teaching and Research, 1750–1815', (Ph.D thesis, University of Toronto, 1985).
59. T. Touchit, *Westminster Journal*, 20 April, 1745.
60. G. Holmes, *Augustan England: Professions, State and Society, 1680–1730* (London: George Allen & Unwin, 1982), 7–8.
61. P. R. Backsheider, *Daniel Defoe: his Life* (Baltimore: Johns Hopkins University Press, 1989), 527.
62. T. Chevalier, *Observations in Defence of a Bill Lately Brought into Parliament for Erecting the Corporation of Surgeons of London into a College* (London: St Paul's Church Yard, 1793), 53.
63. See, for example, William Eamon's 'From the Secrets of Nature to Public Knowledge', in D. C. Lindberg and R. S. Westman (eds), *Reappraisals of the Scientific Revolution* (Cambridge: Cambridge University Press, 1990), 349–55.
64. P. Dear, '*Totius in verba*: Rhetoric and Authority in the Early Royal Society', *Isis*, lxxvi (1985), 145–61.
65. S. Shapin, 'Pump and Circumstance: Robert Boyle's Literary Technology', *Social Studies of Science*, xiv (1984), 487– 94.

66. D. Kronick, *A History of Scientific & Technical Publications. The Origins and Developments of the Scientific and Technical Press 1665–1790,* 2nd edn, (Metuchen, New Jersey: Scarecrow Press, 1976), 21,45.
67. Dear, *op. cit.* (note 64), 146. For an earlier appraisal of 'Bacon's List of Scientific Qualities' as exemplified by surgeons, see James Learmonth's *The Contribution of Surgery to Preventive Medicine* (London: Oxford University Press, 1951), 5–21.
68. For well argued but divergent opinions of Anglo-Franco relations, see J. Black, *Natural and Necessary Enemies: Anglo-Franco Relations in the Eighteenth Century* (London: Duckworth,1986) and R. Porter, 'The Enlightenment in England' in R. Porter and M. Teich (eds), *The Enlightenment in National Context* (Cambridge: Cambridge University Press, 1981), 1–18.
69. R.- J.-C. de Garengeot, *A Treatise of Chirurgical Operations* (London: T. Woodward, 1723), preface.
70. Handley, *op. cit.* (note 6).
71. H.-F. Le Dran, *Observations in Surgery* (London: J. Hodges, 1739), preface.
72. Other contributors of multiple articles include the London practitioners, Claudius Amyand (7 reports), John Ranby (6), John Hunter and Benjamin Gooch (5 each), and William Cheselden, John Belchier, John Huxham, William Hewson and Christopher Warrick (4 each). All but Gooch and Warrick were F.R.S. when they submitted their reports. Further information on Le Cat is found in Theodore Vetter's 'Claude-Nicolas Le Cat. Chirurgien de province au XVIIIe siècle', *Annales Medicales de Nancy*, viii (1969), 433–45.
73. 'Declaration du Roy concernant la communaute des maitres-chirurgiens de la ville de Paris, donnée a Versailles, le 23 avril 1743', in J. Rigal, *La communaute des maitres-chirurgiens jures de Paris au XVIIe et XVIIIe siecle* (Paris: Vigot, 1936), 197–202, as cited by T. Gelfand, 'Empiricism and Eighteenth-Century French Surgery', *Bulletin of the History of Medicine*, xliv (1970), 43.
74. Gelfand, *op. cit.* (note 73), 44.
75. *Ibid.*, 46.
76. Toby Gelfand has lucidly described this use of dissection in the teaching of surgery in Paris in 'The "Paris Manner" of Dissection: Student Anatomical Dissection in Early Eighteenth-century Paris', *Bulletin of the History of Medicine*, xlvi (1972), 99–130.
77. J. Huxham, 'Extraordinary Hernia Inguinalis', *Phil. Trans. Roy. Soc.*, xli (1739–41), 640–1.
78. A. Cunningham, 'The Kinds of Anatomy', *Medical History*, xix (1975), especially 9–11.
79. B. M. Stafford, *Body Criticism: Imagining the Unseen in Enlightenment Art and Medicine* (Cambridge,Massachusetts: The MIT Press, 1991), 12, 49–129.

80. J. Cagua, 'Large Fracture and Depression of the Skull, with a Wound of the Dura Mater and Brain Cured', *Phil. Trans. Roy. Soc.*, xli (1739–41), 495–500.
81. C.-N. Le Cat, 'Two Observations (Hydatids – Hernia with Extraordinary Prolapsus of the Intestine)', *Phil. Trans. Roy. Soc.*, xli (1739–41), 716–24.
82. J. Walthen, 'Method Proposed to Restore Hearing, when Injured from Obstruction of the Eustachian Tube', *Phil. Trans. Roy. Soc.*, xlix (1755–56), 213–22.
83. Stafford, *op. cit.* (note 79), 350.
84. Jacob, *op. cit.* (note 56), 135.

Index

THE HISTORY OF PUBLIC HEALTH AND THE MODERN STATE

Ed. by Dorothy Porter

Amsterdam/Atlanta, GA 1994. VII,439 pp.
(Clio Medica 26)

ISBN: 90-5183-552-3 Bound Hfl. 180,-/US-$ 70.50
ISBN: 90-5183-621-X Paper Hfl. 55.-/US-$ 26.-

Table of Contents: DOROTHY PORTER: Introduction. MATTHEW RAMSEY: Public Health in France. PAUL WEINDLING: Public Health in Germany. CHRISTOPHER HAMLIN: State Medicine in Great Britain. KARIN JOHANNISSON: The People's Health: Public Health Policies in Sweden. SUSAN GROSS SOLOMON: The Expert and the State in Russian Public Health: Continuities and Changes Across the Revolutionary Divide. ELIZABETH FEE: Public Health and the State: the United States. JAY CASSELL: Public Health in Canada. LINDA BRYDER: A New World? Two Hundred Years of Public Health in Australia and New Zealand. DAVID ARNOLD: Crisis and Contradicition in India's Public Health. MARYINEZ LYONS: Public Health in Colonial Africa: The Belgian Congo. MAHITO H. FUKUDA: Public Health in Modern Japan: From Regimen to Hygiene. MILTON I. ROEMER: Internationalism in Medicine and Public Health.